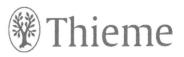

Applied Oral Physiology

The Integration of Sciences in Clinical Dentistry

Robin Wilding, BDS, Dip Pros, M Dent, PhD, MSc
Emeritus Professor
Department of Oral Biology
University of the Western Cape
Cape Town, South Africa

166 illustrations

Thieme
New York • Stuttgart • Delhi • Rio de Janeiro

Library of Congress Cataloging-in-Publication Data

Names: Wilding, R. J. C. 1944- author.

Title: Applied oral physiology : the integration of sciences in clinical dentistry / Robin Wilding.

Other titles: Applied oral physiology (Thieme)

Description: New York : Thieme, [2020] | Includes bibliographical references and index. | Summary: "Applied Oral Physiology: The Integration of Sciences in Clinical Dentistry by prosthodontist, biologist, and educator Robin Wilding integrates basic science topics traditionally taught separately, enabling readers to understand the interconnected relationship between the scientific and clinical aspects of dentistry. On the broadest level, this well-researched, readable, and easy-to-study book brings together related elements of anatomy, physiology, microbiology, and biochemistry. Integration of these areas helps students comprehend the different elements of dental science, thereby improving their ability to understand and treat patient problems. For example, understanding how saliva influences oral health is vital information every dentist needs to know"– Provided by publisher.

Identifiers: LCCN 2020010618 (print) | LCCN 2020010619 (ebook) | ISBN 9781684201792 (hardcover) | ISBN 9781684201808 (ebook)

Subjects: MESH: Mouth–physiology | Mouth–physiopathology | Tooth–physiology | Tooth–physiopathology

Classification: LCC QP146 (print) | LCC QP146 (ebook) | NLM WU 102 | DDC 612.3/1–dc23

LC record available at https://lccn.loc.gov/2020010618

LC ebook record available at https://lccn.loc.gov/2020010619

Thieme Publishers New York

333 Seventh Avenue, New York, NY 10001 USA

+1 800 782 3488, customerservice@thieme.com

Georg Thieme Verlag KG

Rüdigerstrasse 14, 70469 Stuttgart, Germany

+49 [0]711 8931 421, customerservice@thieme.de

Thieme Publishers Delhi

A-12, Second Floor, Sector-2, Noida-201301

Uttar Pradesh, India

+91 120 45 566 00, customerservice@thieme.in

Thieme Publishers Rio de Janeiro,

Thieme Publicações Ltda.

Edifício Rodolpho de Paoli, 25º andar

Av. Nilo Peçanha, 50 – Sala 2508

Rio de Janeiro 20020-906 Brasil

+55 21 3172 2297

Cover design: Thieme Publishing Group

Cover image: A scanning electron microscope image (magnification × 300) of calcified plaque (calculus) which was etched to remove all the organic material. The remaining calcified material reflects the structural organization of the living biofilm just as a piece of dried coral is a relic of the living reef. The insert (magnification × 1000) reveals laminations and channels which bacteria have constructed to define a variety of habitats within the plaque biofilm.

Typesetting by DiTech Process Solutions, India

Printed in USA by King Printing Company, Inc.   5 4 3 2 1

ISBN 978-1-68420-179-2

Also available as an e-book:

eISBN 978-1-68420-180-8

Important note: Medicine is an ever-changing science undergoing continual development. Research and clinical experience are continually expanding our knowledge, in particular our knowledge of proper treatment and drug therapy. Insofar as this book mentions any dosage or application, readers may rest assured that the authors, editors, and publishers have made every effort to ensure that such references are in accordance with **the state of knowledge at the time of production of the book.**

Nevertheless, this does not involve, imply, or express any guarantee or responsibility on the part of the publishers in respect to any dosage instructions and forms of applications stated in the book. **Every user is requested to examine carefully** the manufacturers' leaflets accompanying each drug and to check, if necessary in consultation with a physician or specialist, whether the dosage schedules mentioned therein or the contraindications stated by the manufacturers differ from the statements made in the present book. Such examination is particularly important with drugs that are either rarely used or have been newly released on the market. Every dosage schedule or every form of application used is entirely at the user's own risk and responsibility. The authors and publishers request every user to report to the publishers any discrepancies or inaccuracies noticed. If errors in this work are found after publication, errata will be posted at www.thieme.com on the product description page.

Some of the product names, patents, and registered designs referred to in this book are in fact registered trademarks or proprietary names even though specific reference to this fact is not always made in the text. Therefore, the appearance of a name without designation as proprietary is not to be construed as a representation by the publisher that it is in the public domain.

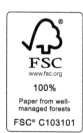

"There is quite enough substance, and depth, in the various fields of oral biology to satisfy even the most stringent requirements for dental students to have a sound scientific background"

J.W. Osborn 1984

Contents

Appendices

Preface

Learning is an enjoyable travel companion on the lifelong journey that dentists go on. They select, and add to their collection along the way, an easy and useful balance of dental science, technology, and clinical skill. It is not possible to acquire all this learning and wisdom during the period of formal training at dental school. In spite of this reality, some schools offer the dental science component of this body of skill in full measure and separate it into disciplines. This titration is not evidence-based and is not effective. The problem is simply too much information. The recently qualified dentist discovers an imbalance between the substantial knowledge mastered at dental school and her, or his, clinical skill. The ability to reveal and assess the key elements of a problem, make appropriate decisions with the patient in relation to the options, and summon the technical skills to put plans into effect, does not receive the foundation as promised by the traditional dental curriculum.

A more appropriate measure of dental science knowledge is achieved in schools which use self-directed learning based on clinical cases. In this style of learning, the contribution made by dental sciences is integrated and on a need-to-know basis. Some dental academics will demur that this style of learning can neither be thorough nor comprehensive. However, they are not preparing students to become clones of themselves; their students are to become clinicians.

Dentists who attend continuing education courses have a good idea of what they need and want to learn. They are surely in a good position to assess the value of course content; as academics, we should be learning from them about the lifelong process of growth as a dentist. If we do listen, we will hear repeatedly that an exhaustive understanding of dental science is not useful in the practice of dentistry. This is not a denial of science, but a preference for applied science, which will be at the core of those who practice evidence-based dentistry.

I hope that this book will serve as an introduction to applied oral physiology and will also enable students or practicing dentists to find what they need to know. More expert-based sources can be found in the suggested reading section. Some information which may be beyond the "need-to-know," but may be of interest, has been included in appendices. There is a glossary for those unfamiliar with some terms.

This book is a work in progress. I hope that it will evolve by way of suggestions and corrections from readers as well as new insights and developments in dental science.

Robin Wilding, BDS, Dip Pros, M Dent, PhD, MSc

Acknowledgments

The presentation of certain views, and the mix and essence of information I have made is personal in nature, but it has been significantly influenced by others. Jeff Osborn was the inspiration for the development of a department of Oral Biology at the University of Western Cape (UWC). The new department helped shift the emphasis of preclinical course work from medical science toward topics relevant to clinical dentistry. Professor Osborn visited UWC where, apart from his support for a change in the preclinical curriculum, he left a legacy of his own particular interests. One of this was the importance of studying the evolution of the jaws and teeth in order to understand its current function in humans. Another was the application of mechanics and mathematics in understanding the dynamics of the temporomandibular joint. Echoes of this legacy are particularly resonant in Chapters 1 and 9 of this book and the short tribute to D'Arcy Thompson in the Appendix.

Other significant sources of inspiration for this book came from leading experts and heads of Oral Biology Departments. I was given invaluable advice on the preclinical curriculum by Gerald Roth from the Kentucky School of Dentistry, Don Burnett of the University of British Columbia, and Barry Sessle and Richard Ten Cate from the University of Toronto.

I have attempted to acknowledge the sources I have used throughout the book, but if I have not been adequately thorough, I apologize in advance and ask readers to let the publishers know of any omissions, so that corrections can be made in subsequent editions

I would like to express my sincere thanks to Delia DeTurris, the acquisition editor of Thieme publishers, for her belief in this project and her quiet but invaluable advice. I would also like to thank Gaurav Prabhuzantye, the project manager of the production team at Thieme, for his care and patience in dealing with my manuscript.

Finally, I would like to thank my patient wife, Carrie, who has put up with my long periods of silence, when my mind was in my book.

Robin Wilding, BDS, Dip Pros, M Dent, PhD, MSc

About the Author

Robin Wilding grew up in Zimbabwe and obtained bachelor and master's degrees in Dentistry, with a diploma in Prosthodontics, from the University of the Witwatersrand in Johannesburg, South Africa. He spent 7 years in private practice as a Prosthodontist in Cape Town before joining the staff of the University of Western Cape as Professor of Dental Prosthetics. An interest in oral biology led to the development of a separate department in that school, and he was eventually transferred to the position of Professor and Chairman of Oral Biology. He was awarded a PhD for his thesis on the factors which determine chewing efficiency. He completed a master's degree in Holistic Science at Schumacher College. He has a number of research publications in international journals which have attracted over 500 citations. He has lectured undergraduates, postgraduates, and practitioners in South Africa and the United Kingdom. Robin was registered in the United Kingdom as a Specialist Prosthodontist until his recent retirement. He was the course organizer for the Prosthetics course offered by the Bristol University Open Learning for Dentists.

1 The Origins of Teeth

Abstract

Mammalian teeth have evolved over many millions of years in response to the particular requirements of warm-blooded animals to catch and kill or graze and browse their food. Mammals like the hyena are able to crush bones with their teeth to get at the nutritious marrow. The elephant crushes shoots and leaves. While humans are not capable of such feats, we do have the essential equipment for cracking nuts and crunching raw vegetables. The design of mammalian teeth gives them strength to resist fracture and the sharp edges to slice, grind, and grate through fibrous foods. The strength of teeth comes from the contribution of two quite different materials. One, enamel is very hard but brittle. The other, dentin is softer but very tough. The combination provides what we recognize now as a composite material such as fiberglass. The sharpness of teeth comes from the fractured edges of enamel. For these edges to be exposed, some of the enamel coating on the tooth has to become worn away. In fact, wear is a prerequisite for optimal function of mammalian teeth. This chapter sets out the origins of teeth in mammals, which offer useful insights into the function of the jaws and teeth in modern man.

Keywords: origins of teeth, evolution, teeth as tools, composite structure, tooth strength, tooth design, tooth wear mesial drift

1.1 Evolution

"Man is a fraction of the animal world. Our History is an afterthought, no more tacked on to an infinite calendar. We are not so unique as we would like to believe. And if man in a time of need seeks deeper knowledge concerning himself, then he must explore those animal horizons from which we have made our quick little march." These words were written by Robert Ardrey in his book *African Genesis*. In order to understand the origins of teeth, it is worth reviewing their process of evolution.

The origins of teeth can be traced to dermal scales around the mouth which became modified to grasp food. For some animals, it was necessary to reduce the size of a piece of food in order to be able to swallow it. Smaller food particles are also easier to digest and offer rapid access to food energy essential to fuel the active metabolism of small mammals. It was the early mammals who used teeth in this way for the first time (*see Appendix A.1 Mastication and Mammals*). The work which a mammal's teeth are required to perform can be compared to

tool use in a workshop. There are different processes used in food preparation and the type of teeth required (*see Appendix A.2 The Mechanics of Tooth Use*).

1.2 The Teeth as Tools

1.2.1 Tooth Strength

The mammalian tooth is particularly well designed to be used as a tool. The surface enamel is the hardest substance produced by any living organism. The brittle nature of the enamel makes it vulnerable to cracking, but this tendency is reduced by the core of underlying dentin which provides the compressive strength and resilience that a solid enamel tooth would lack. The collagen fibers of the dentin run at right angles to the enamel prisms which further discourages the propagation of an enamel crack throughout the tooth. So, the two materials complement each other to form a composite material which is both very hard and resilient (*see Appendix H.1 Cracks, Composites, and Teeth*).

1.2.2 Tooth Design

Two major requirements of a chewing tool are firstly, that each tooth has sharp cutting or grinding edges and secondly, that it allows the escape of processed food away from the cutting edges to avoid clogging. The mammalian enamel is characterized by long slender prisms which run from the amelodentinal junction to the surface. This is in contrast to the reptilian enameloid which is an amorphous crystalline structure; enameloid has, as a result, a higher compressive strength than enamel. The advantage of the mammalian enamel as a tooth tool is that when it wears, instead of just a few crystals being dislodged, a whole prism fractures away leaving a freshly sharp square edge behind (▶ Fig. 1.1).

The second major requirement of a chewing tool is that it allows the shredded food to escape without build-up, so allowing the cutting surfaces to continue working against each other. The escape of processed food is achieved in the mammalian tooth by the contribution of a hard cutting edge adjacent to a softer, but tougher material which wears at a faster rate. The design feature which provides this function in a variety of mammalian teeth is the cusp. A cusp is a raised ridge or elevation of the enamel surface supported by an inner core of dentin. When the cusp wears sufficiently for the dentin to be exposed,

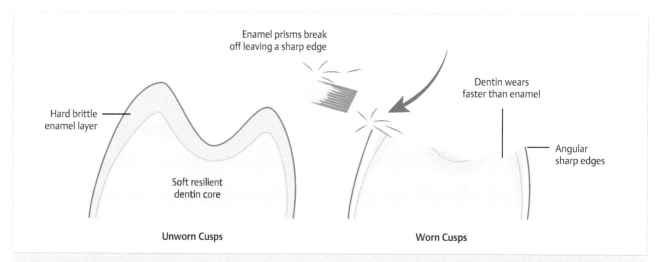

Fig. 1.1 A diagrammatic representation of the influence of cusps on tooth wear. A cross section of a premolar tooth before wear reveals the core of dentin within each cusp. When the cusp has become worn and the dentin exposed, the dentin wears faster than the enamel and prevents clogging with food debris by providing an escape way for reduced food particles. The enamel edges are kept sharp by wear, as entire enamel prisms break away from the enamel surface leaving a sharp edge. The cusps provide an alternating surface of sharp enamel, and an escape way for food.

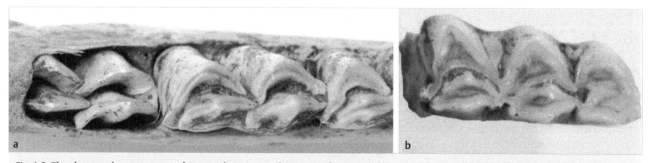

Fig. 1.2 The shape and arrangement of mammalian cusps, when worn, determine the required composite chewing surface. (a) The unerupted molar of this immature sheep (*left*) has several steep and curved cusps. They are not functional chewing elements until they begin to wear down (*right*). **(b)** The adult sheep's molar has worn down to a flat composite shredding surface which does not clog and is self-sharpening.

the tool is ready for use. The softer exposed dentin core of the cusp wears at a faster rate than the enamel covering of the cusp. There is, therefore, always a depression next to the cutting edge of enamel, formed by softer dentin, into which food can escape. In this way, the tool does not clog up with cut debris. The design of the mammalian tooth has evolved in a variety of cusp formations which provide either the scissors-like function of carnassial teeth, or the grinding-like function of the molar teeth of an herbivore. Cusps are formed during the development of the tooth by the formation of folds in the tooth crown. In the unerupted sheep molar, these folds may be seen as pointed, smooth, and rounded cusps. As the tooth begins to function, surface wear causes a series of sharp grating surfaces which shred tough grass fibers (▶ Fig. 1.2). Occlusal wear is so vital to the preparation of the mammalian tooth that some animals, such as guinea pigs, start wearing their teeth in utero so as to emerge into the world ready to chew.

1.2.3 Tooth Wear in Man

The teeth of modern man usually show little evidence of wear. This is because our modern diet does not require chewing hard

foods, and contains little that is rough and fibrous. Dentists have come to accept our unworn dentition as normal, so that when we find tooth wear, which exposes the dentin in our patients, we are concerned. Wear is not necessarily abnormal in a subject who has lived on a course diet, although it may be cosmetically undesirable (▶ Fig. 1.3). There are significant advantages to tooth wear in man. Occlusal wear removes or reduces the enamel fissures between cusps. The occlusal surface is not the only site on the tooth where wear occurs. During chewing, there is a component of the bite force which drives all the teeth forward in an anterior (mesial) direction. This component can be readily illustrated by a simple experiment. A steel shim is placed between any of the posterior teeth. The force to withdraw the shim is measured (also called contact point tightness). The subject then bites firmly with the teeth in maximum intercuspation. The force to withdraw the shim is again measured and will be found to be several times greater than the resting force. The experiment proves that there is a component of the bite force which acts in a mesial direction. This mesial component of the bite force causes the teeth to rub against each other and wears away the approximal (interproximal) surfaces. The approximal contact, which at first is just a point where the two curved surfaces meet, becomes a flattened area of contact between the teeth. This process reduces the area of stagnation between the teeth which is the second most common site for bacteria to accumulate and for dental caries to occur. Occlusal and interproximal tooth wear reduces the risk of caries.

As each tooth loses some approximal enamel, it becomes slightly narrower. A space would develop between the teeth were it not for the mesial component of the bite force which drives the molar and premolar teeth forward like train trucks (*see Chapter 7.7.6 Tooth Displacement and Cell Rests of Malassez*). This *mesial drift* may be insignificant in an individual whose diet consists mainly of soft foods which require little masticatory force. In an individual whose diet is course and unrefined, the drift may be as much as 6 mm in the young adult, enough extra space to accommodate the emerging third molar. So, approximal wear can provide sufficient space in the dental arch to prevent overcrowding of the teeth, a major source of malocclusion (▶ Fig. 1.4).

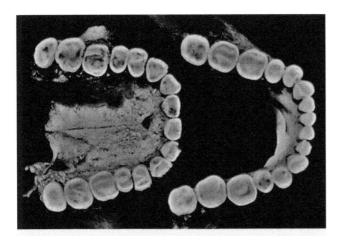

Fig. 1.3 The dentition of a middle-aged hunter–gatherer whose diet was unrefined. Occlusal wear has removed the occlusal fissures, and approximal wear has effectively shortened the dental arch to accommodate all the teeth without crowding. Secondary dentin has been laid down over years of gradual wear to prevent pulpal exposure and the formation of periapical abscess.

Tooth wear reduces the steepness of cusps, which in turn, alters the way the jaw moves during chewing. Wear allows a more lateral, side-to-side chewing movement than the more vertical chewing movement required by unworn cusps. These changes in the pattern of jaw movements, which accompany wear, are reflected in remodeling of the articular eminence of the temporomandibular joint (*see Chapter 9.1.3 Joint Stability*).

The mammalian tooth is an achievement in tool design. It is a self-sharpening, nonclogging, lifelong, and multipurpose aid to food processing. Wear of the tooth surface is essential to prepare the tool for use. When paleontologists are uncertain whether a fossil is reptile or early mammal, they look for the telltale signs of tooth wear on the outer surface of the mandibular teeth and the inner surface of the maxillary teeth. They are looking for the hallmark of the mammalian tooth.

Key Notes

The teeth of mammals have evolved to provide the essential function of preparing food. A feature common to all generic types of teeth is cusps. The purpose of cusps is to provide, when worn, a suitable pattern of composite surfaces for a particular type of chewing function.

Review Questions

1. How does the structure of the mammalian tooth provide for both hardness and strength?
2. How does the structure of the mammalian tooth enable it to remain sharp and avoid clogging?
3. What are the functions of cusps in the mammalian tooth?
4. What are the benefits of tooth wear in the human dentition?

Suggested Reading

Kaifu Y, Kasai K, Townsend GC, Richards LC. Tooth wear and the "design" of the human dentition: a perspective from evolutionary medicine. Am J Phys Anthropol 2003 Suppl 37:47–61

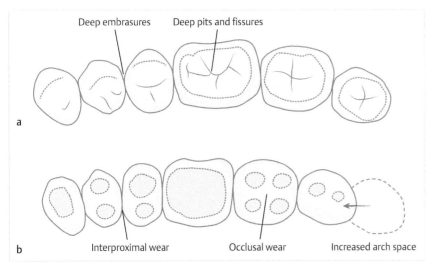

a

b

Fig. 1.4 A diagrammatic representation of the effects of tooth wear. (a) The unworn dentition has occlusal fissure and deep embrasures which trap food and bacteria. There is insufficient space for the teeth and some may be blocked out of the arch. **(b)** Tooth wear of a young adult has removed fissures and exposed dentin (*yellow shaded*). The approximal wear provides enough space to accommodate all the teeth in the arch.

2 Dental Hard Tissues

Abstract

This chapter covers a wide range of topics in order to link the structure of a tooth with its vulnerability to bacteria and their products. The hard tissues of teeth are not merely passive participants in their destruction. There is a constant ebb and flow of demineralization which is dependent on macroscopic conditions, such as the diet and level of oral hygiene, but equally on the microscopic environment of the tooth such as the presence of pits and fissures in enamel. Some demineralization of dentin is prevented by the defense barriers set up by living cells of the pulp–dentin. A knowledge of the natural defense capacity of enamel and dentin to resist destruction by bacterial products allows us to rethink orthodox restorative practices. The use of low-intervention clinical procedures has arisen through awareness of the capacity of the dental hard tissues to resist destruction and repair. The search for minimally invasive procedures must continue while too many teeth are not saved by dentistry but are caught up in a downward spiral of treatment and retreatment until they are eventually beyond further repair.

Keywords: enamel structure, ameloblasts, hydroxyapatite, enamel prisms, etching enamel, early enamel caries, arrested caries

2.1 Enamel: Clinical Aspects

2.1.1 Enamel Minerals

Enamel is about 95% mineral by weight but 87% by volume. Most of this mineral is hydroxyapatite, but there are other apatites and other minerals (magnesium and carbonates), so the mineral phase of enamel is not pure hydroxyapatite. The less mineralized the enamel is, the whiter and more opaque it is; the more mineralized, the more translucent enamel allows the yellow color of the underlying dentin to show through. Examples of white, poorly mineralized enamel are the enamel of deciduous teeth and chalky patches of fluorosis and early carious lesions in adult teeth. Enamel crystals are about 10 times thicker and much longer than the apatite crystals of bone or dentin; the volume is about 1,000 times greater. The surface area is therefore relatively low, and this factor makes enamel crystal less reactive and soluble to acids than are apatite crystals of bone or dentin. The crystal also contains very little of the more soluble carbonates and magnesium salts found in dentin and bone. The enamel crystals are highly orientated and tightly packed. These factors account in part for the greater hardness of enamel in comparison to dentin and also for its resistance to acid demineralization. In addition, enamel has a lower percentage of organic material than dentin (*see Appendix B Table B.1*).

Enamel crystals are packed into larger units, the enamel prism, which is the structure made by each ameloblast as it lays down enamel during development. The prisms are about 100 crystals wide but are very long and may run uninterrupted from the dentin to the tooth surface. Both crystals and prisms have their long axis parallel to each other and are directed toward the surface of the tooth. However, at the prism boundaries, the crystals tend to turn outward and face their neighboring crystals. In this interprismatic zone, the enamel crystal orientation is slightly less ordered, and there is a little more space between them (▶ Fig. 2.1). This makes the interprismatic regions slightly weaker and more easily disrupted by tooth wear. During wear, whole prisms break off leaving a sharp edge to the enamel which is needed to shred food (▶ Fig. 2.2). During preparation of a cavity for a composite or amalgam restoration, the margins of enamel must be prepared so that all the enamel prisms are supported. This prevents their chipping off later and causing a failure at the margins of the restoration (▶ Fig. 2.3) (*see Appendix B.1 Physical Properties of Enamel and Dentin*).

2.1.2 Enamel: Non-Minerals

The non-mineral phase of enamel consists of proteins and water. This phase is not mixed randomly within the mineral but surrounds the large mineral crystals which are packed tightly together. The minute spaces in between the enamel crystals account for the slight porosity of enamel. During tooth development, the first formed enamel is very poorly mineralized. It appears chalk like and is dissolved readily by acids. As the newly formed enamel matures, proteins are removed and the enamel becomes more resistant to dissolution by acids (*see Appendix B.2 Enamel Proteins*).

2.1.3 Enamel Etching

The disorientation of crystals in the interprismatic zone makes it more susceptible to acid demineralization than the well-orientated crystals of prismatic enamel. It is the interprismatic zone which first demineralizes due to early caries. However, the

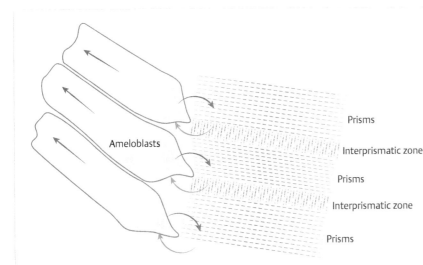

Fig. 2.1 A diagrammatic representation of the formation of enamel prisms during tooth development. Ameloblasts secrete enamel prisms parallel to each other with the enamel crystals orientated in the same direction. In the interprismatic zone, the crystals turn outward. The enamel matrix is secreted and mineralized by the ameloblast (*red arrow*), and the protein then resorbed (*blue arrow*).

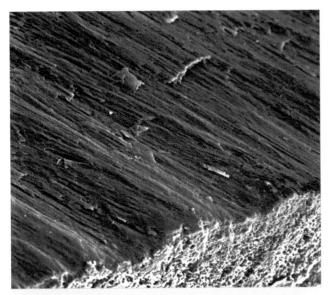

Fig. 2.2 A magnified view of a fractured enamel surface reveals parallel prisms packed together. Scanning electron microscope (SEM) image (magnification × 300) of an enamel surface, prepared by fracture in the direction of the enamel prisms. The fractured surface reveals enamel prisms stacked like the grain in a log of wood. The surface of the tooth was etched to reveal the ends of the enamel prisms.

dissolution pattern varies when organic acids are used to etch enamel. Etching enamel is a routine procedure when using restorative resins, because the resin bonds to a roughened surface better than to a smooth one. The two common etching patterns are etching of the prism center and etching of the interprismatic substance (▸ Fig. 2.4).

2.1.4 Early Enamel Caries

Plaque is an aggregate of bacteria in a sticky matrix which forms on the surface of enamel. Acid which has been formed as a product of bacterial metabolism may dissolve the surface enamel. If the surface breaks down, it may form a visible defect in the enamel which under normal light appears as a white patch. Early enamel caries seen under polarized light reveals

four distinct zones of mineralization (▸ Fig. 2.5). The outer surface zone is well mineralized by replacement ions from plaque and saliva. However, the body of the lesion is poorly mineralized. Deeper to the body of the lesion, a darker zone represents some remineralization, while the deepest zone is yet again demineralized. These zones of demineralization and remineralization illustrate the dynamic series of events which are occurring in the early lesion. Caries is not simply a process of continued demineralization.

2.1.5 Arrested Enamel Caries

The early lesion in enamel may be reversed and remineralized if plaque is removed. Ion exchange on the surface of enamel is a dynamic process which is occurring all the time. It is influenced by the degree of saturation of calcium and phosphate salts in plaque and saliva and the level of fluoride in the enamel and the adjacent plaque fluid. If the fluid surrounding the early lesion is highly saturated, crystals of apatite may form on the outer surface zone and remineralize the enamel of the early lesion. However, minerals in saliva may also block further penetration of calcium ions into the deeper layers of the lesion. If remineralization takes place slowly, and in the presence of fluoride, extensive mineralization occurs throughout the lesion.

The major contribution of fluoride in caries prevention appears to be in the process of arresting early lesions and preventing their progression into irreversible enamel loss and the formation of a cavity. Fluoride is concentrated in arrested enamel lesions and at the margins of actual enamel cavities. This may be due to the breakdown of the enamel surface at the center of an early lesion and the subsequent massive loss of mineral in the center, leaving the margins relatively intact with high fluoride levels.

Arrested enamel lesions are often seen on an approximal surface some time after an adjacent tooth has been extracted. Simply by improving the self-cleansing of the approximal area, the extraction of a neighboring tooth helps to reduce plaque mass. The lesion is recognizable by a brown stain, sometimes surrounded by a halo of chalky white enamel. Fluoride accumulates in remineralizing enamel, making the enamel more resistant to subsequent acid attack. So, an arrested enamel lesion is more resistant to acid demineralization than it was originally, as

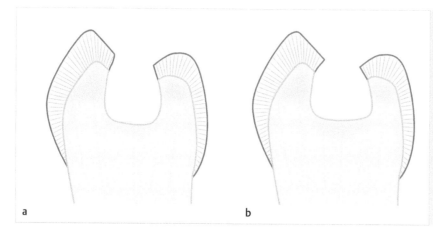

Fig. 2.3 Diagrammatic representation of the orientation of enamel prisms of a tooth illustrating the importance of avoiding leaving undermined enamel prisms during cavity preparation. (a) During cavity preparation it is important to ensure that angle of the cavity wall is prepared along the axis of enamel prisms. (b) Undermined margins leave fragments of prisms behind, which may fracture away from the cavity wall leaving a defect between the restoration of the tooth surface.

a   b

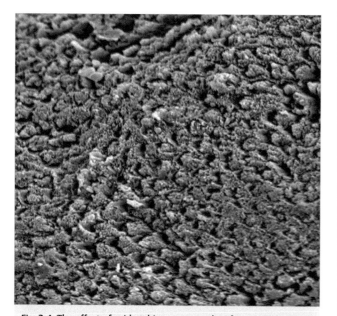

Fig. 2.4 The effect of acid etching an enamel surface. An SEM image (magnification × 1,000) of enamel surface after acid etching reveals that the interprismatic enamel has dissolved more rapidly than the prism core leaving a raise projection. In other areas, the core of the enamel prisms has dissolved more rapidly leaving a pitted surface, which provides mechanical retention for adhesive resins such as fissure sealants.

SZ: Surface zone

B: Body of the lesion

DZ: Dark zone

TZ: Translucent zone

Fig. 2.5 A diagrammatic representation of the layers which can be defined in an early caries lesion which illustrate the dynamic nature of demineralization and remineralization. The early enamel lesion consists of four zones of alternating levels of mineralization. The surface zone (SZ) is remineralized but blocks the passage of calcium ions into the body of the lesion (B) which remains demineralized. It may have to be removed to allow the lesion to become arrested. The dark zone (DZ) is well mineralized, but the translucent zone (TZ) is yet again demineralized. (Adapted from Kidd and Joyston-Bechal 1987.)

each cycle of demineralization leaves the enamel stronger than it was before (▶ Fig. 2.6).

Sometimes, the lesion progresses in spite of the availability of calcium and fluoride ions (▶ Fig. 2.7). This may be due to the presence of the barrier in the superficial zone, which we have noted above, restricts the movement of calcium and fluoride ions into the demineralized zone. This barrier may be due to plugging of the spaces between enamel crystals with salivary proteins.

Replacement minerals cannot get to the damaged site, but if the enamel surface is treated with a deproteinizing agent, remineralization occurs more readily. Remineralization may also be achieved by the removal of this superficial zone of the early lesion. This of course is more destructive than deproteinizing the surface, but there is evidence that tooth wear may be a significant process in arresting enamel lesions. If white lesions return to normal-looking enamel, either after orthodontic band removal or acid etching, it appears to be due to abrasion of the weakened enamel crystals by food and brushing. If remineralization does not occur as fast as the demineralization of enamel, eventually normal enamel structure is lost and a cavity develops.

Key Notes

Calcium hydroxyapatite ions are dissolving from and precipitating onto the enamel surface all the time. By reducing the acidity of the fluid surrounding the enamel surface, the balance toward mineralization instead of demineralization may be sustained. Even established lesions of demineralization may be reversed by fluoride treatment and careful oral hygiene.

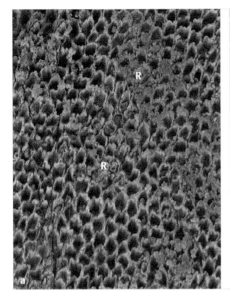
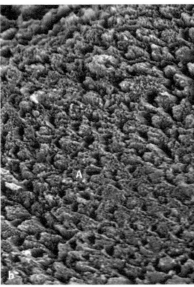

Fig. 2.6 SEM images of enamel reveal remineralization of early caries. A SEM (magnification × 5,000s) of etched enamel surface from an area recognized clinically as arrested caries. **(a)** In the center of the lesion, there are clusters of remineralizations (R) which resisted acid etching during preparation of the specimen. **(b)** Toward the periphery of the lesion, the enamel has become well remineralized and the lesion has become arrested (A).

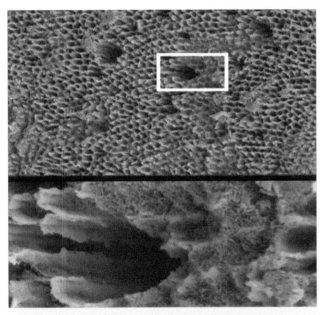

Fig. 2.7 The demineralization of the enamel surface in this SEM image of an early enamel carious lesion would have been irreversible. (Magnification × 300, window × 1,500).

2.2 Pulp–Dentin: Clinical Aspects

The pulp–dentin is a highly vascular loose connective tissue surrounded by a component of calcified connective tissue, the dentin. Although there are very obvious structural differences between pulp and dentin, the following reasons suggest they be treated as an integrated complex.

- During tooth development dentin is formed by odontoblasts of the pulp. After tooth development, peritubular and secondary dentin continue to be formed by the pulp odontoblast.
- The sensitivity of dentin depends on the presence of odontoblasts.
- The capacity of dentin to respond to irritation such as tooth wear, or dental caries, depends on odontoblasts.

- Both sensitivity and response to irritation are directly affected by the state of the entire pulp tissue.
- From an operative point of view, any procedure involving dentin is a procedure involving the pulp; any material or medication placed against dentin is a material or medication placed against the pulp.

2.2.1 Physical Properties

Dentin consists of mainly a collagenous matrix, mineralized to a moderate degree with a variety of apatite salts and magnesium and carbonates. By weight, it consists of 72% mineral, 18% organic matrix, and 10% water. It is less brittle than enamel (the modulus is about one-tenth of enamel), but is softer (about one-fifth of the hardness) and so wears more rapidly (*see Appendix B.1 Physical Properties of Enamel and Dentin*). The physical properties of dentin contribute to two important mechanical functions of the tooth. The first is to provide resilience to fracture. This resilience is due to the presence of proteoglycans. These molecules are resilient and prevent the propagation of cracks. Resilience is also provided by the collagen fibers which are orientated at right angles to a crack which may form in adjacent enamel (*see Appendix B.3 Composites and Resistance to Fracture*). The second important mechanical property of dentin is to provide a composite tooth surface for efficient mastication. Under the influence of a course diet the dentin wears faster than the enamel, leading to the formation of a concave grinding surface surrounded by a sharp cutting edge (*see Chapter 1 The Origins of Teeth*).

2.2.2 Tubules

Dentin is laid down by odontoblasts during tooth development. As the odontoblast retreats away from the secreted dentin, it leaves behind a process of the cell which remains into adult life, inside a fine tube or *tubule*. There is a greater density of tubules in cervical and root dentin than in coronal dentin (▶ Fig. 2.8 and ▶ Fig. 2.9).

The odontoblastic process continues to occupy most of the tubule into adult life. It extends the entire length of the dentinal

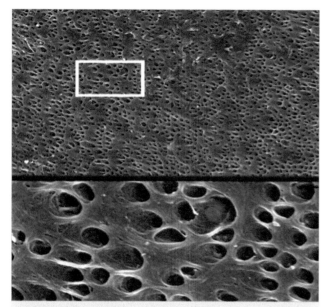

Fig. 2.8 A SEM image (magnification × 300, window × 1,500) of dentin tubules viewed from the coronal pulp. The odontoblasts and their processes have been removed. Note the high density and large diameter of the tubules, which would make this area of the pulp–dentin highly permeability to fluid movement.

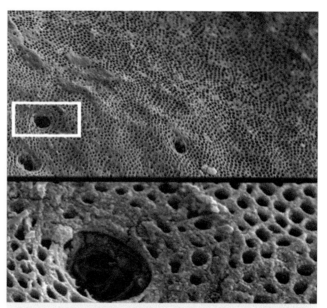

Fig. 2.9 A SEM image (magnification × 300, window × 1,500) of dentin tubules viewed from the root pulp. Note the higher density of tubules in comparison with coronal pulp in the previous image. This high density makes root dentin more permeable and therefore more sensitive to irritants than coronal dentin. The larger apertures are accessories to the apical root canal and may be responsible for spread of infection from the root pulp to the periodontium.

tubule in the crown of the tooth but only about a third of the tubule in dentin around the neck of the tooth. There is less and less recognizable cell content in the tubule as the odontoblastic process gets further away from the cell body and nutrients. Furthest from the cell body the process has no organelles but some microcisterns and microfilaments. There is a space around the odontoblastic process which is occupied by fluid. This fluid is able to flow back and forth along the tubule and may transmit vibrations which convey information to sensors in the body of the odontoblast. Fluid movement within the tubule is thought to cause sensations of pain arising in the nerve endings in the dental pulp. The ease with which fluid is able to move through the dentinal tubules is referred to as *dentin permeability*.

The odontoblastic process secretes dentin around the inner walls which is called *peritubular dentin*. This secretion continues throughout life but occurs more rapidly if there is mild irritation such as wear of the adjacent enamel or dental caries. However, peritubular dentin is also laid down in the absence of attrition, even in unerupted teeth. It is a feature of aging and is used by forensic dentists to determine the age of human remains.

Peritubular dentin reduces the tubule's dimension, and may eventually block it completely (▶ Fig. 2.10). When this happens, the dentin is called *sclerotic*. The high mineral content of sclerotic dentin makes it translucent to light and is easily identified by holding up a ground section of a tooth up to the light.

Peritubular dentin restricts the fluid flow through the dentinal tubule and thus reduces tooth sensitivity from irritants such as wear of enamel and dentin, or loss of cementum covering root surfaces. When peritubular dentin completely blocks the tubule, it protects the pulp from the bacteria and bacterial products occupying more superficial layers of a carious lesion.

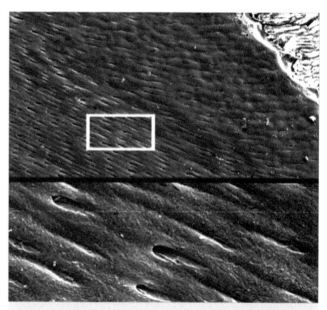

Fig. 2.10 A SEM image of dentin which has been cracked in preparation so as to reveal dentin tubules. The dentin in this image was close to the amelodentinal junction. (Magnification × 300, window × 1,500). There are relatively few open tubules as most have been blocked with peritubular dentin. This zone of the pulp–dentin would have a very low fluid permeability.

As production of peritubular dentin occurs most rapidly in response to irritation, it is most pronounced in the dentin nearest the source of irritation at the tooth surface (caries or tooth wear).

2.2.3 Permeability

Dentin permeability is influenced by the diameter of the dentinal tubule. This diameter varies according to the distance of the tubule from the pulp tissue. The tubules are at their narrowest dimension near the dentin enamel junction (1 μm) and widest nearer the odontoblast, where the average tubule diameter is 2 to 3 μm. The permeability of dentin to fluids is thus greatest near the pulp. The pulp tissue is therefore particularly vulnerable to deep carious lesions or to tooth preparation near the dental pulp (▶ Fig. 2.11). Dentin permeability is also influenced by the amount of peritubular dentin which has been laid down inside the tubule.

After cavity preparation, the permeability of dentin is effectively increased due to the opening of many tubules, 20,000 for every square millimeter of cut dentin. This permeability is reduced within hours of the tooth preparation. This appears to be due to the obturation of the tubule with fibrinogen from the serum.

If dentin is exposed to the oral cavity before peritubular dentin has formed, the tooth becomes sensitive to sweet, hot, and acid foods. These sensations are thought to be due to fluid movement within the tubule which is sensed by the odontoblast or surrounding free nerve endings (*see Chapter 10.4.3 Dentin Sensitivity*). Young adults who have bulimia suffer from enamel demineralization due to the presence of strong stomach acids in the oral cavity. Sensitivity of dentin occurs as peritubular dentin has not formed. Dentin hypersensitivity is also a common complaint in patients with receding gingiva. This sensitivity is caused by the loss of cementum covering the root surface and the exposure of root dentin tubules.

2.2.4 Response to Irritation

When dentin is exposed to oral fluids because of enamel wear, or enamel caries, bacterial products may diffuse down the dentinal tubules and cause a hypersensitive response from the odontoblast to normal stimuli. Cutting or grinding procedures on exposed dentin to remove dental caries is painful and usually requires anesthesia. It has been suggested that a normally cooled preparation of a completely caries-free tooth would not be particularly painful as the dental pulp is not hypersensitive. For obvious reasons this is not routine. The most common clinical sign of dentin hypersensitivity is a painful response of the pulp–dentin to hot and cold foods.

When odontoblasts are subjected to chemical or physical irritants, they increase in size and start laying down new peritubular dentin. They also lay down dentin in the roof of the pulp chamber, called secondary dentin, and retreat from the irritation behind this layer.

2.2.5 Secondary Dentin

Secondary dentin may entirely fill the original pulp chamber in an old and worn tooth. It is a normal physiological process related to tooth wear and aging of the tooth. With age, secondary dentin reduces the diameter of the root canal, causing difficulty in performing endodontic therapy for elderly patients. When secondary dentin is gradually formed, the microscopic appearance differs little from primary dentin. The dentin

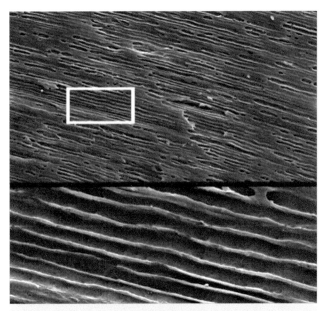

Fig. 2.11 A SEM image of dentin which has been cracked in preparation so as to reveal dentin tubules. This dentin in this image was close to the dental pulp. (Magnification × 300, window × 1,500). There are many open tubules and no peritubular dentin. This zone of the pulp–dentin would have a high fluid permeability.

tubules are less regularly arranged, but they are continuous with the primary dentin. If the progression of tooth wear or dental caries is more rapid, the secondary dentin tubules are quite irregular and not continuous with the primary tubules. So, the new dentin acts like an impermeable barrier wall. This irregular secondary dentin has been referred to as reactionary or reparative dentin. The barrier formed by reparative dentin reduces not only dentin sensitivity but also the responsiveness of the odontoblast to further irritation (▶ Fig. 2.12).

2.2.6 Dental Pulp Hyperemia

If the progress of an advancing carious lesion is rapid, there is insufficient time for secondary dentin to form, and odontoblasts are damaged by bacterial products. Their damage invokes an inflammatory response, with hyperemia, the arrival of inflammatory cells, and the potential for a localized abscess in that part of the pulp closest to the caries lesion. This is a critical point in the progress of pulp damage. If the irritation can be removed by removing the carious dentin and sealing the cavity, pulpal hyperemia may subside. If, however, the hyperemia is extensive and severe, the damage is irreversible and the pulp tissue must be removed by endodontic treatment.

From a clinical point of view, it is difficult to determine whether pulp hyperemia is reversible or irreversible, but there are some guidelines. Firstly, it is suggested that if the sensitivity to stimulation with hot or cold is short-lived, and the pain disappears soon after the stimulus is removed, the situation is hopeful for retaining the pulp tissue. Continual pain after stimulation suggests that the outlook for the pulp tissue is poor and that the pulp damage is widespread. Recall that the pulp is encased in a rigid shell and has a small opening for blood vessels. It is therefore highly vulnerable to vascular congestion and

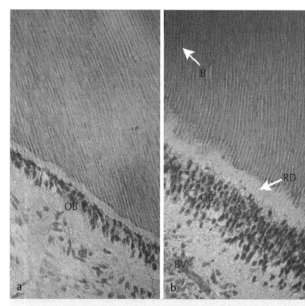

Fig. 2.12 **A histological section through the pulp–dentin of a tooth affected by dental caries.** (a) Normal odontoblast cells in an area of the tooth crown unaffected by caries (magnification × 200). (b) In another part of the same tooth, bacteria (B) in the dentinal tubules seen as fine black stains are advancing toward the pulp. In response to the irritation caused by bacteria, the odontoblasts (OB) and other pulp cells have increased in size and number and there is a greater vascular supply to the tissue (BV). A layer of predentin which will become reparative dentin (RD) has been formed to protect the pulp.

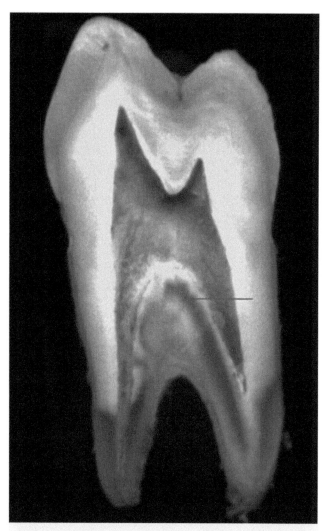

Fig. 2.13 **A maxillary second premolar, sectioned down its long axis in a buccal–lingual plane.** The shape of the pulp chamber follows that of the tooth crown, with a pulp horn under each cusp. The pulp chamber is flattened mesiodistally.

increased tissue pressure. The age of the tooth has a bearing on the outlook for a hyperemic tooth. Younger teeth with open apical foramina allow optimum vascular flow through the pulp, less venous congestion, and therefore greater healing potential than older teeth with narrow apical foramina.

If infected pulp tissue is not removed, further spread may occur into the periodontal ligament through the apex of the tooth and may also communicate with the periodontium via accessory root canals (▶ Fig. 2.9). These routes of communication with the periodontium are responsible for periapical abscess formation and further spread of infection into the alveolar bone. Infected pulp tissue must be removed and the empty spaces of the pulp chamber and root canal sealed up. This process, known as endodontic therapy, requires an intimate knowledge of the anatomy of pulp chambers and root canals. A brief and simplified version is presented below.

2.2.7 The Pulp Chamber and Root Canal

The pulp chamber is largest in the deciduous tooth, so the pulp is rapidly reached by advancing caries. It is also readily exposed during cavity preparation for a restoration, particularly if the operator is determined to remove all softened dentin.

In the permanent tooth, the pulp chamber is largest when the tooth has just been formed, that is before any secondary dentin has been laid down.

Pulp chambers generally follow the shape of the tooth crown. It would be more accurate to say that during tooth formation, the crown shape follows that of the pulp chamber. Thus, the pulp chamber is fan shaped in the incisor teeth, being flattened in a labial–lingual direction. In the canines it is flame shaped, and in the premolars and molar teeth the pulp chamber has peaks, known as horns, which lie under each tooth cusp (▶ Fig. 2.13).

During tooth wear, and aging, it is in these pulp horns that the first secondary dentin appears. In the floor of the pulp chamber, narrow canals lead along the center of each root. So, there are at least as many canals as there are roots and sometimes more. For example, the mesial root of the mandibular first molar is a fusion of two roots. This root, which appears to be single, actually has two root canals, one buccal and the other lingual. A buccal and a lingual canal should also be expected in the maxillary second premolar, even though this root may be appearing to be single. There are other examples of additional canals. The endodontist needs to be familiar with them all.

In the developing root, the root canals are quite wide and funnel shaped at the apex (▶ Fig. 2.14). The apical foramen of the root becomes progressively narrower as the root forms. As we have noted, sometimes there are extra accessory canals in

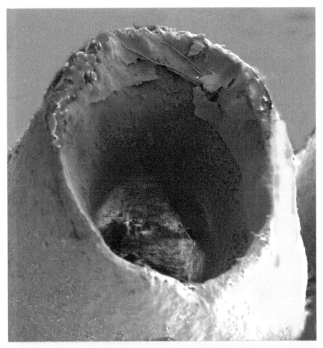

Fig. 2.14 The partially formed root of an unerupted third molar. The root apices do not close until the roots are fully formed.

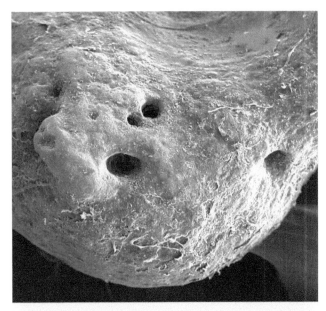

Fig. 2.15 An SEM image of the apex of a fully formed root shows a number of accessory canals. (Magnification × 100). The main apical foramen is not quite at the apex of the tooth but emerges to one side of it. In this example, it is on the left, slightly hidden by an overhang of cementum.

the root, which are difficult to locate, clean out, and fill during endodontic procedures. The apex of the root may also have accessory canals, forming a sort of delta of canals emerging from the root. The apex of the tooth becomes surrounded by cementum, which continues to form throughout life. It may not be obvious exactly where the apex is when examining a periapical radiograph because of this cementum, and accessory canals may not be visible (▶ Fig. 2.15).

Key Notes

Cavity preparation opens thousands of dentinal tubules. As the preparation approaches the dental pulp, the tubules become wider and the fluid flow in response to mechanical, thermal, or chemical irritation increases. Conservative cavity preparations reduce pulpal irritation and postoperative pain.

2.3 Response of the Pulp–Dentin to Caries

The unhindered progress of caries with irreversible damage to the pulp–dentin and periodontium, which has been outlined above, is relatively unusual except in rapidly progressing carious lesions. More commonly, the caries process is gradual, and the pulp–dentin has time to mount some defense. While caries of enamel is clearly a dynamic process of dissolution and precipitation, it is not a vital process in the sense that living cellular reactions occur. In contrast, the pulp–dentin is a vital tissue capable of both a biomineralization process and a physical/chemical process providing some degree of repair to damaged dentin.

The caries process in dentin involves the demineralization of the mineral component and breakdown of the organic

component, and so it is quite similar to the process of destruction which occurs in enamel, except that it progresses approximately twice as fast in dentin. This rapid progress is due to the ease with which organisms are able to migrate down the dentin tubules toward the pulp. These organisms may be seen in a section through a carious lesion. In the advancing front, just a few pioneer organisms are seen in contrast to the more established outer zones where the tubules are full of organisms (▶ Fig. 2.16).

Carious lesions in dentin consist of two distinct layers having different microscopic and chemical structures. The outer layer is heavily infected with bacteria, which are mainly located in the tubule spaces. The dentin collagen fibers are denatured, and so the structural organization disappears and there is no organic matrix to remineralize. The inner layer is more sparsely infected, but it has been demineralized by plaque acid. It still contains high concentrations of mineral salts and may be remineralized (▶ Fig. 2.17).

2.3.1 Bacterial Penetration

A large number of bacterial species have been isolated from dental caries but a few genera are commonly found and predominate (*see Chapter 4.3 The Biofilms of the Oral Environment*). The most frequently isolated from occlusal and smooth surface caries are the members of the *Streptococcus species* and in particular *Streptococcus mutans*, and *Streptococcus sobrinus*, collectively called the mutans streptococci. *Actinomyces species* are the dominant genus in root surface caries. Deep dentin caries has a predominance of lactobacillus organisms with several other gram-positive rods and filaments. Kidd and her coworkers took samples of carious dentin during cavity preparation and cultured the samples so as to count the number of bacteria.[1] As the samples were taken, the dentin was assessed as either soft, medium, or hard, wet or dry, and pale or dark.

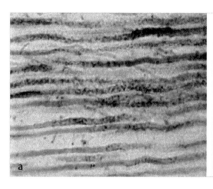
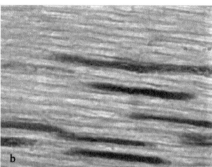

Fig. 2.16 Histological sections of infected and affected dentin from a carious tooth. (a) A section of dentin (magnification × 1,000) toward the surface of a caries lesion with bacteria-like structures packed into the dental tubules. This dentin could be described as infected. **(b)** A section of dentin from the same tooth, closer to the pulp and partly visible in ► Fig. 2.12b. A few dentinal tubules are stained with bacterial debris. This zone of dentin could be described as affected.

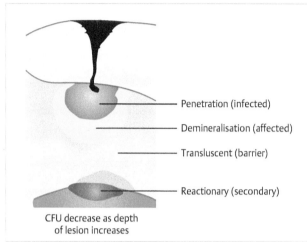

Penetration (infected)

Demineralisation (affected)

Transluscent (barrier)

Reactionary (secondary)

CFU decrease as depth
of lesion increases

Fig. 2.17 A diagrammatic representation of layers within a carious cavity. Dentin caries comprises two main layers. In the outer layer, the dentin is heavily *infected* with bacteria. Both organic matrix and mineral have been lost and the dentin is beyond repair. In the deeper layer, the dentin has been *affected* by plaque acids and demineralized. The number of colony-forming units (CFUs) of bacteria decreases (about 100 times) as cavity preparation proceeds into affected dentin. The damage in this layer is reversible if bacterial metabolism can be halted. A barrier of translucent (well-mineralized) dentin may be formed ahead of the advancing lesion. Reactionary (secondary) dentin forms to protect the pulp from acid irritation. (Adapted from Kidd and Joyston-Bechal 1987.)

The number of bacteria recovered diminished significantly as the caries became dryer and harder and the cavity became deeper. This reduction in numbers of bacteria was not marginal but of the order of 100 times less. There was no significant difference between the number of organisms cultured from medium as opposed to hard dentin. The color of the sample was not associated with the number of bacteria recovered. These findingssuggest that at the stage in cavity preparation, when the wet, heavily infected, soft dentin has been removed, further removal of medium, hard-stained dentin may not contribute to further reduction of infected material and may in fact be unnecessarily destructive. The question arises of the fate of slightly soft dentin when not removed, and whether it is a source of secondary caries.

2.3.2 Secondary Caries

Few dental restorations last a lifetime. Most eventually have to be replaced, either because they break down or because caries recurs. It used to be thought that recurrent or secondary caries was caused by the incomplete removal of all soft, infected dentin during the preparation of the cavity. The first indications that secondary caries may have other causes came from research studies which investigated leakage around the margins of restorations. According to Kidd, there is little evidence that leaving infected dentin behind after cavity preparation would result in caries progression.[2] A review by Ricketts confirmed that the microflora left beneath restorations usually do not grow, although they may survive for several months. Their viability is determined by the degree to which nutrients are excluded by an effective restorative seal.[3]

2.3.3 Conservative Management of Deep Caries

A traditional goal in cavity preparation was to remove all soft dentin until hard dry dentin was reached. In the 1970s, Massler and Pawlak promoted the idea that this was unnecessarily destructive and could often lead to exposure of the pulp in deep cavities.[4] They maintained that soft dentin was not necessarily infected but could be merely affected by plaque acids. They proposed a more conservative cavity preparation, which required the removal of *infected* dentin only, leaving behind soft but not infected, so-called *affected* dentin. Affected dentin could be remineralized if the acid production was halted. These suggestions were at the time supported by little experimental data, but there is now convincing evidence that the pulp–dentin has a significant ability to repair by the formation of reactionary dentin, provided that the heavily infected dentin is removed and the cavity is well sealed from the oral environment. The formation of reactionary dentin is the result of a cellular process involving the mineralization of a supportive extracellular matrix produced by the odontoblast. Demineralized (affected) dentin or enamel may also remineralize by a simple precipitation of mineral salts. The process may take place on the surface of an enamel or dentin cavity which is relatively free of bacteria but at some distance from the odontoblast.

2.3.4 Arrested Caries in Dentin

Arrested caries in dentin is clinically defined by hardness of the dentin surface and a yellow to dark brown color. Arrested carious lesions are found most commonly on lingual and labial aspects of teeth and less commonly in approximal areas. In caries which has become arrested, the dentinal tubules in the area between the soft and hard dentin have been shown to be obstructed by large crystals. It has been suggested that this process appears to occur in a number of stages[5] (► Fig. 2.18).

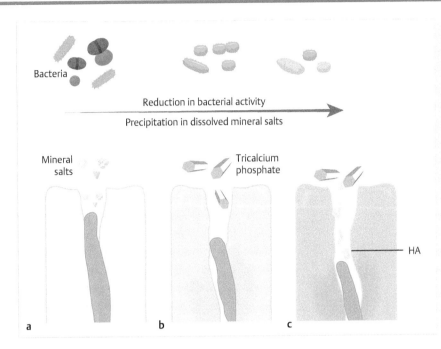

Bacteria

Reduction in bacterial activity

Precipitation in dissolved mineral salts

Mineral salts

Tricalcium phosphate

HA

a   b   c

Fig. 2.18 A diagrammatic representation of the stages in the formation of an arrested lesion in dentin. (a) The dentin tubule contains a high concentration of acid and dissolved mineral salts. **(b)** If bacterial acid production is reduced, and the pH increases, the salts precipitate into large crystals of tricalcium phosphate which temporally block the tubule. **(c)** If further bacterial activity is suppressed, the odontoblast process secretes collagen and calcium salts. Crystals of hydroxyapatite (HA) then form and block the tubule more effectively and permanently. (Adapted from Daculsi et al 1987.[5])

First stage: The acids produced by advancing bacteria have dissolved the mineral in the surrounding intertubular dentin. The tubular fluid becomes saturated with calcium, magnesium, and phosphate ions. The lesion progresses unless the level of metabolic activity of the bacteria is reduced. If acid production is reduced, then the second stage may occur.

Second stage: When the acid levels drop, the saturated solution precipitates, producing large crystals of tricalcium phosphate. These crystals are comparatively soluble but nevertheless block the tubule.

Third stage: The odontoblast process, protected by the large crystals blocking the tubule, secretes collagen into the dentin tubule. Small plate-like crystals of hydroxyapatite accumulate, which are less soluble than tricalcium phosphate and therefore block the tubule more effectively. At the same time, crystal growth occurs in the intertubular dentin. Zavgorodniy and coworkers conclude that the growth of crystals in arrested caries is both a biomineralization process and a dissolution/precipitation mechanism.[6] The dissolution/precipitation mechanism is dependent on the level of acid production by bacteria and the availability of salivary buffers and minerals. These factors determine whether precipitation of minerals or further dissolution will occur. The biomineralization process is dependent on the secretion of collagen by the odontoblastic process, which acts as a scaffold for the precipitation of insoluble apatite crystals.

2.3.5 Regeneration after Pulpal Exposure

A breach in the dentin, which causes exposure of the pulp, may be repaired by a bridge of new dentin provided that the pulp was not inflamed, the exposure was surgical and not carious, and that suitable stimulation was given to the pulpal cells. The stimulation which has been widely used is calcium hydroxide; a more recent material, mineral trioxide aggregate (MTA) has also proved to be successful. The calcium hydroxide is applied as a paste, which applied to the pulpal exposure causes local necrosis and a bridge of scar tissue to form. Calcium is deposited into the scar tissue, and this is followed by the secretion of dentin against the calcified bridge by odontoblasts. The degree of inflammation, the time of irritation and infection, and the location of the exposure must be regarded as decisive factors for the healing of the inflamed pulp rather than the effect of calcium hydroxide as such.[7] This conclusion indicates that the use of calcium hydroxide to induce bridge formation in a carious exposure will have to be a carefully considered clinical decision. Unfortunately, the degree of inflammation of the pulp is difficult to assess as there is a poor correlation between signs and symptoms and the histological state of the pulp. If the pulp tissue stops bleeding without the presence of a blood clot, it does suggest that the hyperemia associated with inflammation is not advanced. The rapid formation of a clot may indicate that a dentin bridge could not form under any circumstances. In view of the considerable time required to perform endodontic treatment on a molar tooth, the possibility of inducing a dentin bridge after removing infected dentin and pulp tissue should be considered (*see Chapter 5.3.3 Healing of a Pulp Exposure*).

2.3.6 The Origin of Replacement Odontoblasts

The odontoblast-like cells which form the dentin-like bridge appear to come from stem cells in the pulp tissue. These cells migrate, divide, and reveal changes which are characteristic of secreting cells, such as an increase in the size of the cytoplasm and nucleus, and the orientation of their cytoskeletal elements (actin and vimentin) toward one side of the cell. They also secrete fibronectin and type II collagen. The cells, which have a terminal process like an odontoblast, secrete a matrix against the wound tissue which becomes calcified. These cells differentiate without the inductive influence of the enamel epithelium, a prerequisite during tooth development. It is thought that the stem cells which remain in the pulp have already been influenced by ectoderm and may be at an intermediate stage of differentiation, between primitive mesenchymal cells and odontoblasts. They are thus responsive to signals in the environment which stimulate their last stage of differentiation.

Key Notes

The aggressive removal during cavity preparation, of all soft dentin, until a hard cavity floor is reached, is the first step in a downward cycle of overtreatment. It increases the risk of pulpal exposure, followed by endodontic therapy, reduction of the tooth crown, which may require pin- or post-retention, and the risk of root fracture, and extraction. The principles of conservation are preferable.

Review Questions

1. How would you account for the hardness of enamel and its resistance to acid attack?
2. What evidence supports the view that enamel caries is a dynamic process, and not simply a progressive demineralization of enamel?
3. Why is there a high concentrated fluoride at the periphery of a carious lesion?
4. Why is it useful to consider the pulp and dentin as one biological unit?
5. What is the clinical significance of the high concentration of dentinal tubules in root dentin?
6. What factors alter the permeability of dentin?
7. What zones of caries have been described in dentin, and how can you account for them?
8. What is the clinical significance of discriminating between infected and affected dentin?
9. How does the pulp–dentin develop a mineral barrier to caries?
10. What is the likely consequence of some bacteria remaining in a sealed cavity?
11. Why does the rate of caries progression in dentin differ from enamel?

12. What is the difference between biomineralization and dissolution/precipitation?

References

[1] Kidd EA, Joyston-Bechal S, Beighton D. The use of a caries detector dye during cavity preparation: a microbiological assessment. Br Dent J 1993; 174(7):245–248

[2] Kidd EA. How 'clean' must a cavity be before restoration? Caries Res 2004; 38(3):305–313

[3] Ricketts D. Deep or partial caries removal: which is best? Evid Based Dent 2008; 9(3):71–72

[4] Massler M, Pawlak J. The affected and infected pulp. Oral Surg Oral Med Oral Pathol 1977; 43(6):929–947

[5] Daculsi G, LeGeros RZ, Jean A, Kerebel B. Possible physico-chemical processes in human dentin caries. J Dent Res 1987; 66(8):1356–1359

[6] Zavgorodniy AV, Rohanizadeh R, Bulcock S, Swain MV. Ultrastructural observations and growth of occluding crystals in carious dentine. Acta Biomater 2008; 4(5):1427–1439

[7] Schröder U. Effects of calcium hydroxide-containing pulp-capping agents on pulp cell migration, proliferation, and differentiation. J Dent Res 1985; 64 (Spec No):541–548

Suggested Readings

Berkowitz BWK, Moxham BJ, Linden RWA, Sloan AJ. Oral biology; oral anatomy histology, physiology and biochemistry. London: Churchill Livingstone; 2010

Brookes SJ, Robinson C, Kirkham J, Bonass WA. Biochemistry and molecular biology of amelogenin proteins of developing dental enamel. Arch Oral Biol 1995; 40(1):1–14

Charadram N, Austin C, Trimby P, Simonian M, Swain MV, Hunter N. Structural analysis of reactionary dentin formed in response to polymicrobial invasion. J Struct Biol 2013; 181(3):207–222

Featherstone JD. The continuum of dental caries—evidence for a dynamic disease process. J Dent Res 2004; 83(Spec No C):C39–C42

Kidd EA, Joyston-Bechal S. The essentials of dental caries. Bristol: Wright; 1987

Pashley DH. Dentin permeability, dentin sensitivity, and treatment through tubule occlusion. J Endod 1986; 12(10):465–474

Sloan AJ, Smith AJ. Stem cells and the dental pulp: potential roles in dentine regeneration and repair. Oral Dis 2007; 13(2):151–157

Stahl J, Zandona AF. Rationale and protocol for the treatment of non-cavitated smooth surface carious lesions. Gen Dent 2007; 55(2):105–111

3 Oral Mucosa and Periodontium

Abstract

Into this chapter are grouped the soft tissues of the mouth and the tooth-supporting tissues. The oral mucosa varies from the thin, fragile lining of the floor of the mouth to the rugged masticatory mucosa of the tongue and hard palate. These tough mucosal surfaces may have to withstand the rigors of masticating hard food. The periodontium which includes the structures supporting the teeth is of great importance to dentists. When it is infected and the tissue destroyed, the teeth may literally fall out. And notwithstanding all the progress in treating periodontal disease, it remains resistant to treatment in many patients. The junction between the tooth root and the supporting tissues provides a potential route of entry of bacteria into the body, which is unusual; all other external openings of the body are lined with epithelium with the exception of the fallopian tubes. The teeth are not held rigidly in their sockets like reptilian or fish teeth. They are able to move slightly in function and have the capacity to reposition as they erupt and drift when unsupported by neighbors or opposing teeth. An understanding of the dynamic structures of tooth support is essential to understanding the response of the periodontium to infection.

Keywords: oral mucosa, oral epithelium, lamina propria, masticatory mucosa, gingiva, periodontium, epithelial attachment, junctional epithelium, cementum

3.1 Structure of Oral Mucosa

The oral mucosa is the tissue lining the mouth. The two major layers of the oral mucosa, the oral epithelium and the lamina propria, are equivalent to the epidermis and dermis of the skin.

3.1.1 Oral Epithelium

The oral epithelium is a stratified layer of squamous cells which may either be keratinized or nonkeratinized. The characteristics of the individual layers (i.e., basal, prickle, granular, and keratin) are similar to those seen in the skin. Most of the cells of the epithelium are keratocytes. As they mature and are pushed to the surface by dividing cells in the basal layer, they will fill with keratohyalin granules and finally keratin.

There are three other types of cell in the epithelium.

- The melanocytes produce pigment and transfer it to the keratocytes around them. The number of melanocytes is no greater in heavily pigmented epithelium, but their activity is increased.
- The Langerhans and other dendritic cells are active in the immune response of the epithelium. They act as sentries, detecting the presence of foreign antigens on the surface of the oral epithelium. They then migrate from the epithelium to local lymph nodes where they present information about surface antigens to T (CD4) lymphocytes. The Langerhans cells do not have desmosome attachments, and so during histological processing the cytoplasm shrinks down around the nucleus producing a clear halo. Hence, these cells are referred to as clear cells.
- The Merkel cell is a mechanical receptor for tactile sensations.

The superficial layers of the epithelium may be both keratinized and nucleated. Keratinized epithelium is almost impermeable, due to a glycoprotein intercellular cementing substance, special cell junctions (desmosomes), and the keratin within the cell. Keratin (*Greek*, kera = horn) is a fibrous protein which is the main constituent in hair, hide, horns and hooves, claws, scales, feathers, and beaks. It is made up of a triple helix in a left-handed coil (contrary to the right-hand coil of collagen). The keratin fibers form a meshwork around the nucleus of the cell and attach to the desmosome plates inside the cell wall. Unlike collagen fibers, they remain within the cell (intracellular), where they provide a scaffolding joining one cell junction to another. The components for synthesizing the keratin molecules come from the constituents of the cytoplasm of the cell itself. As the content of keratin increases, the cell shrinks, shrivels up, dries out, and becomes lifeless but very tough.

The surface ultrastructure is characterized by microinvaginations on the surface side of the flattened squamous cell and microprojections on the deep side (▶ Fig. 3.1). The projections of the cell above interlock like a press stud with the invaginations on the surface of the cell below, providing a strong bond between the cells. Nonkeratinized epithelium is in general thicker than keratinized epithelium. It is slightly more permeable, but only to low-molecular-weight compounds such as glyceryl trinitrate (used to relieve an attack of angina pectoris). The surface ultrastructure lacks a robust interlocking mechanism with the adjacent cells which are readily detached from each other by light mechanical scraping.

3.1.2 Lamina Propria

The lamina propria is a layer of interlocking fibers, which gives strength to the epithelium above. It consists mostly of tough collagen fibers, some elastic fibers, and reticulin. In between the fibers are fibroblasts and other connective tissue cells. Beneath the lamina propria of the mucosa is usually a layer called the submucosa. It is a loose connective tissue containing fat, blood vessels, nerves, and lymphatics. In some areas such as the hard palate, the submucosa is also fibrous and binds the overlying mucosa quite firmly. However, there is no submucosa at all beneath the gingival mucosa. The lamina propria of the gingiva is bound directly onto the periosteum. It is therefore often referred to as a mucoperiosteum (▶ Fig. 3.2).

3.2 Function of Oral Mucosa

The oral mucosa has a protective, secretory, and sensory function.

The protective function is served by its resistance to tearing and compression, which is provided by the tough and yet resilient lamina propria. The oral mucosa is also mostly impervious to the penetration of bacterial toxins. Protection from microorganisms is also afforded by the shedding (desquamation) of the surface layer of cells. Bacterial colonies attached to these surface cells are thus regularly carried away when the surface cells are sloughed off. The cells are themselves flushed away in the saliva and swallowed.

Minor salivary glands in the submucosa secrete via ducts passing through the mucosa. These secretions help to keep the mucosa moist and free of excessive accumulations of bacteria.

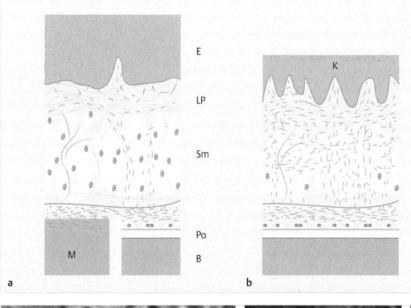

Fig. 3.1 A diagrammatic representation of the components of oral mucosa. (a) The lining mucosa has a relatively thick epithelium which is not keratinized (E), supported by thin lamina propria (LP). The submucosa (Sm) contains blood vessels and minor salivary glands, in a loose connective tissue. The submucosa may be attached to muscle (M) or the periosteum (Po) covering bone. (b) Masticatory mucosa has a keratinized epithelium (K) and a dense lamina propria of collagen fibers, which attach the epithelium directly to the periosteum covering bone (B).

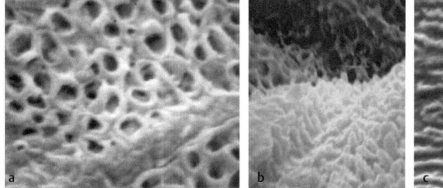

Fig. 3.2 A scanning electron microscope (SEM) image of the surface epithelial cells from oral mucosa (magnification × 2,000). (a) The surface membrane of each cell has invaginations. (b) These interlock with projections in the adjacent cell. (c) Nonkeratinized epithelium has microplications, and each cell is less firmly attached to its neighbor than keratinized cells.

The secretions of minor salivary glands contain the same antibacterial elements as those from the major salivary gland and contribute to the control of bacterial growth on the oral mucosal surfaces. There are also sebaceous glands sometimes seen on the inside of the cheek (also called Fordyce's granules). They have no function but are important to recognize as being normal.

The mucosa provides a suitable site for sensory nerve endings, such as those associated with pain, touch, temperature, and the taste receptors of the tongue and palate. Some of these receptors are important in the initiation of reflexes like swallowing or jaw opening.

3.2.1 Rates of Turnover of Oral Mucosa

The rate of cell division (mitosis) of the basal layer of cells normally keeps pace with the rate of desquamation from the surface. The time taken for a recently divided basal cell to reach the surface and exfoliate is the turnover time for one cell. The rate of mitosis is reduced with increasing age but increased by stress, infection, and changes in the levels of female hormones. Apart from these influences, the rates of turnover vary according to skin and mucosa types. The cells of a keratinized epithelium exfoliate after about 60 days for skin and after 45 days for gingiva. In comparison, the nonkeratinized lining mucosa turns over in 25 days. However, even this is a short period compared to the gut epithelium, where cells only last 10 days. The junctional epithelium around the cervical margin of the tooth is very fragile and turns over in 4 to 6 days. The rate of turnover of epithelium is related to its functions. Those which are primarily protective (skin) have a tough layer of impervious keratin and turn over relatively slowly. Mucosa, which must be flexible and stretch during function, is not protected by keratin but is quite thick. The shedding of the surface cells is an important protective device which compensates for the lack of a protective keratin layer. Mucosa which must be permeable to allow for food absorption (e.g., gut) or to allow secretions of fluid to combat bacteria (e.g., junctional epithelium) must be very thin and is therefore easily damaged. Its turnover rate is high.

3.3 Regional Variation of Oral Mucosa

The oral mucosa may be divided into three types, each of which has a different structure related to its function. The three types are masticatory mucosa, lining mucosa, and gustatory mucosa (▶ Fig. 3.3). The gingiva, while forming part of the masticatory oral mucosa, is also intimately related to the periodontium or supporting structures of the tooth. The periodontium consists of the gingiva, periodontal ligament, cementum, and alveolar bone.

3.3.1 Masticatory Mucosa

Masticatory mucosa is a descriptive term for the mucoperiosteum, which forms most of the gingiva and covers the hard palate. It is hard enough to resist the abrasion of coarse and rough food particles. It is also firmly attached to the alveolar bone and teeth so that little displacement occurs when a tough food bolus slides down the tooth. Edentulous patients, who have no dentures, are often able to chew directly onto their masticatory mucosa covering the residual alveolar ridges without causing any damage; they also make such frequent use of the tongue against the palate that the tongue becomes larger and more muscular than usual.

Gingiva: The part of the masticatory mucosa which covers the alveolar bone around and in between the teeth is firmly attached to the underlying bone and therefore referred to as *attached gingiva*. The part of the gingiva which encircles the teeth but is not attached to either tooth or bone is known as the *free gingiva*. The attached gingiva is usually keratinized, but if it becomes inflamed, it may become nonkeratinized. The more effectively the teeth and gingiva are cleaned, the greater is the tendency for the gingiva to be keratinized. The width of the attached gingiva varies between 4 and 8 mm but is on the average wider in older people. The gingiva is paler pink in color than the mucosa lining the mouth, due to its opacity, but also

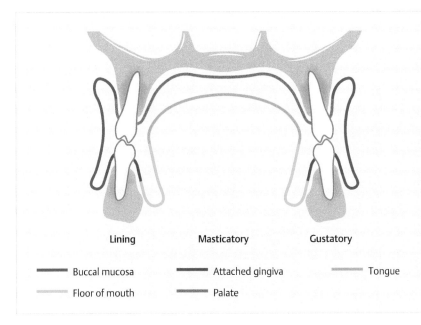

Fig. 3.3 A diagrammatic representation of the distribution of lining, masticatory, and gustatory mucosa.

Lining	Masticatory	Gustatory

Buccal mucosa — Attached gingiva — Tongue

Floor of mouth — Palate

may be more heavily pigmented with melanin. The junction between the gingiva and the mucosa lining the vestibule and cheeks is noticeable. This mucogingival junction forms a scalloped line around the root eminence of each tooth (▶ Fig. 3.4).

There is a shallow sulcus (about 2-mm deep) between the free gingiva and the enamel of the tooth, and this sulcus is lined with nonkeratinized epithelium. A probe can normally be inserted into this sulcus to measure the depth without causing bleeding. This sulcus epithelium is continuous with the

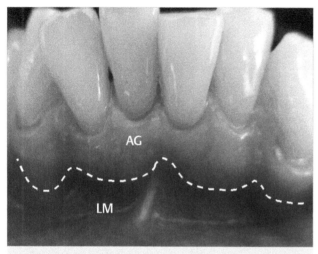

Fig. 3.4 Healthy oral mucosa. The attached gingiva (AG) reveals the contour of the underlying alveolar bone. The broken line marks the mucogingival junction between the attached gingiva and the lining mucosa (LM).

junctional epithelium, which is a physical attachment or junction between the tooth and its gingiva. When viewed in histological sections, the gingival epithelium has long rete pegs, which represent long and tall ridges penetrating deeply into the lamina propria (▶ Fig. 3.5).

Most of the fibers of the oral mucosa are irregularly arranged, but there are some recognizable gingival fiber groups associated with the fibers of the periodontal ligament (▶ Fig. 3.6). They are named simply by their orientation. Thus, there are a group of fibers connecting the gingiva to the tooth, the so called *dentogingival* fibers. The ends of the fibers are anchored into the root by being included into cementum. The *alveolar crest* fibers bind the gingiva to the crest of the alveolar bone surrounding the tooth socket. Another *circular* group surrounds the tooth and the *interdental* fibers run between the buccal and lingual papilla between the teeth.

The attached gingiva has a finely pitted or stippled surface due to the insertion of fiber bundles which help bind the lamina propria to the fibers of the periosteum and periodontal ligament.

Collagen fibers are the most essential component of the gingival fiber complex. Reticulin fibers are numerous in the tissue adjacent to the basement membrane and in the tissue surrounding large blood vessels. Oxytalin fibers are present in the connective tissue of the periodontium and appear to be concerned with vascular support. Elastic fibers are only found in gingiva and the periodontium in the connective tissue associated with blood vessels. In the lining mucosa, however, elastic fibers are numerous.

Hard palate: The mucosa of the hard palate is continuous with the gingiva on the palatal side of the maxillary teeth. A pattern of ridges with varying size and shape occurs toward the

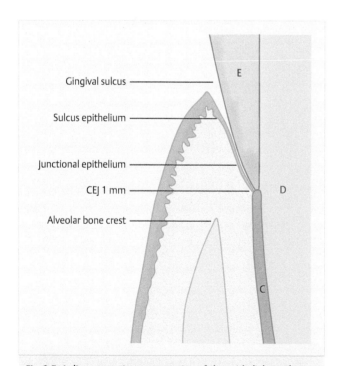

Fig. 3.5 A diagrammatic representation of the epithelial attachment to the tooth. The junctional epithelium is a continuation of the sulcus epithelium but is physically attached to enamel by hemidesmosomes. Note the relationship between the cementoenamel junction (CEJ) and the crest of the alveolar bone. C, cementum; D, dentin; E, enamel.

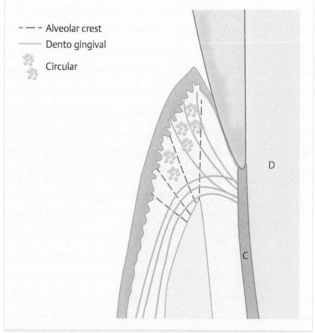

Fig. 3.6 A diagrammatic representation of the gingival fiber attachment to the tooth and alveolar bone. The dentogingival fibers are anchored into the root by cementum. The alveolar crest fibers secure the gingiva to the alveolar bone. Circular gingival fibers provide a firm cuff around the tooth, holding the attached gingiva to the tooth. C, cementum; D, dentin; E, enamel.

anterior half of the palate. These ridges are known as rugae and may be as characteristic in their pattern as finger prints. The most anterior feature is the incisive papilla which indicates the position of the incisive foramen. The palatal mucosa has no submucosa and is tightly bound to the palatal periosteum except for an area on either side of the midline, where the submucosa contains fat and more posteriorly, the palatine mucous glands. It also contains the palatine arteries, veins, and nerves.

3.3.2 Lining Mucosa

The lining mucosa covers the cheeks, vestibular sulcus, inner surface of the lips, floor of the mouth, and undersurface of the tongue. Most of the lining mucosa lies directly over muscle, and so there is little space for any submucosa. Where the submucosa is more substantial, there are minor salivary glands, vessels, and nerves. The lining mucosa of the floor of the mouth is particularly thin. It provides a useful route of entry for some drugs. Patients who suffer from angina (heart pain) may get relief by placing a tablet of nitroglycerine under the tongue. Recall that it is common practice to place a thermometer under the tongue as it is in close contact with blood vessels.

3.3.3 Gustatory Mucosa

The dorsal surface of the tongue is covered with a specialized mucosa which has both taste and masticatory function. Taste buds lie within the epithelium over the surface of the tongue, the soft palate, and epiglottis. The tongue is divided into two parts, an anterior two-thirds and a posterior third, by a V-shaped groove, the sulcus terminalis. The epithelium of the tongue is highly keratinized with pointed projections of keratin with a core of lamina propria. The keratin at the tip is extended into a short spiky process. These fine projections are known as *filiform papillae*. The tongue may appear fury if during illness this keratin is not worn away. The purpose of these papilla in man is uncertain. They probably serve a similar function as in other mammals where they protect the surface of the tongue from the abrasive action of rough foods. They also serve to provide a grip on slippery foods in order to form a bolus and to cleanse the oral surfaces of food debris. There are larger, less thread-like papillae of the tongue called *fungiform papillae* from their resemblance to a mushroom. They are scattered singly over the tongue but concentrated near the tip. The epithelium of fungiform papillae contains taste buds. The *vallate papillae* are prominent features, just anterior to the sulcus terminalis. There are only about 12 vallate papillae and they do not project above the surface. The furrow contains numerous taste buds and the openings of the serous glands of von Ebner. The *foliate papillae* are projections around the side of the tongue and have no special function.

Taste buds are oval structures within the epithelium of the tongue. They consist of elongated cells packed together whose ends open out into a pit below an opening in the epithelium. Not all the cells are active, but some may be either supportive to, or precursors of, active cells. The number of taste buds diminishes with age. The sensory supply to the anterior two-thirds is via the lingual branch of the mandibular nerve. The taste sensations are carried via the chorda tympani branch of the facial nerve. The posterior third receives its sensory supply

from the glossopharyngeal nerve. The motor supply to all muscle of the tongue except the glossopharyngeus is the hypoglossal nerve.

The *periodontium* is a term used to describe the supporting and investing structures of the tooth. These comprise the alveolar bone, periodontal ligament, cementum, and the gingiva, an important component of which is the gingival attachment to the tooth by the junctional epithelium. We have reviewed the structure of the gingiva and gingival attachment, so what follows are the other components of the periodontium, the alveolar bone, cementum, and periodontal ligament.

> **Key Notes**
>
> A removable dental prosthesis may have to derive occlusal support from the residual alveolar ridge. The thickness, and resilience to displacement, of the mucosa overlying the residual ridge exhibits regional variation. This variation may limit the ability of the mucosa in certain regions to resist compression caused by masticatory forces. These limitations may determine the patient's ability to tolerate the prosthesis.

3.4 Alveolar Bone

The roots of the teeth are held in a ridge of bone which is called the alveolus. Dense bone (cortical plate) covers the outer surface and lines the interior surface of each tooth socket. The dense appearance when seen on a radiograph, of the cortical plate around the tooth root, gave rise to the term *lamina dura*. Foramina (holes) in the outer cortical plate and the lamina dura allow for the passage of blood vessels and nerves. Within the dense bony plates covering the alveolar bone is a less dense network of bone trabeculae. These trabeculae are like inner girders, which are frequently remodeling in response to the changes in directions of the stresses and strains occurring in the bone during forces applied by the teeth during function. A thin septum of bone separates adjacent teeth and roots of multirooted teeth. The level of alveolar bone around each tooth is surprisingly constant in the unworn dentition at 1 to 2mm below the level of the cement-enamel junction (CEJ). If this distance is greater than 1 to 2mm, it is an indication that the bone has been resorbed or remodeled due to disease of the periodontium (chronic periodontitis). This distance does, however, increase quite normally in individuals who experience tooth wear, reflecting another compensatory mechanism, continued eruption (*see* ▶ Fig. 8.14). Radiographs of the teeth reveal the difference in density between the cortical plates and trabeculae and the level of bone around the roots of each tooth. If for any reason the teeth should not develop, the alveolar ridge of bone is absent. The alveolus gradually resorbs following the loss of teeth due to extraction. There is some evidence that alveolar bone can be distinguished from the rest of the bone of the mandible or maxilla, which is then described as basal bone. Elephants' teeth erupt surrounded by a shell of alveolar bone, which is quite separate from the jaw bone until eruption occurs.

There is a clinically important regional variation in shape and thickness of the alveolar bone which is determined by the size and shape of the tooth roots and their position in the arch.

Maxillary alveolar bone: In the maxilla, alveolar bone is thinnest around the labial aspect of the maxillary incisor roots.

Here, the cortical plate and the lamina dura fuse together without any intervening trabecula bone. The bone becomes progressively thicker toward the molar teeth but particularly so on the palatal side of the roots. Sometimes, there is very little bone separating the apex of the roots of the maxillary posterior teeth and the floor of the maxillary antrum. The thinness of the labial/buccal alveolar bone covering the maxillary roots has important clinical application when anesthetizing the teeth to allow cavity preparation to be carried out painlessly, or a tooth to be extracted. If local anesthetic is injected under the lining mucosa, next to the thin buccal bone of the maxillary teeth, it infiltrates through to the periodontal ligament and dental nerve where it blocks nerve transmission to the tooth allowing painless restorative or surgical procedures. The thinner buccal bone of the maxillary teeth also permits the tooth socket to be expanded sufficiently to allow extraction of the tooth in a buccal direction. The proximity of the molar roots to the maxillary antrum may be a clinical hazard. During efforts to remove a fractured molar root fragment, it may be pushed into the antrum, with resulting clinical complications.

Mandibular alveolar bone: As in the maxilla, the mandibular alveolar bone is thinnest around the labial aspect of the mandibular incisors' roots and thicker around the molar roots. The lingual plate of bone supporting molar roots is usually thinner than the buccal plate. This should not encourage the clinician to extract mandibular teeth by expanding the socket toward the lingual plate as the lingual nerve and artery may be damaged. The root apices of the third molar may be close to the inferior dental nerve which makes surgical removal of third molar roots potentially hazardous.

The cortical plate of bone of the mandible is thicker than that covering the maxilla. A clinical consequence of this thick cortical plate is that anesthetic solutions do not readily filter through it. Infiltration anesthesia for mandibular teeth is usually ineffective. The alternative is to block the mandibular nerve by depositing anesthetic solution close to the nerve before it enters the mandible on the mesial aspect of the ramus.

Histology of alveolar bone: The cortical plates and lamina dura of alveolar bone consist of circumferential and concentric (haversian) lamellae (*see Chapter 7.3.4 Intramembranous Bone Formation*). The bone intervening between the lamella has the same basic histology, but as a result of resorption, it has been remodeled into a honeycomb-like system of trabeculae (struts). The histological appearance of trabecula bone is misleading as it gives no indication of their three-dimensional structure (*see* ▶ Fig. 7.6). The spaces between the trabeculae are occupied by red marrow (hematopoietic tissue) in the young, but this is replaced in the adult by fatty tissue. Fibers run through the alveolar bone, connecting the roots of neighboring teeth. Fibers embedded in the cementum of the roots are also embedded in the lamina dura of the tooth socket and are known as Sharpey's fibers.

Alveolar bone, like all other bones, contains no sensory nerves except those conveying impulses along C fibers which are concerned with healing. The extraction of a tooth is painful due to damage to the nerves supplying the dental pulp, periodontal ligament, gingiva, and periosteum. When the osteotomy (bone removal) site for an implant fixture is prepared, the only tissue with a nerve supply is the periosteum, which may be anesthetized using a local infiltration. This is of clinical importance, as it allows an osteotomy to be prepared in the mandible, without administering a nerve block to the inferior dental nerve. This nerve therefore remains sensitive and reactive to any damage which might occur during the osteotomy procedure by the operator cutting too deep into alveolar bone. Inferior dental nerve damage is a serious complication of implant placement, which can be avoided by leaving the inferior dental nerve responsive, so that the patient may warn the operator before serious damage to the nerve occurs.

Key Notes

During the extraction of a tooth, the potential for expansion of the socket and displacement of the root is greatest where the alveolar bone is thinnest. A knowledge of the patterns of variation in thickness of the alveolar bone supporting the roots of teeth is therefore of clinical importance.

3.5 The Periodontal Ligament

The periodontal ligament is the connective tissue which lies between the roots of teeth and the lamina dura of the alveolar bone. The periodontal ligament is continuous with the lamina propria of the attached gingiva at the coronal end of the tooth and continuous with the pulp tissue at the root apex. It is thus vulnerable to the spread of infections from two sources. Firstly, from the gingiva and secondly from the root apex of a tooth if the dental pulp is infected. The periodontal ligament is about 0.2-mm wide, but this varies between individuals and areas of the root. It is wider in people who habitually place greater stresses on the teeth. The periodontal ligament consists predominantly of fibers. The fibers are surrounded by the extracellular matrix, in which cells, blood vessels, and nerve fibers are found. Some elements of the ligament have a rapid rate of turnover.

3.5.1 Periodontal Ligament Fibers

The periodontal ligament fibers are mainly collagen with some reticulin, elastin, and oxytalan fibers. Many of the collagen fibers are gathered together in bundles (the so-called principal fibers). These fiber bundles have been divided into groups on the basis of their direction and site. We can recognize apical, oblique, horizontal, alveolar crest, interradicular, and transalveolar fibers (▶ Fig. 3.7). It should be recalled that the fibers of the gingiva also contribute to the collagen fibers of the periodontal ligament. They ensure the firm but resilient attachment of the gingiva and teeth to the alveolar bone.

Oxytalan fibers are unlike collagen in that they are not banded, but they do consist of fibrils running parallel to the long axis of the fiber. They are more numerous nearer the tooth than the alveolar bone. They seem to be more numerous in teeth which are under heavy loads such as those supporting fixed partial prosthesis. The means whereby oxytalan fibers contribute to tooth support are controversial, but their association with blood vessels has led to the suggestion that they may maintain patency of vessels even during the moments of compression of the ligament.

The elastin fibers are confined to the walls of the blood vessels and the reticulin fibers to basement membranes.

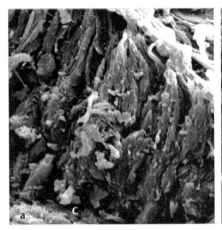
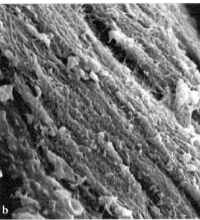

Fig. 3.7 SEM images of the two separate areas of periodontal ligament remaining attached to an extracted tooth (magnification × 2,000). **(a)** The collagen fiber bundles in this area of the PDL are orientated between the cementum surface (*C*) and the outer surface of the ligament which has separated from the tooth socket, estimated by the *broken line*. **(b)** The fiber bundles in this area of the periodontal ligament (PDL) are longer and appear to run in an oblique direction.

3.5.2 Response of the Periodontal Ligament to Loading

Teeth are not fixed in the tooth socket but are displaced by even light forces. A maxillary incisor moves about 10 μm when a horizontal load of 0.5 N is applied. The tooth becomes progressively firmer as the load continues (*see Appendix C.1 Tooth Displacement*). The fibers of the ligament may suspend the tooth in the socket and so come under tension when the tooth is intruded. However, it is likely that other forms of support are also involved, as intrusion of an incisor tooth causes expansion of the alveolar plates of bone on either side. This observation suggests that the tooth is also supported by compression of the ligament (*see Appendix C.2 Tooth Mobility*).

3.5.3 Cells of the Periodontal Ligament

The periodontal ligament is highly cellular. The predominant cell is the fibroblast which occupies about 50% of the volume. Fibroblasts are usually fusiform in shape, but they may, when especially active, become disk shaped. The fibroblasts of the periodontal ligament are mostly of this disk-like shape. This active form of the cell is testimony to the rapid secretion and resorption of collagen and ground substance. Breakdown of collagen used to be thought to be an extracellular process, but there is evidence that collagen fibers are phagocytosed into the cytoplasm of the fibroblast and then broken off into small fragments to be degraded within lysosomes. Fibroblasts can be both phagocytosing part of a collagen fibril at one end and secrete new fibrils at the other. This degree of activity would most likely be found in a young erupting tooth and less conspicuous in older teeth. The turnover of collagen in the ligament is one of the most rapid of any connective tissue. The half-life of collagen in the rat molar is just 1 day. Half-life is an expression which represents the speed with which a substance is altered. Thus, in 1 day, half the collagen has been replaced.

Epithelial cell rests (ECR) of Malassez are remnants of the epithelial root sheath of Hertwig and form a sparse network around the root (▶ Fig. 3.8). Lindskog and coworkers have shown that tissue cultures of the ECRs appear to inhibit the formation of bone by osteoblasts.[1] The zone of inhibition is similar to the width of the periodontal ligament. They suggest that the ECRs, having epithelial origins, have the capacity to prevent ankylosis of the bone to the tooth. More recent studies have supported this work, concluding that ECRs are involved in maintaining the periodontal space.[2] It is therefore possible that

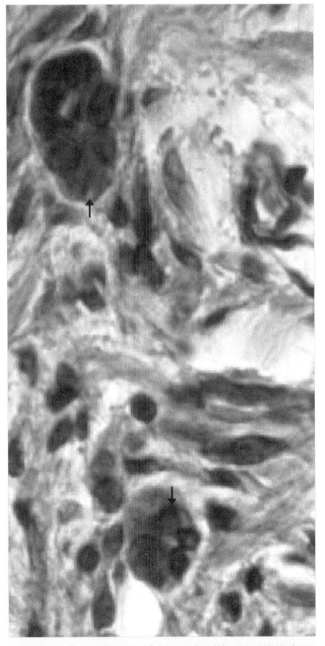

Fig. 3.8 A histological section of the periodontal ligament (PDL) close to the cementum surface showing two nests *(arrows)* of epithelial cell rests of Malassez (magnification × 1,000).

when the tooth is displaced in the socket, it is the reduced distance between the ECRs and bone which causes bone resorption, rather than, or perhaps as well as, tissue compression (*see Chapter 7.7 Bone Remodeling*).

Osteoblasts or osteoclasts may be found on the surface of the tooth socket, depending on the state of activity at the time of observation. Osteoclasts are derived from monocytes and are responsible for resorption of the alveolar bone. On the cementum surface of the root, cementoblasts may be found. Mast cells, macrophages, and undifferentiated mesenchymal cells may occur in small numbers in the periodontal ligament.

3.5.4 Vascular Supply of the Periodontal Ligament

The vascular supply to the ligament is via the gingiva, alveolar bone, and apical vessels. The periodontal arteries enter through a series of Volkmann's canals from the lamina dura of the alveolar bone and join those entering at the apex of the socket with the pulpal vessels (▶ Fig. 3.9). The vessels from each source branch and anastomose with each other to form a plexus around the tooth and form a cuff around the neck of the tooth, which consists of a strange glomeruli-like structure. Human incisor teeth undergo small pulsations toward the labial side, which coincide with the arterial pulse.

3.5.5 Functions of the Periodontal Ligament

The periodontal ligament provides the following functions:
- Attachment of the tooth to the socket allowing for resilience to impact and slight displacement during function.
- A mechanism for repositioning of the tooth in the socket during eruption and later in response to occlusal and approximal wear.
- An effective site for mechanoreceptors which provide sensory information about the direction and magnitude of forces applied to the tooth during function.
- To prevent ankylosis (bony fusion) of the root to the socket and prevent root resorption.

Teeth, which have been accidentally knocked out (avulsed), may be reimplanted, but the inevitable death of periodontal ligament cells, due to the disruption of their blood supply, has long-term consequences. In the absence of vital cells and also in a bacterially contaminated environment, the ligament repairs with a fibrous scar. Eventually, the scar tissue calcifies and the root becomes fused or ankylosed to the alveolar bone. Recall that bone is constantly being resorbed and reformed. The root may then be included in the resorption process, but of course it is replaced with new bone, not root dentin. The capacity of the ligament to prevent bony ankylosis to the root may be a function of the ECRs of Malassez, or there may be some characteristic of periodontal ligament fibroblasts, which secrete a type of collagen which inhibits calcification.

> **Key Notes**
>
> The periodontal ligament is a crucial source of feedback to direct accurate and powerful jaw movements that will ensure effective tooth contacts during mastication. Tooth loss deprives the masticatory system of this feedback and is one reason for the significant limitations in restoring the dentition with a dental prosthesis.

3.6 Cementum

Cementum is a bony tissue which covers the root and sometimes part of the crown and forms attachment for the fibers of the periodontal ligament.

3.6.1 Functions of Cementum

- Cementum provides a means of attachment and reattachment of periodontal fibers to the tooth root. During continued eruption and drift the periodontal fibers have to be removed and reattached into the cementum. Cementum is also a key role player in the reattachment of periodontal ligament fibers to the tooth during healing of a periodontal pocket.
- Cementum protects the underlying dentinal tubules from exposure to oral fluids and bacteria. If the epithelial attachment to the tooth root migrates apically, cementum may be exposed. It is softer than enamel and easily abraded during overzealous scaling or incorrect tooth brushing techniques. If the underlying root dentin is exposed in this way, it may become sensitive and cause discomfort which can be difficult to reduce.
- Addition of new cementum around the apex of the root compensates for tooth wear on the occlusal surface and provides a means of continued eruption of the tooth. Continued eruption may also be caused by alveolar bone growth.

Cementum forms a thin uneven layer over the root surface. It is thinnest at the cervical (toward the neck) end of the tooth and

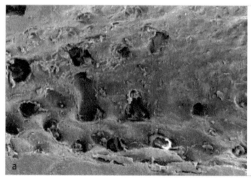
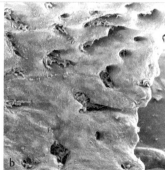

Fig. 3.9 SEM images of the inner surfaces of a tooth socket (magnification × 500). (a) The apical part of the tooth socket (toward the left of the micrograph) is perforated with a number of foramina for blood vessels and one or two larger ones near the apex for the bundle of nerves and vessels entering and leaving the pulp through the apex of the root. (b) The gingival part of the tooth socket is also perforated by many large foramina through which blood vessels supply the periodontal ligament and the free gingiva.

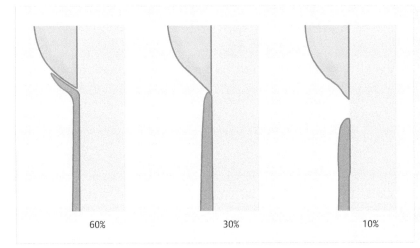

In 10% of subjects, dentin at the CEJ may be unprotected by either enamel or cementum. The configuration of the CEJ may vary within individuals.

60%   30%   10%

thickest at the apex. At the CEJ, cementum may either overlap the enamel (in about 60% of teeth) or meet edge to edge. It may also be deficient in meeting the enamel leaving a zone of exposed dentin which may become sensitive during tooth brushing (▶ Fig. 3.10).

It is possible to recognize different types of cementum based on the presence or absence of cells and fibers. Afibrillar (no fibers) cementum is uncommon but may be seen overlapping the enamel for a short distance at the CEJ. Most cementum contains fibers from two sources. Intrinsic fibers are thin and sparse and laid down as part of the ground substance. Extrinsic fibers come from the periodontal ligament and are trapped in the cementum as it forms. These extrinsic fibers provide an anchor of attachment between the periodontal fibers and the root of the tooth. The cells which form cementum are not evenly distributed but are more common toward the apex of the root surface, where there is active formation of new cementum (▶ Fig. 3.11).

Cementum shows incremental lines which correspond to periods of inactivity. Mostly, there is apposition of cementum which continues throughout life; in fact, cementum thickness is a useful indication of the age of a tooth (*see Chapter 11 Ageing*). Cementum rarely seems to resorb under natural conditions but may do so in response to excessive forces used during orthodontic tooth movement. Sometimes, cementum accumulates in unusually thick deposits (hypercementosis), and this may make extraction of teeth difficult as the bulbous apex locks the tooth into the bony socket.

3.6.2 Origins of Cementum

Cementum is formed by cementoblasts which may be derived from the dental epithelium, but there is also a view that their origins are from the dental follicle. There is a close relationship between mature enamel and cementum. In the teeth of herbivores, such as elephants and cows, cementum is deposited against enamel between the cusps of the tooth and contributes to the composite surface of the tooth when wear has exposed dentin. This association of cementum may be found in its origins. There is evidence that cementoblasts are derived from remnants of the enamel epithelium under the inductive influence of cells from dental mesenchyme.[3] On the cell membranes of cementoblasts and osteoblasts, there are specific receptors (integrins) for an adhesion molecule in the matrix of mineralizing tissue, called bone sialoprotein (BSP). Just before the first layer of cementum is formed on the developing root surface, the dental follicle cells

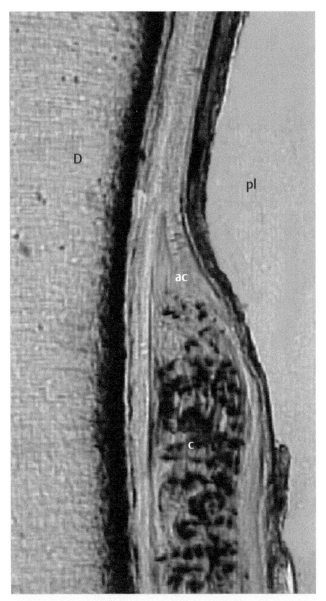

Fig. 3.11 A undecalcified section through the root of a molar tooth (magnification × 500). The image has been selected from an area halfway toward the root apex showing the transition between acellular (ac) and cellular (c) cementum. The periodontal ligament (pl) has been removed during processing D, dentin.

produce BSP which is subsequently found in mineralizing cementum. This suggest an important role played by BSP in the differentiation of cementoblasts prior to mineralization. While the participation of dental follicle cells is necessary, the progenitor cell of the cementoblasts appears to be derived from the dental epithelium. The epithelial cell rests described by Malassez have, in tissue cultures, been found to be essential for cementum formation. They synthesize a protein, amylin, which is localized to the area of cementum formation. The epithelial cell rests also appear to induce the formation of the fibrous attachment between root surface and adjacent bone. Between the cementum and dentin there is an intermediate, highly calcified layer. It has been called intermediate cementum, but there is evidence that it is not produced by cementoblasts or odontoblasts. This layer contains enamel proteins and may be a very thin layer of enamel. The conclusions from many studies is that the epithelial cell rests retain their potential to differentiate into mesenchyme stem–like cells capable of secreting both bone, collagen, and cementum and thus may be the progenitor cells of cementoblasts.[4] It has also been argued that cementoblasts are not derived from either Hertwig's root sheath or ECRs but from mesenchymal cells of the dental follicle under the influence of ECRs.[5] The epithelial cell rests may play an important role in periodontal regeneration.

3.6.3 Changes in Cementum with Aging

We have noted that continued eruption of the tooth, to accommodate for occlusal wear, may occur due to the deposition of new cementum to the root apex. This thickening of apical cementum appears to occur even if there is little tooth wear. It is a feature of aging and is one of the more reliable features used by forensic pathologists in estimating the age of a tooth or the body in which it is found.

3.6.4 Cementum Formation in Healing

The specific morphology of tooth support requires that fibers, embedded in the bone of the tooth socket, are also embedded in cementum covering the tooth root. Periodontal ligament fibers cannot adhere to the tooth root if the surface is covered by epithelium. Downgrowth of the junctional epithelium onto the surface of the cementum thus prevents fiber attachment to the root surface. If the tooth root is cleaned and the epithelium removed, it grows back during healing, faster than new cementum can form. Surgical techniques have been developed which prevent this downgrowth of epithelium. An artificial membrane is placed over the bone and root surface with the intention of preventing downgrowth of epithelium while healing occurs. This technique, called *guided tissue regeneration*, may promote the deposition of new cementum onto the root surface. The principle of guided tissue regeneration has been successfully applied in encouraging new bone formation around a dental implant, although the evidence for its success in regenerating periodontal ligament reattachment is less secure.

The new cementum is dependent on the differentiation of cementoblasts from cells dormant in the periodontal ligament. Only after new cementum is laid down against the root surface are fibers able to become incorporated in the new cementum and reattach the root to the alveolar bone. New bone then forms in the tooth socket, which traps the periodontal fibers, and a structural ligament is once more created.

The stimulus for the differentiation of new cementoblasts is provided by enamel matrix protein produced by epithelial cell rests. A derivative of these proteins from pigs has been shown to induce the differentiation of cementoblasts, fibroblasts, and osteoblasts. Clinical trials have shown that enamel matrix proteins are able to increase the success rate of reattachment of the tooth to the bony socket.[6]

Tooth displacement by an orthodontic appliance is followed by resorption of bone lining the tooth socket. This resorption is effected by osteoclasts. These are large multinucleate bone cells which appear to remove a *lacuna* (*Latin lake*) of bone around them. Once the tooth has repositioned, healing occurs first by migration of fibroblast-like cells into the resorption lacunae. After 3 weeks, new bone appears in the resorption defects. Associated with new bone formation after physiological tooth drift in rats are the noncollagenous bone proteins, osteonectin, osteopontin, and osteocalcin. It is likely that all three proteins are influential in controlling the balances of resorption and deposition of mineral in bone remodeling and healing (*see Chapter 7.7.4 Tooth Repositioning*).

> **Key Notes**
>
> Following periodontal disease, the reattachment of collagen fibers to the root surface is an essential step in repair of the entire periodontium. It is impossible without the regeneration of cellular cementum in which new fibers may be embedded. This regeneration cannot take place while the root surface is covered by a downgrowth of the epithelial attachment.

3.7 Junctional Epithelium

The junctional epithelium is an extension of the epithelium of the gingival sulcus but has some important differences. Firstly, unlike the epithelium of the gingival sulcus, it is physically attached to the surface of the tooth (▶ Fig. 3.12). Further, it is nonkeratinized, lacks the prominent rete ridges of gingival epithelium, and has no granular or keratin layer. The basal cells of the junctional epithelium are cuboidal and attached to the external basal lamina. The layer of epithelial cells above the basal lamina varies in thickness but is not more than about 20 cells thick. The unusual feature of junctional epithelium is that the surface cells are also attached to an internal basal lamina which in turn is attached to the enamel (or cementum) of the tooth. This attachment is achieved by hemidesmosomes at intervals along the basement membrane. This internal basement lamina is a product of the underlying cells and requires synthesis just as the synthesis of keratin would in the epithelium of attached gingiva.

The junctional epithelium forms a cuff of attachment around the tooth and is therefore of key importance as a barrier to the entrance of bacteria down the tooth surface and into the periodontium. We have seen the value of rapid turnover in epithelia, which allows regular shedding of the surface cells, along with any organisms that have obtained a foothold. The junctional epithelium exploits this process and turns over in just 4 to 6 days (in marmosets). The cells are not shed against the tooth surface but migrate through the layers above and emerge at the junction of the tooth and gingival sulcus. The junctional epithelium exploits other features of its structure to control the

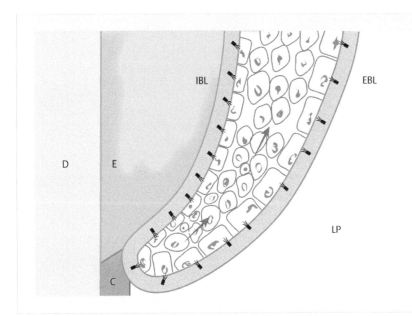

Fig. 3.12 A diagrammatic representation of the junctional epithelium. The basal cells are attached to the external basement lamina (EBL) by hemidesmosomes. The inner basement lamina (IBL) forms the epithelial attachment to enamel, also via hemidesmosomes. The central cells of the epithelium are loosely attached and allow gingival fluid to flow outward into the gingival sulcus. C, cementum; D, dentin; E, enamel; I-break/>LP, lamina propria.

microorganism of dental plaque. The individual cells are not held close together (fewer desmosomes), and this allows neutrophil leukocytes to patrol in between the cells. Lymphocytes and monocytes may also occasionally be seen in the junctional epithelium. They are seen in much greater numbers if the gingiva becomes inflamed. Lastly, to help sweep away and disable microorganisms invading the junctional epithelium, a fluid exudate flows between the cells of the junctional epithelium and emerges into the gingival crevice (*see Chapter 4.2.4 Gingival Crevicular Fluid*).

If the junctional epithelium is surgically removed, a new junctional epithelium forms and attaches to the tooth. It is presumably derived from the epithelium of the sulcus.

3.7.1 Loss of Epithelial Attachment

If plaque accumulates on subgingival surfaces of the tooth, there is a shift in the balance of microorganisms toward more gram-negative organisms which are anaerobic and proteolytic. They are capable of penetrating into the gingival lamina propria and junctional epithelium where they break down collagen and other proteins. They produce endotoxins to which the immune system responds with an infiltration of neutrophils into the damaged epithelium and submucosa. The neutrophils engulf the bacteria which are then killed by enzymes inside lysosomes within the cell. The neutrophil may itself die and break up releasing the toxic content of lysosomes into the tissue which do further damage. A colorful metaphor describes this situation, as a battlefield littered with and polluted by the dead, both defending soldiers and enemy. The initial clinical manifestation of this shift in the dominance of some organisms is inflammation, redness, and swelling of the marginal gingiva. If a periodontal probe is inserted into the gingival sulcus, light bleeding occurs. This sign, bleeding on probing, is an important marker of gingivitis.

The breakdown of the junctional epithelium causes loss of its hemidesmosomal attachment to enamel. Loss of attachment is not readily recovered. It may allow progress of

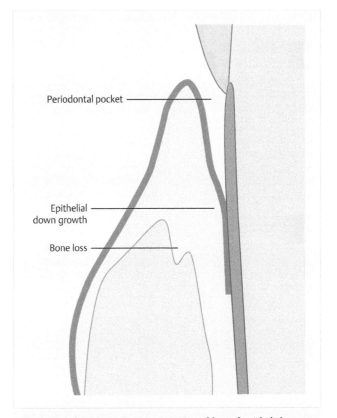

Fig. 3.13 A diagrammatic representation of loss of epithelial attachment to the tooth and the development of a pocket with loss of periodontal ligament attachment to cementum. There has been bone loss from the crest of the alveolar bone. The junctional epithelium has grown down into the pocket preventing reattachment of periodontal fibers.

pathogenic bacteria into the periodontal ligament and damage the periodontal ligament and surrounding bone. The clinical manifestation of this progression is the presence of a pocket between the tooth and the periodontium (▶ Fig. 3.13). If the depth of the gingival sulcus is now measured, an increase beyond the normal 2 mm may be found. Deep pockets of over 4-mm depth indicate some loss of bone height and may lead to tooth mobility and eventual tooth loss.

The oral bacteria associated with the development of inflammation in the periodontium are thought to be a consortium of organisms, which interact to cause periodontal disease together. They include *Porphyromonas gingivalis*, *Treponema denticola*, and *Tannerella forsythia* (*see Chapter 4.3.6 From Symbiont to Pathobiont*).

3.7.2 Influence of Female Hormones

At puberty, the ovaries begin a cyclic production of estrogen and progesterone in response to secretion of gonadotrophic hormones from the pituitary gland. The main functions of these hormones are the control of the menstrual cycle. However, they also affect many other parts of the body including the oral cavity. The early teens are associated with an increase in gingival bleeding. It can be demonstrated that this is the result of an increase in a number of bacteria known to cause gingivitis. These include gram-negative anaerobes such as members of the consortium already described and include *Prevotella intermedia*. The increase in these bacteria may be due to their ability to use estrogen and progesterone as substitutes for vitamin K, an essential growth factor.

During pregnancy, there is a sustained increase in both estrogen and progesterone levels, above even the cyclic peaks which occur just before the end of each menstrual cycle. The changes in the oral cavity during pregnancy are therefore more pronounced and common. In addition to the effect on bacteria already mentioned, there are vascular, cellular, and immune changes which are collectively responsible for the condition known as pregnancy gingivitis. The immune changes include a reduction in the migration of inflammatory cells. There is also an increase in a subset of CD4, cells which kill B lymphocytes, the cells responsible for producing antibodies to some of the very bacteria which are thriving in the high levels of the estrogen and progesterone. Progesterone causes increased vascular permeability and release of prostaglandins, both factors which support inflammation. Progesterone also reduces the production of collagenases, so the balance of collagen turnover between secretion and resorption is upset, allowing the collagen content of the gingival lamina propria to increase. These influences may lead to the development of a mass of healing (granulation) tissue in the gingiva. This mass is called a pregnancy epulis. It is quite harmless and regresses as does the gingivitis, after the birth of the child.

The onset of menopause is due to age changes in the ovaries, which fail to respond to pituitary hormones. The decrease in estrogen and progesterone contributes, along with other factors, to cause osteoporosis, a decrease in bone mass. There is no evidence that osteoporosis is linked with severe periodontal disease which also involves loss of bone around the teeth. Menopause is, however, associated with a decrease in mucosal secretions, including saliva. Dry mucosa is easily damaged and affects the comfort and retention of dentures.

Key Notes

The junctional epithelium must perform the functions of a barrier to infection and call up resources, if the barrier deteriorates into a battleground. In this thin layer of epithelium, all the defense mechanisms of the immune system may be recruited, including the special defenses of antibodies, neutrophils, macrophages, and complement. The conditions which initiate this deterioration, from what is normally a commensal relationship, into a full-scale defense against pathogens, are vital to uncover.

Review Questions

1. What causes the extraction of molar teeth to be more difficult than incisor teeth?
2. Does the periodontal ligament support the tooth like a hammock (under tension) or like a cushion (under compression)?
3. What are the functions of the periodontium?
4. Why is it important to place an avulsed tooth back in its socket as soon as possible?
5. What similarities and differences are there between cementum, dentin, and bone?
6. What features of the junctional epithelium provide a barrier to the progress of plaque microorganism into the periodontal ligament?
7. What is the nerve and blood supply of the periodontium?
8. How is the periodontium affected by changes in the level of female hormones?
9. What evidence suggests that cementum formation may be induced by cells of epithelial origin?
10. What are the functions of cementum?
11. What role do epithelial cell rests have in preventing ankylosis?
12. Why is the formation of new cementum essential during healing of the periodontal ligament?

References

[1] Lindskog S, Blomlöf L, Hammarström L. Evidence for a role of odontogenic epithelium in maintaining the periodontal space. J Clin Periodontol 1988; 15(6):371–373

[2] Fujiyama K, Yamashiro T, Fukunaga T, Balam TA, Zheng L, Takano-Yamamoto T. Denervation resulting in dento-alveolar ankylosis associated with decreased Malassez epithelium. J Dent Res 2004; 83(8):625–629

[3] Xiong J, Mrozik K, Gronthos S, Bartold P. Epithelial cell rests of Malassez contain unique stem cell populations capable of undergoing epithelial mesenchymal transition. Stem Cells Dev. 2012; 21 (11):2012–25

[4] Luan X, Ito Y, Diekwisch T. Evolution and development of Hertwig's epithelial root sheath. Dev Dyn 2006 May; 235(5): 1167–1180

[5] Harahashi H, Odajima T, Yamamoto T, Kawanami M. Immunohistochemical analysis of periodontal reattachment on denuded root dentin after periodontal surgery. Biomed Res 2010; 31(5):319–328

Suggested Readings

Amar S, Chung KM. Influence of hormonal variation on the periodontium in women. Periodontol 2000 1994; 6(6):79–87

Berkovitz BK. Periodontal ligament: structural and clinical correlates. Dent Update 2004; 31(1):46–50, 52, 54

Lovegrove JM. Dental plaque revisited: bacteria associated with periodontal disease. J N Z Soc Periodontol 2004; 87(87):7–21

Lyngstadaas SP, Wohlfahrt JC, Brookes SJ, Paine ML, Snead ML, Reseland JE. Enamel matrix proteins; old molecules for new applications. Orthod Craniofac Res 2009; 12(3):243–253

Marsh PD, Martin MV, Lewis MAO, Williams DW. Oral microbiology. London: Churchill Livingstone; 2009

Mineoka T, Awano S, Rikimaru T, et al. Site-specific development of periodontal disease is associated with increased levels of Porphyromonas gingivalis, Treponema denticola, and Tannerella forsythia in subgingival plaque. J Periodontol 2008; 79(4):670–676

Scott DA, Krauss J. Neutrophils in periodontal inflammation. Front Oral Biol. 2012; 15:56–83

Wesselink PR, Beertsen W. The prevalence and distribution of rests of Malassez in the mouse molar and their possible role in repair and maintenance of the periodontal ligament. Arch Oral Biol 1993; 38(5):399–403

Xiong J, Mrozik K, Gronthos S, Bartold PM. Epithelial cell rests of Malassez contain unique stem cell populations capable of undergoing epithelial-mesenchymal transition. Stem Cells Dev 2012; 21(11):2012–2025

4 The Ecology of the Oral Cavity

Abstract

The oral cavity provides a variety of niche habitats for hundreds of species of oral bacteria. There are potential habitats on the teeth, tongue, or gingival sulcus and a constant supply of nutrients from food residues, saliva, and the products of other bacteria. The human host and its bacterial partners in the oral cavity and gut have a cooperative relationship which goes back millions of years. Cooperation between different bacterial species is just as important as competition in conserving this relationship; their interdependence holds together several different species in a consortium, a sort of mutual benefit community. If dental caries or periodontal disease occurs, it is always due to a disturbance in the dominance or hierarchy of bacteria within the consortium, often caused by something as simple as an increase of sugar in the diet, or at the other extreme, malnutrition. All the members of the consortium are well-established residents, so dental caries and periodontal disease are not the result of foreign pathogens but may be classified as noncommunicable diseases. The balance between the efforts of organisms to maintain growth on the oral surfaces, by both competitive and cooperative tactics, and the host's factors which tend to support and tolerate certain commensals, but inhibit potential pathogens, is the theme of this chapter. Oral health strategies, which work best, are those based on an understanding of the principal factors which regulate and maintain a stable oral microbiome.

Keywords: oral environment, oral ecology, salivary pellicle, oral fluids, gingival fluid, dental plaque, calculus, dental caries, diet and caries, nutrition and oral health, fluorides, mucosal immunity, oral tolerance

4.1 Introduction

Ecology is the study of the relationship between living organisms and their environment. An ecosystem is a specific environment in which plant and animal species live in an interconnected web of cooperation and competition. For example, a forest is an ecosystem in which trees, bushes, and smaller plants interact with insects, soil bacteria, birds, small mammals, and reptiles, in fact, a large spectrum of most major classes of living organisms. Within the forest, each tree could be seen as a small ecosystem on its own, as it supports a characteristic collection of interactive bacteria and insects. The complexity and stability of an ecosystem take a long time to develop. If a temperate forest were to be cleared to the ground, it is estimated that it would take 200 years to regain its original rich and varied number of species.

The oral cavity is an ecosystem on a smaller scale, which also requires time to acquire a mature ecological balance of organisms. The time is much shorter than that needed for a forest to mature, as the life cycle of bacteria is faster than trees, and there are only 500 or so species or bacteria in the mouth. However, it still takes 2 weeks before a film of plaque bacteria has reached maturity. The organisms which have established themselves in an ecosystem are those which have been able to adapt to the physical environment and to the other species in the ecosystem.

Not all the members on an ecosystem are of equal importance to its survival. Some, called *keystone species*, have a decisive influence even when they may represent a small proportion of the total numbers of organisms in the ecosystem. Keystone species determine the composition of the ecosystem and control the relative numbers of each species. An example of a keystone species is the sea otter. On the Western coast of North America, the otter keeps down the population of sea urchins which graze on the base of kelp. Without the sea otter the urchins would devour the kelp and destroy the entire ecosystem of the kelp beds.

There are keystone species in communities of bacteria, occurring in the gut and oral cavity, which communicate with their microbial community, via chemical messages, a communication which microbiologists have called cross-talk or *quorum sensing*. The chemical messages induce control of gene expression in the target organism. Communication between bacterial species is also observed in the spread of antibiotic resistance. Genes from bacteria which confer resistance to antibiotics are able to be shared with other species of bacteria.

Stability is a feature of successful ecosystems, and it is dependent on maintaining a balance in the hierarchy of member species of the system. This balance is maintained partly by the stability of the physical environment such as the availability of light, oxygen, and nutrients, but it is also dependent on the population control of each species. This control is achieved through processes of competition for resources and cooperation between species in maintaining a balanced and stable population.

The relationship between different species is not always competitive. In fact, cooperative partnerships are more significant in nature than competitive ones. In the long term (evolutionary length), competition for survival has not been the best strategy, as 99% of all the species that have ever lived are now extinct. However, there are some remarkable examples of cooperation which have lasted 3 billion years. The relationship between mitochondria and all nucleated animal cells started off as a host–parasite relationship. The cell gave shelter to the mitochondria which were able to use oxygen to produce high-energy molecules and thus could be a great benefit to an active cell. The partnership was so successful that it led to the evolution of the eukaryote cell, with nucleus, mitochondria, and cilia. The eukaryote cells enabled an unprecedented surge in evolution of multicellular forms of life. The mitochondria have retained their genetic identity over the millions of years of this partnership and their separate process of reproduction through the female lines of organisms. The relationship is still recognizable as a form of symbiosis, the living together of different organisms. There are many other examples of symbiotic relationships, which, as they are better understood, indicate that they are of significant importance. A close and highly interdependent relationship between bacteria is found in a biofilm. This is a dense aggregate of many species which have abandoned a solitary planktonic life for the benefits of a cooperative community existence.

4.2 The Oral Environment

The following section will describe the features of the oral environment which support and influence the ecology of the mouth. The oral cavity provides a range of fairly stable habitats for microorganisms. There is a plentiful supply of both oxygen and nutrients, and there are physical surfaces for attachment, although some surfaces are more liable to disruption than others. The oral mucosa, including the tongue and exposed tooth surfaces, is exposed to saliva flow and the disruption caused by shear forces which occur during swallowing and mastication. The surface epithelial cells of the oral mucosa are shed (desquamated) when mature and carry off with them any organisms which have colonized the cell's surface (▶ Fig. 4.1). This process is particularly important for the health of the gingival sulcus, one of the most highly populated habitats in the oral cavity. This site provides shelter, and a rich supply of nutrients provided by the gingival crevicular fluid flowing out of the gingival sulcus. The cells of the junctional epithelium and gingival sulcus epithelium desquamate regularly, clearing away colonizing organisms. It has been noted in *Chapter 3 Oral Mucosa and Periodontium* that the turnover period of the junctional epithelium may be only a matter of days.

For those organisms which are able to adhere to the exposed tooth surface, there are large areas to colonize. The sheltered tooth surfaces, such as the approximal areas and occlusal fissures, are more densely colonized than more exposed tooth surfaces, and it is these sites which have the greatest risk of developing dental caries (▶ Fig. 4.2). Oral organisms are unable to attach directly to tooth enamel, but they may adhere via an intermediary layer of proteins, the salivary pellicle.

The presence of a fixed restoration, which has defective margins, and a removable restoration, which covers the oral mucosa, provides a protected environment for organisms which allows the total mass to increase (▶ Fig. 4.3). When the teeth are lost, these habitats disappear and the oral flora is dramatically altered; in general, it is less diverse.

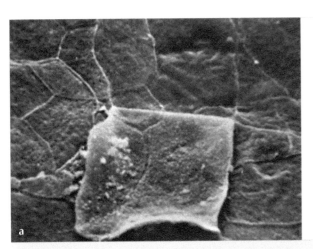
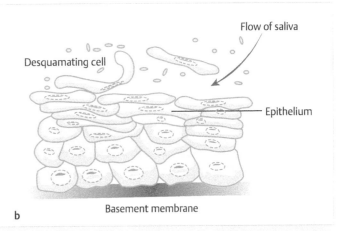

Fig. 4.1 The desquamation of the surface epithelial cells of oral mucosa. (a) A scanning electron microscope (SEM) image of a surface cell which has partly desquamated (magnification × 1,000). **(b)** A diagrammatic representation of the effect of desquamating epithelial cells on the control of colonization of epithelial surfaces by oral organisms.

4.2.1 Salivary Pellicle

Salivary pellicle is a thin layer (10 μm) of various salivary proteins which heap up on top of each other, on the surface of recently cleaned enamel, within a few hours. The smaller-molecular-weight phosphoproteins and sulpho-glycopeptides are the first to adhere to freshly cleaned enamel. Some of the phosphoproteins and calcium-binding proteins form ionic bonds with the apatite crystals of enamel. Other proteins adhere because bacteria have caused them to clump together; they are less strongly bound to the enamel surface. Most of the salivary proteins are rich in the amino acid proline and are collectively described as proline-rich proteins (PRPs). The coverage and composition of the pellicle change during its early formation. After the smaller-molecular-weight proteins, the larger glycoproteins adhere, and this stage is rapidly followed by the adhesion of the first oral organisms. Pellicle has the following influence on the oral environment:

- It protects enamel from demineralization by providing a layer of proteins, which isolates the surface from changes in the acidity of fluids surrounding the tooth.
- It influences the types of microorganisms which will adhere to the tooth surface.
- It lubricates the enamel surface and may therefore reduce the rate of tooth wear (▶ Fig. 4.4).

Given a surface onto which oral organism are able to adhere, a further defining feature of the oral environment is the fluid surrounding the pellicle and bathing all the surfaces in the oral cavity. Oral fluid is a term which best describes the mixture of substances which might be found in a sample of fluid from the mouth. It would mainly consist of saliva from the major and minor glands, each with its characteristic feature. The oral fluid would also contain gingival sulcus fluid, desquamated epithelial cells, bacteria, and some blood cells, mostly neutrophils. It is difficult to detail the exact composition of saliva as the secretions from each gland are not identical, and they all vary with the rate of secretion of saliva.

4.2.2 How Saliva Defines the Oral Environment

The essential functions of saliva are both enabling and protective. Saliva enables mastication and speech as it lubricates the oral structures during function. It also protects enamel from demineralizing and enables a stable ecology of oral organisms to live as *commensals* while excluding more overtly pathogenic bacteria.

Lubrication: Lubrication is provided by mucins (glycoproteins) which are selectively adsorbed to mucosa and enamel. On mucosa, they protect the tissues against drying, irritants, and bacterial enzymes. Together with the water content of saliva, glycoproteins provide lubrication for speech and mastication and preparation of a food bolus which can be readily swallowed. It appears to be the carbohydrate part of the glycoproteins, which is important for lubrication. (*see Chapter 6.2 Glycoproteins*)

Mechanical cleansing: The flow of saliva and subsequent intermittent swallowing provide a flushing system which removes food particles, bacteria, and desquamated cells from

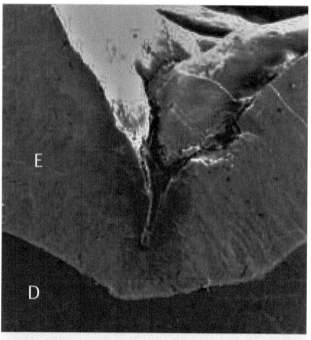

Fig. 4.2 **Oral habitats sheltered from salivary flow become readily colonized by oral organisms.** An SEM image of a buccal/lingual section of a maxillary premolar. A pit in the center of the central fissure is a secluded habitat for bacteria. The proximity of the base of the pit to the dentin is an important factor in the progress of dental caries (magnification × 500). D, dentin; E, enamel.

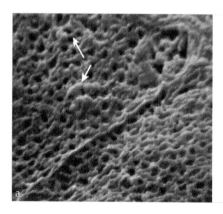
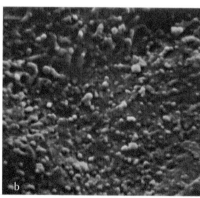

Fig. 4.3 **SEM images of the surface of keratinized oral epithelium, the impact of a restoration. (a)** The superficial squamous cells of the healthy epithelium of the hard palate have a pitted surface into which projections from the overlying cells interlock. The epithelial cells provide a habitat for oral organisms (*arrows*). **(b)** The palate of a complete denture was covering these epithelial cells. The surface microstructure has become altered, and there are large numbers and variety of oral organisms which have colonized this surface (magnification × 10,000).

the mouth. The rate at which this removal occurs is referred to as the *clearance rate*. The more complete the fluid eliminated at each swallow, the more rapid will be the clearance of a substance from the mouth. Clearance will also depend on the flow rate of saliva; it is thus dramatically reduced during sleep (*see Chapter 4.2.3 Rate of Flow of Saliva*). The clinical importance of clearance lies in the rate of elimination of sucrose and fluorides from the oral cavity. A high rate of salivary clearance in individuals has been associated with a reduction in caries prevalence.

Buffering capacity: Calcium apatite crystals on the enamel surface may become ionized and dissolve into the saliva, if the fluid environment drops below a pH of 5.3. Saliva contains *buffers* which tend to restore the pH to neutral or at least safer levels of acidity. The primary sources of the buffering capacity of saliva are bicarbonate ions (HCO_3^-). The products of the acid–bicarbonate reaction are water and carbon dioxide. Phosphates, protein, and urea are buffers of lesser importance. Organisms which are able to metabolize urea may form ammonia (NH_3^+) as an end product. This will raise the pH and tend to neutralize acids. The buffering capacity of saliva becomes greater as the flow of saliva increases.

Antisolubility: Calcium and phosphate ions in the saliva are *supersaturated* due to the presence of certain calcium-binding proteins (*see Appendix D.1 Saturated Solutions*). There is therefore little tendency for calcium ions from the enamel to leave the surface and enter an already saturated environment (▶ Fig. 4.5). The majority of salivary proteins (50–70%) are characterized by the frequency of the amino acid proline in their chain structure.

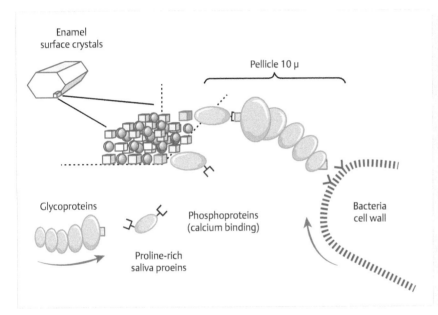

Enamel
surface crystals

Pellicle 10 μ

Glycoproteins

Phosphoproteins
(calcium binding)

Proline-rich
saliva proeins

Bacteria
cell wall

Fig. 4.4 A diagrammatic representation of the role of salivary pellicle in adhesion of oral organisms. Calcium-binding phosphoproteins (*yellow*) bind onto calcium atoms of enamel. Larger glycoproteins bind to the smaller phosphoproteins to form a layer of salivary pellicle. Bacteria bind selectively to certain larger proline-rich proteins in pellicle.

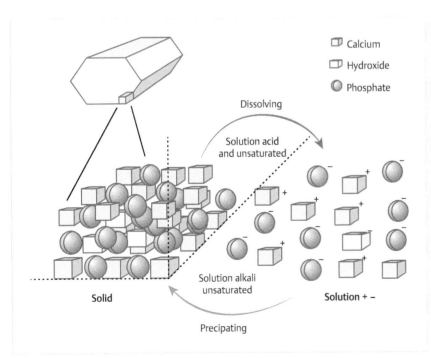

Dissolving

Solution acid
and unsaturated

Solution alkali
unsaturated

Solid

Precipating

Solution + –

□ Calcium

□ Hydroxide

○ Phosphate

Fig. 4.5 A diagrammatic representation of the effect of acidity on the degree of saturation of saliva and the dynamics of mineralization and demineralization. Saliva is a saturated solution of calcium and phosphate ions at a normal pH. If the solution becomes acid, the saliva is no longer saturated and hydroxyapatite ions dissolve (demineralize) and enter solution from the crystal. If the solution becomes alkali, saliva becomes saturated and ions precipitate (remineralize) back onto the crystal.

Proline has a particular affinity for binding calcium. This accounts for the ability of PRPs to maintain a supersaturated solution of calcium in saliva. It also accounts for their ability to bind chemically onto the calcium in the hydroxyapatite of enamel during the formation of pellicle. The attachment of PRPs to enamel not only protects it from being dissolved by acids in the mouth, but in addition, it prevents the deposition of apatite crystal onto enamel. Without this function "secondary" crystal deposits would grow onto tooth surfaces. Crystal growth on enamel is not calculus, which is calcified plaque. The PRPs also bind selectively to microorganisms providing a chain which forms a link between organisms and tooth surfaces via the salivary pellicle. The PRPs cannot bind to organisms before they have been absorbed onto the hydroxyapatite of the enamel. Only then is a special sequence of amino acids revealed to which organisms can attach. The PRPs also bind onto some food proteins, in particular tannins, which would be otherwise be toxic.

Antimicrobial peptides and proteins: Oral fluid has several components (about 45) which are antibacterial to a varying degree. Some of the proteins such as immunoglobulins (Igs), lactoferrin, and lysozyme are thought to have a role in defense although studies have not shown a correlation between the levels of salivary proteins and dental caries. The smaller peptides on the other hand do appear to have a more predictable defensive action on oral bacteria. These are collectively called antimicrobial peptides (AMP). They include defensins (alpha and beta), cathelicidin, and histatins. All are found in salivary gland and duct cells and in gingival crevicular fluid. Their sources in crevicular fluid are the neutrophils that migrate into the oral cavity. One of the AMPs, alpha defensin was found to be significantly lower in children with caries. This finding may lead to a useful measure of caries risk in children. The defensins and cathelicidins are broadly effective against oral microorganisms including *Streptococcus mutans* and *Porphyromonas gingivalis*, but it is difficult to generalize their antibacterial function. It is likely that they act synergistically with other antimicrobials. They also stimulate the acquired immune system and could enhance IgA production.

Lysozyme: Lysozyme is an enzyme present in saliva and tears. Its antibacterial effect is due to the splitting of a bond in the peptide chain of the cell wall of certain gram-positive organisms. The normal flora of the mouth seems to be little affected by lysozyme; it may be more important as a defense against exogenous ("foreign") organisms.

Peroxidaze: Peroxidaze catalyzes the peroxidation of thiocyanate (SCN) to hypothiocyanite (OSCN) which inhibits bacteria metabolism. Peroxidaze is effective in even low concentrations when the pH of plaque decreases.

Lactoferrin: Lactoferrin is an iron-binding protein which inhibits the metabolism of some bacteria.

Immunoglobulins: A secretory component is added to immunoglobulins in the salivary glands, which activate its potential to neutralize bacteria in the oral cavity. These secretory immunoglobulin A (sIgA) do not operate as humeral antibodies, as they are not in a tissue fluid environment. They therefore cannot make a direct attack on an antigen causing agglutination, precipitation, neutralization, or lysis. Neither they can produce any amplification of the complement or anaphylactic system. Immunoglobulins appear to operate in the following ways:

- sIgA neutralizes viruses, and toxins, or enzymes produced by microorganisms. For example, sIgA is able to neutralize the enzyme glycosyltransferase which is necessary for *S. mutans* to synthesis extracellular polysaccharides.
- sIgA blocks the attachment sites for adhesion of bacteria to the mucosal surface. This blocking occurs in two ways: by covering the specific attachment sites on epithelial cells and by covering the part of the bacterial cell wall which is the active site for attachment. Some species of bacteria are more susceptible than others to the blocking effect of sIgA (▶ Fig. 4.6).
- sIgA also cause bacteria to clump together (agglutinate) which facilitates clearance.
- sIgA may bind to the active sites of food antigens thereby reducing the risk of developing an excessive immune response and allergy to certain foods.

The defense mechanism of sIgA is not as effective as might be expected. Certain bacteria (*Streptococcus*, *Bacteroides*, and *Capnocytophaga species*) produce proteases which split the dimer of sIgA into two ineffective parts. These IgA proteases do

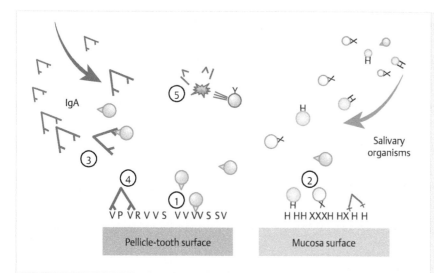

Fig. 4.6 Diagrammatic representation of the action of sIgA on salivary organisms. (1) some organisms are unaffected by sIgA and adhere selectively to salivary pellicle, while others (2) adhere to oral mucosal surfaces. IgA causes clumping (3) of susceptible bacteria and blocks sites (4) of adhesion to other organisms. Some bacteria (5) are able to split the IgA dimer.

in turn elicit antibody production, but they are so weakly antigenic that the response is not effective. This may explain why *Streptococcus sanguis* and *Streptococcus mitior* are able to remain constant members of the oral cavity throughout life. If a patient is treated with immunosuppressive drugs (e.g., used in bone marrow transplants), the secretion of sIgA is reduced, and the oral flora may become invaded with organisms from the gut. The presence of large numbers of gut organisms in the oral cavity causes a mucositis which is difficult to control. This mucositis suggests a wider protective role of sIgA. sIgA may be most effective in controlling the population of exogenous organisms in the mouth (*see Chapter 4.7.3 Antigen Tolerance*).

4.2.3 Rate of Flow of Saliva

The mouth is bathed by a resting flow of saliva which during the day is a total of about 1 L. This ensures that the mouth and throat are kept moist at all times. During sleep the rate of flow is almost unmeasurable and accounts for the dryness of the mouth on waking. In other circumstance, particularly feeding, the rate of secretion of saliva increases. The following factors are important in the stimulation of saliva which is driven by the activity of both sympathetic and parasympathetic nerve pathways.

- *Taste:* Taste is the most potent salivary stimulant. Different modalities vary in their power to stimulate saliva flow. Sour food ranks highest through salt and sweet to bitter tasting foods. One of the functions of the water in saliva is to dissolve and spread food chemicals (*see Chapter 10.6 Taste*).
- *Mastication:* When food is held between the teeth, a little saliva flows from the ipsilateral (same side) glands. As further bite force is exerted, receptors in the periodontal ligament send impulses to the brain and the rate of flow is increased. These events have been described as the masticatory–salivary reflex.
- *Touch:* Stimulation of nerve endings in the oral mucosa, particularly by spicy or irritating substances, produces an increase in flow rate of saliva. Hot or cold water also has a stimulating effect. In some areas of the oral cavity, such as the soft palate, even light touch causes an increased flow of saliva. This may be a response to enable swallowing and a protective response to the onset of retching.
- *Sight, smell, and thought:* The presence of food, or even the thought of it, increases salivary secretions. Some foods like lemons or onions have a particularly strong effect even at a distance from the mouth.
- *Nausea and vomiting:* Copious amounts of saliva are released during vomiting. This may be a protective reflex, protecting the oral cavity from stomach acids which are sufficiently concentrated to damage the oral mucosa and etch tooth enamel.
- *Nutrition:* Malnutrition causes irreversible damage to the salivary glands of rats if it occurs during infancy. During later years, malnutrition in human children has been shown to reduce the rate of saliva secretion and the protein content.
- *Drugs:* Several drugs which are mood altering (antidepressants and tranquilizers) reduce salivary secretions.
- *Ageing:* During ageing all mucosal secretions are reduced, and this may lead, in the oral cavity, to the onset of root surface caries.
- *Radiation:* One of the undesirable side effects of radiation treatment for oral tumors is damage to the acinar cells of the salivary glands. The xerostomia (dry mouth) which develops is usually permanent and requires special preventive measures to be put in place in order to prevent caries in patients who have had radiation treatment.

Saliva is an active secretion from both major and minor salivary glands. The three major salivary glands are the parotid, submandibular, and sublingual glands. The composition of saliva varies according to the types of secretory gland (*see Appendix D.2 Salivary Gland Secretion*).

4.2.4 Gingival Crevicular Fluid

Filter paper inserted into the gingival sulcus soon becomes saturated with crevicular fluid. This fluid derives from the connective tissue of the gingiva, passes through spaces in the junctional epithelium, and enters the gingival sulcus. The rate of flow and composition of the gingival crevicular fluid (GCF) are influenced by the following factors:
- The fluid flow is minimal in the morning and reaches a maximum at the end of the day.
- GCF flow is increased by tooth brushing and mastication.
- Pregnancy causes the rate of GCF to increase. There is an increase in gingival inflammation represented by a tendency for gingival bleeding during pregnancy.
- Fluid flow is minimal during the middle of the menstrual period.
- GCF flow is increased in diabetics.
- One of the earliest signs of gingival inflammation is an increase in GCF flow. There is some correlation between the rate of flow and the severity of the gingival inflammation.

The spaces between the cells of the junctional epithelium comprise 18% of its volume. These spaces are large enough to allow the passage of large molecules and cells (*see Chapter 3.7 Junctional Epithelium*). Thus, bacteria and their toxic products and other antigens may enter the gingival connective tissue through the junctional epithelium. This constant minor invasion causes a mild inflammatory state in the lamina propria of the junctional epithelium. Hence, neutrophils which have migrated into the junctional epithelium in response to the presence of bacterial products are flushed out into the GCF fluid. From this route, 25,000 neutrophils enter the mouth every 15 minutes. Other cells found in the GCF are desquamated epithelial cells.

In health, the GCF is neither exactly like serum or an inflammatory exudate. There are slightly higher concentrations of inorganic ions than in serum and higher levels of carbohydrates. The serum immunoglobulins, IgG, IgM, and IgA, are all found in GCF (not the secretory version of IgA which is found in saliva). Their presence may regulate the entrance of bacteria into the epithelium. One of the functions of antibodies is in triggering the complement cascade of reactions which produce enzymes capable of inflicting damage to the cell walls of bacteria. These enzymes are also capable of damaging host cells, and this may be another reason for the inflammatory state of the lamina propria under the junctional epithelium. The enzymes found in GCF are evidence of the battle between invading bacteria and the defending neutrophils. For example, there is acid phosphatase (from cell breakdown), glucuronidase, lysozyme, hyaluronidase, and collagenases.

Review Questions

1. What do you understand by the term keystone organism?
2. What features of the oral cavity make it possible to describe it as an ecosystem?
3. What makes saliva supersaturated?
4. How does pellicle protect the tooth?
5. How does sIgA control the growth of oral organisms?
6. What factors cause a decrease in saliva flow?
7. What is meant by salivary clearance and how does it affect oral health?
8. What factors affect the rate of flow of gingival crevicular fluid?
9. What are the essential differences between GCF and saliva?

4.3 The Biofilms of the Oral Environment

The oral flora is established from birth by organisms which are passed from the mother to the child. Many bacteria in the air and in food also have access to the oral cavity but do not survive. The oral flora is therefore a specific and, in health, a fairly stable bacterial community. There are, even in healthy mouths, huge numbers of microorganisms. Saliva contains 100 million organisms per milliliter, but the gingival sulcus supports 100 billion bacteria per milliliter. This massive population of the gingival sulcus is possible because the oral organisms have adopted a communal existence. They have formed biofilms, in which a variety of species live in a densely packed mass. The oral biofilms depend on the establishment of a symbiotic relationship with their host and a symbiotic relationship between species, in order for their ecosystem to thrive.

4.3.1 Biofilms

Slime is an everyday description of the slippery film, which covers surfaces which are always wet. Slime collects on the inside of water pipes, the bottoms of ships, artificial heart valves, the lining of the gut, rocks, and plants in ponds, rivers, and sea. The word slime tells us that is slippery but not that is made up of living organisms, so biofilm is a more accurate description. Biofilms have a most interesting characteristic, in that the different species of bacteria show levels of interaction, cooperation, and organization not found in their free-swimming or planktonic forms. The collective behavior of organisms creates a microecosystem. Over time, a stable hierarchy and balance between the different species develop. As we have noted in other ecosystems, some organisms, the keystone species, have a disproportionate influence. These organisms may influence the structure of the biofilm, and if it is in a symbiotic relationship with a host, the keystone species determine the biofilms' relationship with the host.

The deeper layers of a biofilm have a lower concentration of oxygen than the surface layer. These oxygen-depleted layers provide a suitable microenvironment for *anaerobic* organisms which are unable to survive in the oxygen-rich (*aerobic*) environment of the oral cavity. The deeper layers of the biofilm would also have lower concentrations of nutrients were it not for channels which are maintained for the transport of nutrients through the mass of organisms.

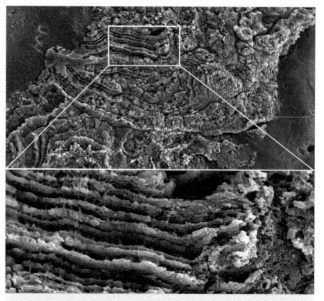

Fig. 4.7 A SEM image (magnification × 300) of calcified plaque (calculus) which was etched to remove all the organic material. The remaining calcified material reflects the structural organization of the living biofilm just as a piece of dried coral is a relic of the ecosystem of the living reef. The insert (magnification × 1000) reveals laminations and channels which the organisms have constructed to define a variety of habitats within the plaque biofilm.

These channels may be seen in an oral biofilm which has calcified (calculus), a process which mineralizes the soft matrix and preserves its architecture (▶ Fig. 4.7). The gradients of substrate concentration, oxygen availability, and pH in the complex structure of the biofilm provide a wide variety of habitats for microorganisms. The structural organization and functional coordination of organisms in a biofilm and the specialized role of some species, which orchestrate the behavior of other species bring biofilms close to the realms of a single organism.

The external environment has at first a decisive influence on the early colonizing species of a biofilm. As the biofilm matures, the cooperative influence of the early colonizers creates an inner structural and functional organization. The biofilm begins to create its own inner environment which supports organisms that would not otherwise survive in the external environment. This dynamic, in which organisms create a purpose-defined environment for the benefit of their own and other species, requires a review of accepted evolutionary theory. This orthodox view places the organism within an environment to which it must adapt or die. The restriction has not provided for the organism to create its own environment by cooperation with other species. Cross-talk between organisms, now known as quorum sensing, would have been ridiculed just 50 years ago. It is about 50 years ago an idea, suggested by James Lovelock, that the biosphere regulated itself was also ridiculed. The theory was unfortunately given a mystic name Gaia (earth mother), but it was supported by serious scientists. The more that is understood of the structural and organizational microenvironments created by biofilms, the more likely it becomes that the Gaia theory of biosphere self-regulation is a manifestation of an upscaled version of the self-organization found in biofilms (see *Appendix D.3 Gaia Theory*).

4.3.2 Calculus

Saliva is saturated with calcium and phosphate ions which may precipitate in an alkaline environment. If the precipitate occurs within plaque, it forms a firm, chalky deposit called calculus (Fig. 4.7). Plaque may become alkaline due to the activity of some oral bacteria which release ammonia during their metabolism of salivary urea. Calculus which is supragingival is generally white and chalky, whereas calculus which is subgingival is darker and harder. The precipitated calcium is either soft brushite (supragingival) or harder whitlockite (subgingival, perhaps from calcium in the crevicular fluid). The submandibular gland saliva has a higher concentration of calcium than other glands and has a relatively high pH. This may explain the rapid accumulation of calculus on the lingual surfaces of the lower incisors. Deposits of calculus have been implicated as a cause of gingivitis and periodontitis. Removal of calculus by prophylaxis has long been thought to help prevent periodontal disease although recent evidence challenges this assumption.

4.3.3 Growth of a Biofilm

Growth of a biofilm occurs in three distinct phases (▶ Fig. 4.8).

Adherence to a substrate is the first phase. Generally, hydrophilic (water-loving) surfaces encourage bacterial attachment and hydrophobic surfaces encourage their detachment. Many species of oral organisms produce biosurfactants, which decrease the surface tension of the substrate surface, causing it to become hydrophilic. These biosurfactants are of universal benefit to all species of adhering organism, so the production of them has communal value. The attachments made by organisms onto oral surfaces are either by specific protein adherent sites (*ligands*) on the bacterial cell membrane or nonspecific polysaccharide attachments via *fibrils*. Of these two forms of attachment, the fibrillar attachments, though less specific, are stronger than the rather weak but specific ligand connections.

Aggregation is the second phase of growth in which organisms clump together to form a complete layer. Aggregation may involve the adhesion of different species to each other. Two species which adhere to each other are *P. gingivalis* and *Streptococcus gordonii*. They also have significant levels of intercommunication which share changes in gene expression which prepare for a community existence in the biofilm. The partnership of these two species may become significant in orchestrating the early stages of gingivitis and periodontal disease.

The third phase of biofilm growth is the rapid increase in number of organisms. The concentration of organisms in a biofilm is likely to be 10,000 times greater than their concentration in planktonic form. This shift between a solitary planktonic existence, and a dense biofilm, requires some major adaptations of the bacteria which are achieved by *gene regulation*. This gene regulation is triggered by chemical messengers from other organisms, an example of quorum sensing (*see Appendix D.4 Gene Regulation in Biofilms*).

The benefits of existence in a biofilm as distinct from a floating (planktonic) existence in water are significant. The biofilm provides shelter, accommodation, food sharing, stability, and continuity. Planktonic bacteria are vulnerable to quite low concentrations of toxic chemicals (disinfectants). Bacteria in a biofilm are protected by the outer layers of organisms and very resistant to even high levels of disinfectant. The biofilm is only reliably disrupted by mechanically scraping or brushing it of the surface it is attached to (*see Appendix D.5 Strategies for Controlling Biofilms*).

4.3.4 Dental Plaque

Dental plaque is a biofilm which forms on oral surfaces. It is formed by a variety of oral organisms which form an aggregate within an adhesive matrix of salivary and bacterial polymers.

If a tooth surface is thoroughly cleaned, a layer of salivary pellicle forms within hours. Individual bacteria may soon be found attached to the pellicle (▶ Fig. 4.9). The early colonizers are mostly cocci and small rods which stain gram-positive bacteria (*See Appendix D.6 Gram Staining Bacteria*). Later colonizers are filamentous organisms which form a meshwork and may themselves become the site of attachment for smaller organisms. Adhesion to each other may improve the chances of survival where there is competition for surfaces. When viewed with a scanning electron microscope (SEM), these aggregates of organisms were described by Listgarten as "corn cobs." A similar arrangement has occurred between some rod-shaped organisms and filament-shaped bacteria which has already attached to the pellicle. These aggregates have been called "bottle brushes." The attachment of the filamentous organisms to the pellicle is by specific ligands, whereas the interbacterial attachments are by fimbriae. It is not clear what the relationship is

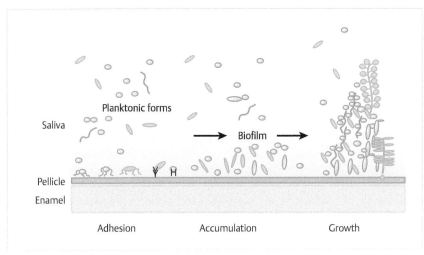

Fig. 4.8 A diagrammatic representation of the stages in development of a biofilm. Note that as the biofilm develops, there is increasingly some organization of microorganisms, which is not present in the planktonic forms or microorganisms.

Planktonic forms

Saliva

Biofilm

Pellicle

Enamel

Adhesion   Accumulation   Growth

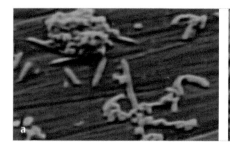
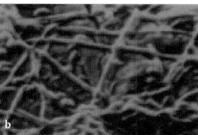

Fig. 4.9 SEM images of the early colonization of an enamel surface with oral organisms (magnification × 5,000). (a) Coccal and rod-shaped organisms are visible on enamel after 24 hours. **(b)** Filamentous organisms begin to create an interwoven mesh of organisms after 48 hours.

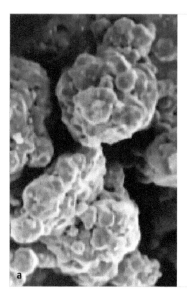
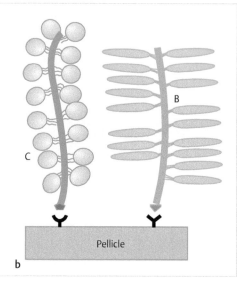

Fig. 4.10 Plaque organism unable to adhere to an oral surface may attach to organisms which are able to adhere. (a) A SEM image of a corn cob aggregation (magnification × 10,000). **(b)** A diagrammatic representation of the adhesion between different species of bacteria which gives rise to corn cob (C) and bottle brush (B) aggregates. These adhesive arrangements illustrate cooperation between certain species of cocci and filamentous bacteria.

between the two species of organisms in these aggregates, but it is likely that there is mutual benefit (▶ Fig. 4.10).

Successful adhesion to oral surfaces will depend on the preference for different surfaces. *Streptococcus salivarius* has a preference for the oral mucosa of the cheek, while *S. mutans* and *S. sanguis* attach more readily to the tooth surface pellicle. This species preference for sites is due to the presence of receptor sites on the bacteria and on the oral surface, which are complimentary to each other.

After 7 to 10 days, the plaque is mature and is a complex mixture of species containing gram-negative bacteria and spirochetes. The environment within the plaque changes as bacterial products accumulate and as the deeper layers are isolated from the influence of saliva. Channels in the biofilm are created which allow nutrients, oxygen, and bacterial products such as the chemical messengers of quorum sensing to permeate throughout the biofilm (▶ Fig. 4.7).

Several oral organisms produce polysaccharides, which are secreted from the cell and stored outside the organism. There are different types of extracellular polysaccharides, but they have, in common, the ability to help organisms to bind together and also to provide a means of food storage, which the organism can utilize in time of need. Thus, bacteria are able to sustain acid production, up to an hour after a sucrose-containing meal, by metabolizing the glucans they produced while the sucrose was available.

The mature microenvironments of plaque, formed by structural organization and specific competition and cooperation between species, provide a niche for over 200 species (▶ Fig. 4.11) (*see Appendix D.7 Microenvironments*).

4.3.5 Variations in Plaque

Plaque in different sites has different characteristics. For example, the plaque found on maxillary incisors may have a lower pH than the mandibular incisor plaque. The reason for this difference is due to the exposure of the anterior teeth to the drying effect of air flow around them. The reduction in saliva flow surrounding these teeth diminishes the buffering effect of saliva, and the plaque becomes relatively acidic. The proximity of the lower incisors to the duct openings of the sublingual and submandibular glands ensures an abundant supply of salivary buffers to the plaque on lower incisors, reducing its acidity. The deposits of calculus on mandibular anterior teeth are due to the higher resting pH level, higher calcium levels, and reduced ionic strength of submaxillary saliva. On the other hand, the labial surfaces of the maxillary incisors are infrequently in contact with saliva, and so plaque pH may drop to below the critical level for dissolution. This may account for the tendency for caries to develop in the maxillary incisors before the mandibular incisors.

A measure of the oxygen supply is the oxidation potential (Eh) and is an important factor in the environment for anaerobic organisms. Areas with high Eh values are the exposed surfaces of the teeth and oral mucosa and are unsuitable for anaerobic organisms. Areas with low Eh values are the stagnant areas far from atmospheric oxygen such as the interproximal embrasures, occlusal fissures, and gingival sulcus. These structural habitats may be modified by the other environmental factors, such as the amount of sugar in the host diet, the level of oral hygiene, and flow of saliva.

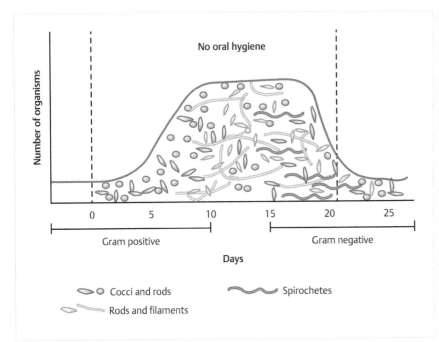

Fig. 4.11 A diagrammatic representation of the diversity of organisms in mature plaque. Gingivitis develops after a 20-day period during which there is a cessation of oral hygiene. As the plaque matures, the number of organisms increases and the biofilm becomes more diverse.

Some oral organisms such as the motile rods and spirochetes are quite fastidious and need particular nutrients. These nutrients may only be produced by other organisms in the gingival sulcus.

It is of clinical importance to be able to measure the amount of plaque on the teeth as it is an indication of the effectiveness of oral hygiene. While plaque is visible as a white coating on the teeth, it is more readily seen if a stain is used. There are several methods of measuring plaque, but most use an index which records a score of how many surfaces are covered with plaque. Of perhaps even greater importance than the plaque index (amount of plaque) is the rate at which it forms. The rate of plaque formation is surprisingly not influenced by the plaque index but by the position of the tooth in relation to the lips; the rate increases with distance from the lips and is highest on the buccal surfaces of maxillary molars and lowest on the mandibular incisors.

4.3.6 From Symbiont to Pathobiont

A biofilm may form on suitable surface of a host, which provides moisture, food, and shelter, without doing the host any harm and may even contribute to the welfare of the host. The organisms of such a biofilm may be described as symbionts. This symbiosis has been established over many millions of years in the guts of a large variety of animal species from termites to man. How does this symbiont biofilm remain, for the most part benign, but yet clearly able to switch into a pathogenic mode?

Our commensal gut organisms not only keep out a more pathogenic flora, but contribute to the full development of our immune system and provide us with some nutrients such as vitamin K_2. However, if there are even slight changes in the environment, which includes changes in the health status of the host, the balance between species may be disturbed. Certain species may become more dominant than others, and no longer be as harmless to the host. From being symbionts, they become pathobionts.

A distinction needs to be made between pathogens and pathobionts. Pathogenic organisms are understood to be capable of causing disease when introduced into a susceptible host. Pathobionts which have shifted from a symbiotic relationship to a less benign one become damaging to the host, but only when part of a consortium of other organisms have made the same shift. For example, *Treponema denticola* is a symbiont in the healthy gingival sulcus. It may become a pathobiont with other species causing gingivitis, but if introduced on its own to a susceptible host such as germ-free mice, gingivitis does not occur. It will only occur in the mice if the whole consortium is introduced. Pathobionts, unlike pathogens, may return to a symbiotic relationship if the balance of the ecosystem is restored to a state of health.

If broad-spectrum antibiotics are taken for any length of time, one of the side effects is disruption of the balance of resident gut organisms, which are not the target of the antibiotic. This disruption causes a shift in dominance of organisms such as *Clostridium difficile*, which cause diarrhea. Doctors advise patients who are taking antibiotics to eat yoghurt, which helps rebalance the intestinal flora. A more dramatic treatment for patients whose gut flora is unbalanced (e.g., Crohn's disease) is to administer fecal transplants containing a less pathogenic spectrum of gut bacteria. It is considered by some microbiologists that most chronic, noncommunicable diseases are linked to a disordered microbiome. The term *dysbiosis* is used to describe the inbalance of a microbiome which leads to a shift to pathobiotic bacteria.

The most common oral diseases include dental caries, gingivitis, periodontal disease, alveolar abscess, pulpitis, periapical infection, peri-implantitis, and denture stomatitis. They are all caused by bacteria endogenous to the oral cavity, which have transformed from symbionts to pathobionts. In view of the origins of the causative organism, these oral infections should be described as noncommunicable. From this perspective, it may be useful to revisit the role of cross-infection control in dentistry.

4.3.7 Cross-Infection Control

It is instructive to consider the surgical classification of wounds according to the level of contamination. This classification ranges through four progressive levels of contamination, starting with *clean* and increasing through intermediary levels, *clean/contaminated, contaminated/dirty,* to *dirty*. According to these criteria, oral surgery wounds would be classified as *clean/contaminated*. The endogenous nature of most oral diseases therefore suggest that cross-infection would be most effective when directed toward intraoral control of potential pathobionts. For example, the importance of using a rubber dam barrier, to exclude salivary organisms during endodontic treatment, has been well established and is considered a best practice by endodontists. The use of a barrier rubber dam has also been recommended for restorative procedures when attempts are made by the operator to remove all infected caries, leaving a sterile cavity to restore.

There are other measures which have been recommended, which reduced the burden of endogenous contamination. For many years, it has been considered as the best practice to remove the plaque around the root surface of a tooth before extracting it. The purpose of this measure is to reduce the amount of dental plaque forced into the socket during application of the extraction forceps. In view of the endogenous origins of bacteria which cause an infected (dry) socket, a pre-extraction prophylaxis is a sensible precaution (*see Chapter 5.3.2 Healing of a Tooth Socket*). A similar preparation of a surgical site has been a recommended practice by many implant surgeons. An incision into the gingival sulcus, when creating a surgical flap for the placement of an implant fixture, releases orders of magnitude more pathobionts into the surgical site than might enter on the blade of the scalpel on which some airborne organisms may have alighted. For this reason, prophylaxis of teeth adjacent to a planned surgical site should proceed any surgery so as to reduce the unintentioned spread of plaque organisms.

The term cross-infection may deserve an expanded interpretation, as the non-communicable diseases of the oral cavity are not caused by foreign organisms transmitted from other individuals, or indeed by any single species of organism. Viral infections such as herpes, Epstein-Barr and AIDS are communicable via the oral cavity, though in quite specific conditions of transmission.

The trend toward central sterilization in an effort to reduce cross-contamination in the operating area should be seen in context with the threat to infection by endogenous pathobionts. It might be well to recall the Roman writer Cicero's warning that "The enemy is within the gates... it is our own criminality that we have to contend with."

4.3.8 Single Organism or Consortium

The traditional theory of organisms causing diseases was defined by Koch in his isolation of *Mycobacterium tuberculosis* as the cause of tuberculosis. This theory stresses the vital role of the single organism and makes the isolation of pure cultures essential for proper diagnosis. However, diseases are also caused by communities of organisms which are for the most part endogenous or common symbionts of the body. In these conditions, it is necessary to culture at least a consortium of likely organisms as

no single organism produces the disease. The diversity of organisms in the collective consortium is essential for the system to exert its effect. Marsh was the first microbiologist to culture a consortium of organisms in the investigation of dental caries and periodontal disease. This break with tradition led to the development of variations in artificial mouth simulations which have led to great advances in understanding the complexity of these diseases. We now know that we should not be looking for a single organism responsible for either caries or periodontal disease, but a group whose interdependence may be crucial to their success as pathobionts.

4.3.9 Dental Caries

A shift in the oral environment, such as an increase in dietary sugar, causes an imbalance in the dominance of some key organism in the dental plaque, which has accumulated on enamel surfaces. A sudden supply of sugar causes those bacteria to flourish, which have a particular ability to uptake and metabolize sugar rapidly. Species such as the mutans streptococci along with other *Lactobacillus species* produce lactic acid as a by-product of metabolism (*aciduric*). This lactic acid may cause the pH of the dental plaque to fall below 1.5, a critical level, which begins to demineralize enamel crystals. This demineralization may be the beginning of dental caries, but of course such an outcome is purely associative, and of no apparent benefit to the pathobionts casing it. Of greater impact on the biofilm environment, of the rise in lactic acid, is the inhibition of other plaque organisms which are acid sensitive.

Dental plaque which is associated with dental caries has twice as much lactic acid and larger numbers of *S. mutans* than noncarious plaque (NCP). ▶ Table 4.1 summarizes these and other differences between NCP and carious plaque (CP). It should be noted that the change from NCP to CP is not due to one single organism, nor does it require the arrival of a new species, but merely a change in the hierarchy of organisms already present. There is a consortium of organism, which is at the forefront of the shift toward greater acidity of the biofilm, and they include the group of mutans streptococci, *S. mutans*, and *Streptococcus sobrinus* and lactobacilli. *Actinomyces* species are also involved in root caries. *S. mutans* is a keystone species which orchestrates these changes. From the data which come from artificial mouth experiments it seems as if the slight shift toward acidity promotes a shift in this hierarchy which rapidly gathers momentum.

4.3.10 Periodontal Disease

A cessation of oral hygiene also brings about a shift in the oral environment, which alters the balance of plaque organisms in the gingival sulcus. These sulcus organisms are more anaerobic than plaque organisms of the enamel surface, and their source

Table 4.1 A comparison between five key features of noncarious plaque (NCP) and carious plaque (CP)

	NCP	CP
Lactic acid	+	+ +
Streptococcus mutans	+	+ +
Streptococcus sanguis	+ +	+
Actinomyces	+ +	+
Sucrose metabolism	+	+ + +

of nutrition contains a greater proportion of proteins from the gingival fluid. If plaque of the gingival sulcus is not regularly removed by oral hygiene, the GCF flow increases, the pH increases, and there is a shift toward more anaerobic, gram-negative, non-sugar metabolizing (*asaccharolytic*) species. These include *P. gingivalis*, spirochetes, *Fusobacterium nuclea-tum*, and *Tannerella forsythia*. The resultant inflammation of the gingival tissues may progress to periodontitis, an inflamma-tion which involves loss of the epithelial attachment to the tooth and destruction of bone. Although *P. gingivalis* is not present in large numbers, it functions as a keystone species. It achieves the orchestration of other symbionts in the shift toward pathobionts in the following ways:

- It produces isobutyric acid which stimulates the growth of the spirochete *T. denticola.*
- It releases proteases which degrade the proteins of the GCF making them available as nutrients for other members of the consortium.
- It interferes with cross-talk between complement and neu-trophils so as to ensure its own survival.
- It manipulates and depresses the host immune response by entering neutrophils in the lamina propria, preventing their killing ability, thus preserving itself and other bacteria.

The progressive tissue damage to the periodontium is brought about in part by the host's own defense mechanisms. In response to lipopolysaccharides on the cell membrane of *P. gingivalis*, neu-trophils migrate into the junctional epithelium and phagocytosis the bacteria. Their own subsequent death and autolysis cause the release of lytic enzymes which further damage the gingival sul-cus tissues. The inflammation caused tends to further increase the exudate into the gingival sulcus of nutrients which further gives support to the pathobiont organisms in the consortia. In addition to *P. gingivalis*, these include *Prevotella intermedia*, *Tannerella forsythia*, and *Treponema denticola*.

The resultant inflammation of the gingival tissues may prog-ress to periodontitis, an inflammation which involves loss of the epithelial attachment to the tooth and destruction of bone.

The presence of destructive periodontal disease allows blood-borne migration of *P. gingivalis* and colonization of brain and car-diovascular tissues. *P. gingivalis* has recently come under scrutiny as a cause of cardiovascular diseases and Alzheimer's disease. The capacity of *P. gingivalis* to enter and survive within immune cells and, to some extent, alter the behavior of these cells may explain its ability to colonize distant tissues such as the coronary arteries and to bypass the blood–brain barrier and enter brain tissue. After some years, during which it has infected neurons and spread along nerve axons, it may emerge out of the host cell and release toxic proteases such as gingipains. These enzymes break up tau and ubiquitin proteins which are essential supporting elements of neural tissue. Ubiquitin stabilizes amyloid protein thereby pre-venting the accumulation of malformed amyloid precursor pro-teins which are associated with Alzheimer's disease. There is evidence that the progression of Alzheimer's disease and vascular sclerosis of coronary arteries, is caused by *P. gingivalis* which has gained access into the blood from infected periodontal pockets. Attention to oral hygiene appears to have a wider preventive role than previously thought.[1]

Marsh proposed the "ecological plaque hypothesis" which concludes that "Disease is a result of undesirable changes in the microbial balance, metabolism, and composition of dental biofilms."[2] There are several factors which might alter the microbial balance including diet and level of oral hygiene. These two factors are clearly important in influencing the balance of bacteria with a specific ability, such as the mutans streptococci, to exploit an increase in the availability of dietary sugars. Diet-ary factors and oral hygiene can therefore explain a shift in the microbial balance of plaque toward initiating dental caries. It is also clear that the level of oral hygiene is a significant factor associated with the prevalence of periodontal disease. The risk factor of developing periodontal disease has been found to be around five times higher in individuals with poor oral hygiene.[3] This does not imply that poor oral hygiene is a cause of perio-dontal disease but that it is a contributing risk factor. There are individuals who suffer from periodontal disease but maintain a high level of oral hygiene. There are studies which have revealed that even those with very poor levels of oral hygiene have no periodontal disease.[4]

The "undesirable changes" which Marsh suggests would appear to be due to other, so far illusive factors.

Key Notes

Biofilms are microbiomes which exhibit an advanced level of functional and structural organization. This organization is due to the intimate interrelationships of different species which are characterized by symbiosis. Slight changes in the environment may cause symbionts to become pathobionts. This imbalance in the microbiome is called dysbiosis.

Review Questions

1. What example can you think of which illustrates coopera-tion between oral organisms?
2. Why do planktonic bacteria have to switch on 80 genes in order to take up residence in a biofilm?
3. What suggests that biofilm life is more supportive for organisms than planktonic life?
4. What could be the value to plaque organism of secreting extracellular polysaccharides?
5. How is the oral flora influenced by the arrival of the first teeth and by fixed and removable restorations?
6. What comparisons could be made between maturing plaque and a maturing forest ecosystem?
7. Why is it that calculus appears most commonly near the openings of salivary glands?
8. How could you account for the increased prevalence of dental caries in maxillary incisor teeth?
9. How would you distinguish between the term pathogen and pathobiont?
10. What features of the organism *P. gingivalis* define it as a keystone organism?

4.4 Oral Ecology and Dental Caries

Dental caries results from a combination of a dietary disorder in which excessive amounts of sugar are consumed and the consequent disruption of the ecological balance of bacteria in dental plaque. Of all the mammals, man alone is affected. Other

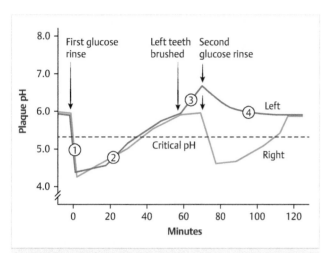

Fig. 4.12 **A plot of the pH of plaque before and after a glucose mouth rinse.** At (1), the pH of plaque drops due to acid produced by bacteria fermenting the sucrose. At a pH of 5.3, enamel begins to dissolve. At (2), the pH rises due to the buffering action of plaque and saliva. At (3), one side of the arch is brushed, and the pH rises to neutral value of 7.0. At (4), a second glucose rinse causes the plaque pH on the unbrushed side to again drop below 5.3. The brushed side also drops, but not below the critical pH level. (Adapted from Stephan RM, Miller BF. A quantitative method for evaluating physical and chemical agents which modify production of acids in bacterial plaques on human teeth. J Dent Res 1943;22:45–51.)

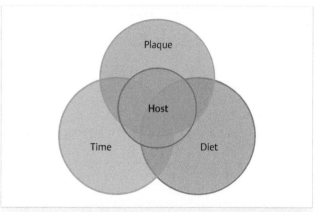

Fig. 4.13 **Diagrammatic representation of the four essential factors in the onset and progress of dental caries.** Changes in either factor, but particularly in diet, may either increase or decrease the risk of caries. Some parts of the tooth environment are more susceptible than others. For example, caries tends to occur in the fissures of the tooth and at the approximal surfaces, before it occurs on smooth accessible surfaces. If the period of time that plaque pH decreases to levels which cause demineralization short, remineralization may occur. If the dietary intake of sugar is high and the level of oral hygiene poor, caries may advance rapidly.

mammals do not suffer from caries (laboratory or domesticated mammals may be the exceptions). Dental caries may cause only microscopic damage to a tooth, or it may completely destroy it. The necrosis of the pulp–dentin leads to spread of bacteria to the tooth socket and the formation of an alveolar abscess. We have noted in the previous section that there are many factors at work in maintaining a stable oral ecology. Dental caries is far more complex than a bacterial infection. It is caused by interaction between oral bacteria, their access to fermentable carbohydrates, and vulnerable parts of the tooth. This relationship can be illustrated by a graph, which bears Stephan's name, and has become a classic of dental science. It shows the rapid drop in plaque pH after a glucose rinse (▶ Fig. 4.12). The drop in pH is the result of fermentation of the sugar by some plaque bacteria, which produce lactic acid as a by-product. The gradual return of the pH is the result of buffers present in plaque and saliva. Provided the pH does not drop below 5.3 the enamel remains intact, but below this critical level, crystals of apatite dissolve (demineralize).

Fortunately, both plaque and saliva are saturated with calcium and phosphate ions, so that if the pH returns fairly rapidly above the 5.3 level, ions will go back into the enamel and recrystallize (remineralize). Acid environments favor demineralization and occur when there is a plaque biofilm, a supply of sugar which bacteria metabolize, and limited amounts of saliva. Neutral or alkali environments favor remineralization and occur when there is no sugar available, good oral hygiene, and abundant saliva. The presence of fluoride ions in the tooth or in the plaque also help remineralization to take place. While caries results from a dietary disorder, the damage to the tooth is not done directly by the excess of sugar, but by the shift it causes in

the dominant organisms in the biofilm. The duration of the shift and the tooth environment are also factors (▶ Fig. 4.13).

Caries becomes established in the fissures of the teeth more readily than it does on smooth surfaces. This is because the fissures trap food and are less accessible to all the protective functions of saliva. For similar reasons, the approximal areas of the teeth are at risk. In general (with the exception of the mandibular incisors), the pattern of caries attack is related to the eruption sequence of the teeth. The longer a tooth has had a permanent neighbor, the more at risk its approximal surface. Hence, a vulnerable period for the permanent dentition is from 6 to 13 years of age. Teeth which are far removed from a source of saliva are at greater risk than teeth which are constantly bathed in saliva. So, the maxillary anterior teeth (especially the approximal areas) are more inclined to become carious than the mandibular incisors, around which saliva collects, as it enters the oral cavity from the submandibular and sublingual salivary ducts. The most common sights for dental caries in the permanent dentition are the first molars and the maxillary incisors.

4.4.1 Diet and Control of Dental Caries

Given that modern man is more vulnerable than his ancestors, there are some features of our diet which may increase or reduce caries risk.

A high-fiber diet: The diet of a hunter–gatherer was high in vegetable fiber and lacked refined carbohydrates. The consequence of such a diet was a certain amount of tooth wear. Occlusal wear removes the deep occlusal fissures which trap plaque. Approximal wear flattens the point of contact between each tooth which reduces the stagnant areas for plaque to accumulate. Approximal wear also reduces the width of the teeth and so allows them to be accommodated into the arch without being crowded. We have also noted that chewing hard food increases the rate of secretion of saliva, which has many protective roles in maintaining oral health. If the total outflow of saliva can be increased, there is a greater chance of protection of all the teeth in the arch.

Increase in saliva flow: Some foods, like cheese, stimulate the flow of saliva. Sugar is also a good stimulator of saliva, but, of course, also provides a rich source of nutrients for plaque bacteria. However, sugar substitutes, which are of no nutrient value to bacteria, are effective saliva stimulants, as is the mere act of chewing. Chewing a gum, which is artificially sweetened, makes biological sense and indeed has a role in arresting caries. The flow of saliva is reduced at night, making the oral environment particularly susceptible to plaque acids. Allowing children candy or sweet beverages at bedtime thus has a far greater impact on acid production during the night, than it would during the day. The Vipeholm study was a landmark in caries research, though today it would not be permitted on ethical grounds. The study involved observing the cariogenic effects of taking carbohydrate snacks in between meals and the influence of different food consistencies. Both sugar levels and sticky consistency were found to increase the prevalence of caries (*see Appendix D.8 The Vipeholm Study*).

Refined carbohydrates: Carbohydrates of the simple type like sucrose, glucose, and fructose are more cariogenic than the larger starch molecules. This is because starchy foods are not so readily broken down by plaque organisms into simple fermentable sugars. The capacity of plaque to produce acid from sugars is reduced in patients who are being fed on a gastric tube. It seems that unless the plaque organisms can get access to sucrose, the acid-forming capacity does not develop. Sucrose also provides the substrate for *S. mutans* to form insoluble extracellular polysaccharides, which provide a nutrient source when dietary levels fall; they also have unique adhesive properties.

Unrefined carbohydrates: Unrefined carbohydrates may contain some protective factors such as phytates or other inorganic phosphates. Fats in the diet seem to be beneficial in small amounts by increasing the ease with which food is removed from oral surfaces. They seem therefore to complement the lubricating influence of salivary glycoproteins. It may be observed that communities living on a simple unrefined diet have some degree of resistance to caries. This may occur, but it is not due to any nutritional virtue of an unrefined diet, in fact, such communities often show signs of nutritional deficiencies. It is rather the absence of refined carbohydrates which confers protection against oral disease.

In summary, there is an ebb and flow of minerals into and out of the enamel. It is only when remineralization fails to keep up the pace of repairing the damage caused by acids that the caries process destroys tooth structure, and there is a net loss of mineral into the environment. Dental caries may be prevented by restricting the intake of dietary sugars and removing plaque; at least these are the methods promoted by dentists in their own families. These simple habits seem to have worked, as dentists' children have less caries than the general population.

4.4.2 Risk Factors in Predicting Dental Caries

This chapter has reviewed some of the factors which contribute to the complex balance between the organisms of the oral cavity and the host. It is useful in managing the treatment of caries on a public health scale to be able to identify those individuals in a community, particularly young children, who are most at risk. Measuring all, or even some, of the factors involved in the shift from health to disease in order to estimate the caries risk of an individual has been attempted, but it is a time-consuming exercise and impractical for assessing the risk for entire communities. The awareness of the members of the community in particular parents and their commitment to oral hygiene and control of dietary factors will also be essential factors in any meaningful risk assessment. The most useful risk assessment is one that includes an individualized program of prevention and management with minimal clinical intervention, rather than restoration.

Dental Caries Management by Risk Assessment (CAMBRA): CAMBRA includes an assessment of risk and an individualized program for children up to 5 years old, which is designed to control dietary factors and institute a program of hygiene. There are three main assessment factors:
- Risk factors, such as going to bed with a bottle.
- Preventive factors, such as use of a fluoride-containing tooth paste.
- Clinical factors of which the three most important are as follows:
  - Recent new caries lesions in the prime care giver.
  - Existing caries in the child.
  - White lesions or signs of enamel decalcification.

This assessment can be accomplished by dental or medical providers of care. It should be followed by a demonstration of proper toothbrush technique and then a fluoride varnish application. Finally, an outline of goals for the entire family is drawn up which includes dietary control, effective oral hygiene, and the use of fluoride-containing toothpaste and gum.

4.4.3 Dental Caries, Infection, or Dietary Disorder?

Dental caries is described by public health dentists as a dietary disorder. Microbiologists prefer the description, infectious disease, as without the component of microorganisms, dental caries does not occur. The bacteria involved are therefore an essential cause.

The preference for the term dietary disorder is based on the view that unless the diet contains refined carbohydrates, caries does not or very rarely occurs. It is also observed that the organisms which cause caries are not true pathogens but pathobionts, which have become opportunist at metabolizing sugar, the product of which is lactic acid, which by accident happens to damage tooth enamel. Dental caries is a noncommunicable disease which further clarifies the contrasts with an infectious disease, in which there is an essential role of a single pathogen. Those who prefer the term dietary disorder are also focusing on the prevention of dental caries in the population. Prevention is more productive when focused on dietary modification and oral hygiene than it is when focused on antimicrobial therapies. It may also be of benefit to educate the public to the reality that they are not victims of a microbial infection. They have to take responsibility for a dietary habit, which many agencies are reminding them, that may lead to a variety of health issues which include caries, diabetes, and obesity.

There is no doubt, however, that the professional view must be inclusive of all the factors which contribute to causing dental caries.

Key Notes

It is useful to consider caries a dietary disorder as this perspective directs clinical dentistry toward prevention. Known risk factors are poor oral hygiene, consuming sugar in between meals, and for young children, going to bed with a bottle containing a sweetened beverage.

Review Questions

1. How does an unrefined diet reduce the risk of dental caries?
2. How does Stephan's curve help us to understand the process of dental caries?
3. What factors apart from diet are essential in causing caries?
4. What parts of the tooth are at greatest risk of becoming carious?
5. Which teeth in the mouth are at greatest risk?
6. What did the Vipeholm study show?
7. To what extent is dental caries a one-way process?
8. What are the best predictors of caries risk?
9. Should dental caries ever be described as a dietary disorder?

4.5 Nutrition and Oral Ecology

The term nutrition refers to the availability of nutrients to the cells of the body. It is thus dependent on the needs of the body, the absorption of food from the gut, and an adequate diet.

Primary malnutrition: Primary malnutrition occurs when there is a severe shortage of all food types. It has also been called protein–calorie malnutrition, which is a term used to describe a collection of nutritional diseases. These include kwashiorkor, caused by insufficient protein, and marasmus, which results from a lack of all food types.

Secondary malnutrition: Secondary malnutrition occurs when in spite of an adequate diet, the demands made by chronic disease or malabsorption leave insufficient nutrition for daily activity. For example, a 12-year-old who has malaria will be malnourished unless she or he has additional food. This is because during a bout of malaria fever, the body needs more than double the normal supply of food energy. It is estimated that 20% of the food energy available in developing nations is taken up in sustaining the burden of human parasites. Despite community services and available medicines, the prevalence of whipworm in preschool children was found to be 75% in a rural African town. Treatment requires more than medication but must include nutritional support as well, for at least 3 years, to compensate for impaired growth.

Malnutrition tends to be cumulative, that is, each generation becomes progressively affected. A mother who is not well nourished tends to have less well-nourished daughters, whose own children in turn are severely malnourished. Poorly nourished children tend to be susceptible to chronic diseases such as parasitism or tuberculosis, in which case they suffer from both primary and secondary malnutrition. The combination of disease and hunger work together in a downward spiral which ends in death. The marvels of medicine, especially antibiotics, took us a giant leap forward during the second half of the 20th century. However, in developed nations, the life span was already increasing and the infant mortality dropping during the first half of the 20th century. Diseases like dysentery, cholera, plague, and tuberculosis were on their way out before antibiotics were discovered. This occurred because poverty was reduced; there was good sanitation, clean water, and abundant food, all the major factors in protecting communities from chronic infectious diseases.

Malnutrition is the most common and important cause of suppression of the immune system and slow healing. It also affects growth and development, both of which require the full complement of nutrients in the diet. If a child goes through a period of malnutrition, it may be possible for it to catch up the lost growth provided an adequate nutrition is restored. However, there is a crucial period during which malnutrition does permanent damage, which cannot later be undone. Malnutrition during the last trimester of pregnancy and the first year after birth may cause loss of intellect and physical stunting which is permanent. Babies, who are underweight have greater risk of disease in later life and hence shorter life expectancies than babies of average birth weight and length.

4.5.1 Oral Manifestation of Malnutrition

The development of the teeth occurs primarily during fetal life and in childhood. It is during this period that the fetal requirements for nutrition are greatest. The nutrition of the fetus is dependent on the mother's nutrition. If the mother becomes ill or malnourished during the period of her pregnancy when the fetal teeth are calcifying, from the fourth month of pregnancy, they may be seriously affected. The formation of the permanent teeth, which begin to calcify at birth, may also be seriously affected by early malnutrition or childhood diseases. Signs of childhood malnutrition or disease may be seen as pits and irregularities on the surface of the enamel, once the tooth has erupted. These enamel irregularities provide a natural habitat for plaque and are at risk of developing caries. The malnourished child has another more serious risk of poor oral health. All the antibacterial qualities of saliva are dependent on the availability of proteins or peptides. The levels of the PRPs which bind calcium, lactoferrin, peroxidaze, and not least, salivary immunoglobulins are all lower in malnourished children.

One of the immediate consequences of this "malnourished" saliva is that it cannot support the normal oral flora. If the complex oral ecosystem is upset, more pathogenic organisms, such as yeasts, become dominant. A study in Peru found that the deciduous teeth of children who had suffered an episode of malnutrition during infancy were more susceptible to caries at ages between 3 and 4 years than those who had been well fed as infants. This study illustrates the permanent damage to salivary glands that occurs due to malnutrition during the critical window of time which includes infancy.

The increased incidence of acute necrotizing ulcerative gingivitis (ANUG) and candidiasis is higher in malnourished children and older patients. ANUG is particularly dangerous in malnourished children as it may progress to noma, a life-threatening and destructive oral infection.

4.5.2 Trace Elements, Minerals, and Vitamins

Fluoride is such an important trace element that it is discussed separately. However, there are other trace elements in a natural diet which seem to give some protection against caries. Some elements which may give such protection are molybdenum, aluminum, and titanium.

Calcium, phosphorus, and magnesium appear to be incorporated into dentin and enamel at the expense of bone and are not retrievable later in times of dietary shortage of these elements. So, the teeth of a pregnant or lactating mother are not weakened by calcium loss, though the bones may be.

Vitamin A has an important effect on the differentiation of ectodermal cells and in allowing the synthesis of the mucinous glycoproteins. Deficiency is rare but may cause keratinization of the salivary ducts and impaired secretion of mucin.

The vitamin B group has a key influence in mitosis and therefore is vital for tissues whose cells have a rapid turnover. Deficiency reduces the replacement rate of epithelial cells, and they therefore become thin, inflamed, and infected. The tongue and cheeks may become sore or "burning" and cause discomfort in eating and swallowing.

Vitamin C is necessary for the formation of collagen and some connective tissue constituents such as chondroitin sulfate. A scorbutic diet (one that causes scurvy) in rats causes breakdown of collagen fibers in the periodontal ligament, atrophy of alveolar bone, and gingival bleeding. Vitamin C appears to be important for tissue of mesodermal origin.

Vitamin D deficiency in young rats and dogs produces rickets and osteomalacia, an excess of osteoid in bone. Enamel and dentin are thinner and poorly calcified. The enamel becomes hypoplastic, and because of the uneven surface may be more prone to caries.

4.6 The Influence of Fluorides on the Oral Ecosystem

4.6.1 Distribution of Fluoride in Teeth

Fluoride concentrations are much higher (500–2,000 ppm) in the surface, 20 µm of enamel than they are deeper inside (20 ppm). Fluoride is concentrated at the margins of early caries. This illustrates the importance of fluorides in the remineralization of teeth (▶ Fig. 4.14). In view of the short period during which dentin and enamel are being formed, it would seem that the crucial years for fluoride uptake would be during childhood, when the teeth are being mineralized. However, it is clear that fluoride can be absorbed onto the surface of the tooth during adult life and that high concentration of fluoride can accumulate. It is strange that surface levels of fluoride are just as high in unerupted teeth (although the layer of high fluoride-containing enamel is much thinner) (*see Appendix D.9 Fluoride Availability, Toxicity, and Fluorosis*).

4.6.2 Fluoride Protection of Enamel

The hydroxyl ion in the apatite crystal is held by electrostatic forces to the calcium inside the lattice of hydroxyapatite. It is mobile and reactive. When the hydroxyl ion is replaced by a fluoride ion, a stronger hydrogen bond forms; the fluoride locates accurately into the crystal space, the hydroxyapatite is more stable and dissolves less readily (▶ Fig. 4.15). The result of this interaction is the formation of fluorapatite. The new fluorapatite crystal is not only less easily dissolved, but also it is larger in size. This increased volume effectively reduces the surface area of the crystal exposed to acids. It is thus possible,

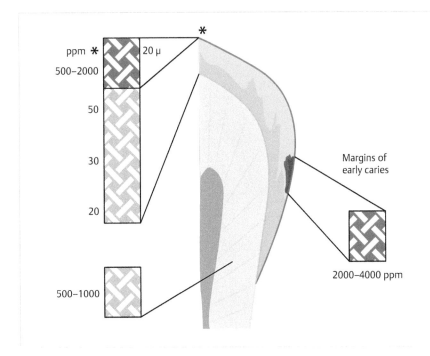

Fig. 4.14 A diagrammatic representation of the concentration of fluoride at different depths and sites on the enamel. Fluoride is concentrated in the surface 80 µm of enamel, which is approximately one-fiftieth of the full thickness. In the deeper layers of enamel, it drops to less than one-tenth of the concentration in this layer. Fluoride concentration in dentin is almost as high as it is in the enamel surface layers. Fluoride is concentrated around early caries lesions in enamel.

Margins of early caries

2000–4000 ppm

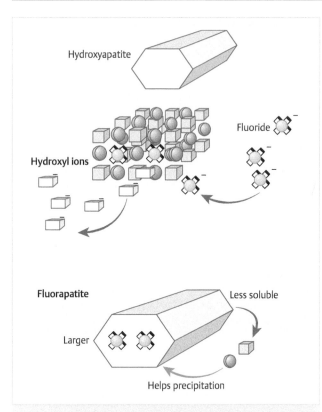

Fig. 4.15 A diagrammatic representation of the mechanism whereby fluoride ions decrease the solubility of enamel. Incorporation into the calcium apatite crystal of fluoride ions creates a larger fluorapatite crystal, which is less soluble than hydroxyapatite and so inhibits demineralization and facilitates mineralization.

even in the fully formed tooth, to alter the composition of the hydroxyapatite crystal on the surface of the enamel by applying fluoride to the tooth. Fluoride defends enamel against dissolution, primarily by acting at the site of an early caries lesion, because it favors apatite crystals to reform if they have been dissolved by plaque acids. Fluoride also encourages remineralization for a completely different reason. It is antibacterial, and so suppresses the activity of plaque bacteria. It does this in two ways:

- It inhibits the transport of glucose through the cell membrane of the bacteria.
- It blocks the enzyme enolase, which is necessary for pyruvate production, and formation of adenosine triphosphate (ATP). Plaque concentrates fluoride ions. Mostly, the increase is a result of high levels inside the organisms.

In summary, the role of fluoride in reducing caries may be as follows:

- Improving the stability of the crystal by forming less soluble fluorapatite.
- Increasing the rate of remineralization.
- Increasing the crystal size and reducing the surface area.
- Inhibiting plaque organisms.

4.6.3 Administration of Fluoride

It is of greatest value for fluoride to be available while the enamel is being formed. The fluoride must therefore be taken into the body as part of the diet. Deciduous teeth begin calcifying during the last 3 months of pregnancy. However, it is of no value to give the mother fluoride tablets, as the fluoride levels in plasma are always low, and they are even less in the placenta and still less in the fetus. The permanent teeth begin to calcify at birth, so as soon as possible (about 6 months) fluoride can be added to baby foods and later taken as a tablet. Fluoride tablets remain a useful supplement to the diet provided that the local water levels are not adequate. Enamel formation of the second molars is complete by the time the child is 6 years old, so after this, there is no point in taking fluoride tablets.

It is also of value for fluoride to be available in the oral cavity when it is referred to as topical fluoride. The most common source of topical fluoride is in toothpaste. Fluoridated toothpaste may have been responsible for the decrease in dental caries seen in the developed nations, though there are other important factors as well. Fluoride may also be applied to the teeth in polishing pastes and in gels which are held around the teeth in customized trays; unfortunately, fluoride is cleared from the mouth fairly rapidly, so the benefit of such topical applications is short-lived.

The most widely available source of fluoride is in drinking water. Adding fluoride to a water supply, however, is expensive and may not be cost effective unless the population of the town is of a suitable size. In small towns and villages, fluoride tablets and fluoridated toothpaste may be more appropriate. The evidence suggests that fluoridated water not so much prevents dental caries as it retards its progression by encouraging remineralization of lesions.

An increasingly important vehicle for fluoride application is in restorative materials. The glass ionomer cements contain fluoride, which leaches out into the area surrounding the restoration. It appears that very small concentrations of fluoride are effective, if they are constantly maintained.

Key Notes

Malnutrition of the fetus in the last trimester and of the infant in the early childhood may cause damage to the development of the teeth and salivary glands. Fluoride supplementation may be a useful defense against caries, but the administration needs to be carefully controlled.

Review Questions

1. What is the difference between diet and nutrition?
2. How can malnutrition be cumulative?
3. At what stage in the child's development is malnutrition most likely to cause permanent damage?
4. What are the oral manifestations of malnutrition?
5. Why are the teeth of a pregnant woman not affected by the fetal demand for calcium?
6. What is the fluoride level of the water in your area?
7. What is an optimal amount of fluoride in water to prevent caries?
8. What is the distribution of fluoride in teeth?
9. How does fluoride change the hydroxyapatite crystal?
10. What effect does fluoride have on plaque?
11. Should fluoride be given to the pregnant mother?

12. Does fluoridated water supply prevent new carious lesions developing?

4.7 Mucosal Immunity and Oral Ecology

4.7.1 General Barriers to Infection

Skin is clearly a most important barrier to invasion by microorganisms; one of the major risks of skin burns which covers a large area is an uncontrollable infection. Other barriers to infection, which are less obvious, but much more extensive, are the mucosae, which line the alimentary canal, the respiratory tract, and urogenital tracts. While skin covers an area just less than 2 square meters, there is 400 square meters of mucosa lining internal surfaces which is vulnerable to invasion. In addition to this larger area, mucosal surfaces are further at risk as they do not have the surface layer of insoluble keratin, which protects skin. Finally, to complicate the defense problems of mucosa, the alimentary tract, from oral cavity to rectum, supports thriving populations of microorganisms. It is therefore not surprising that mucosal surfaces are equipped with specialized strategies for controlling the colonization and invasion of microorganisms. The most important form of defense has been to develop a long-standing symbiotic or at least commensal relationship with organisms which are nonpathogenic.

In order for these organisms to remain symbionts, they must either evade or be tolerated by the host's immune system. It is now clear that not only are the oral and gut microbiota tolerated, but they also contribute to harvesting energy, minerals, and bioactive components from food. They also have an essential role in the development and maturation of the immune system. These resident organisms also exclude more overtly pathogenic varieties in the same way that a landlord benefits from peaceful tenants who keep out the criminal element. Even though there will be organisms living on mucosal surfaces, their numbers are limited by another defense mechanism. This is the regular shedding of the surface epithelial cells. Before colonies can become established, they are dislodged with the cell and flushed away. This occurs on a large scale; shed cells and dead organisms account for most of the bulk of feces. In case, all this is not adequate, secretions from the glands under the epithelial surface contain antibacterial enzymes and antibodies.

4.7.2 Mucosal Immunity

The mucosal antibodies are a special group of secretory immunoglobulins (sIgA) formed next to submucosal glands and secreted onto the mucosal surface. Mucosal or secretory IgA is a dimer made up of two units, each the size of the serum molecule. In addition, it has a secretory component which is contributed by the secretory cells of the glands of the mucosa. The immunoglobulin's secreted in tears, saliva, milk, gastric, and respiratory secretions are all of this sIgA type. sIgA, like all other antibodies, is specific to antigens encountered by lymphocytes of the immune system. These antigens may have come from the cell walls of microorganisms, or their enzymes and products, or they may be from food and drug proteins.

An antigen which is ingested with food, or which is part of the resident oral flora of the mouth, may be presented by dendritic cells in the mucosal epithelium, to T lymphocytes in the lamina propria. Most of these presentations will occur in the gut-associated lymphoid tissue (GALT). From the GALT, antigen-sensitive cells reach the bloodstream via the thoracic duct, and then preferentially seed to subepithelial secretory sites. They home directly to the salivary glands, where they can be found close to the secretory acinar cells.

At these subepithelial sites, these B lymphocytes differentiate into plasma cells and produce IgA which is specific to the ingested antigen. The IgA produced by the subepithelial plasma cells cannot be transported through the epithelial acinar cells of the gland until it is bound to a secretory component produced by the epithelial cells. The precursor of this component is a glycoprotein, polymeric immunoglobulin receptor (pIgR). Once pIgR has bound to IgA, the sIgA bundle is then transported through the epithelial acinar cell and out into the duct and into the saliva.

The level of sIgA secreted in saliva is dependent on the stimulation of the acinar cells to produce the secretory component. This stimulation is regulated by inflammatory mediators, such as the lymphokines interferon, tumor necrosis factor (TNF), and interleukin-2 produced by helper T lymphocytes (CD4 cells).

The distinction between the processes of IgA production and the production of the secretory component is well illustrated in HIV infection. In subjects who are HIV positive, there is an increase in the rate of sIgA secretion. In AIDS sufferers, there is a decrease in sIgA, which is not due to inability to produce the specific IgA antibody but due to a lack of CD4-type lymphocytes. The CD4 lymphocytes are essential to stimulate the production of the secretory component. The inability of the host to sustain sIgA secretion may be a determining factor in the onset of symptoms of immune deficiency.

At first glance, the antibacterial components of salivary glands appear to be unimpressive. They certainly allow huge populations of oral organisms to thrive. The first microscopist Anton van Leeuwenhoek observed "there are more animalcules (sic) living on the scum of man's teeth than there are men in a kingdom." What sort of antibacterial forces do we have to allow this "kingdom" of plaque? The answer is that after millions of years of coevolution, a select microbiota has established a symbiotic relationship with mammals, which tolerate and benefit from their partnership. There is evidence that immune cells of the gut are influenced by "cross talk" with the commensal bacteria of the gut which, amongst other influences, benefits host tolerance. Some bacteria produce a ligand which binds to the cell membrane of innate lymphoid cells and stimulates the secretion of IL-22. This cytokine promotes resistance to gut pathogens. Changes in the balance of gut flora (dysbiosis) may cause changes in the levels of immune cell response.

4.7.3 Antigen Tolerance

Antigens given by mouth (including food antigens) often result in a decreased serum antibody response. There is a degree of tolerance which prevents a hostile response of the immune system to the antigen. This tolerance occurs due to reduced amounts of antibody produced by B lymphocytes and reduced activity of CD4 T-cells to the antigen. A particular type of T-cell has been found to control this suppression. These are known as regulatory T-cells (Tregs). They produce TGFβ and IL4 cytokines which are well known for their suppression of CD4 T-cell activity. This loss of systemic reactivity to foreign antigens taken by mouth protects the body from an allergic reaction to food antigens. How does this tolerance develop?

There is increasing evidence to support the role of nonpathogenic bacteria during the early years of the colonization of the gut flora. Early workers noticed that those who worked with hay rarely suffered from hay fever. There is a growing understanding that exposure to environmental antigens and nonpathogenic bacteria trains the infant immune system to tolerate commonly encountered antigens such as pollen without treating them as pathogens.[5] The incidence of asthma is lower in those children raised in a rural farming environment.

Colonization of the infant's microbiota with those bacteria, which have had a long evolutionary history of symbiotic relationships with humans, appears to be essential for the proper maturity of the immune system. It has been observed that the main source of this microbiota is the infant's mother. Children born by C-section never encounter the flora of the vagina, and so miss a window of opportunity in infancy to establish a tolerance to a spectrum of the mother's commensal flora. A large study in Sweden found that babies born by C-section had 20% higher risk of developing food allergies later in life than those born via the birth canal.[6] Trials are taking place to determine whether seeding infants born by C-section with vaginal microbes may be beneficial.

The loss of tolerance to commensal organisms in the gut may cause Crohn's disease and ulcerative colitis. Downregulation of pIgR has been found in Crohn's and ulcerative colitis patients, which suggests that the normal communication between gut organism and the epithelial secretory cells may have broken down. Loss of tolerance to food antigens may be the cause of celiac disease.

The process whereby the immune system develops a tolerance to food antigens and commensal organisms is complex, although it is clear that it depends on acquiring in early life, encounters with the symbionts, which are going to colonize the gut.

The tolerance to food antigens and commensal oral bacteria is in contrast to the development of antibodies to some bacteria known for their pathogenic potential. T cells specific to *P. gingivalis* have been found in the serum of patients suffering from periodontal disease. The exact mechanism by which harmless symbionts are distinguished from pathogens is not yet clear enough to direct interventions which may be beneficial.

4.7.4 A Caries Vaccine

In the search for a method of controlling caries, attempts have been made to develop a vaccine that would stimulate IgA, which was specific to *S. mutans*, as this organism is reliably found in caries lesions. Such progress has been made in laboratory animals which are inoculated with *S. mutans* and fed on high levels of sucrose in order to induce caries. Neither of these steps to induce caries represents the human condition in which it is clear that caries is caused by a variety of resident organisms. It would be impossible to control caries in human subjects, unless IgA antibodies could be raised for

all potential pathogens. This would require the reversal of a long-standing tolerance to many oral organisms. The relationship between host and commensal oral organisms is an old and well-established one, which is usually extremely successful and protective; yet, dental caries affects almost all of us. The reason for this "fall out" between host and organisms is no reflection on the immune system, but on our dietary preferences.

An indication of the effective role of sIgA in the oral cavity is illustrated by observing the effect of suppressing the immune response. Children with bone marrow transplants receive immunosuppressive drugs which reduce sIgA secretions. An unwelcome complication is the development of an oral mucositis. This is not due to an overgrowth of oral organisms but an invasion of gut organisms. It would therefore appear that salivary antibodies effectively exclude gut organism which could be pathogenic, but the normal oral flora is tolerated. In view of the common diseases caused by oral commensals, this might seem a poor performance for a protective mechanism. However, the consequences of a more alert and aggressive response to oral antigens would clearly cause more food allergies than we already seem to suffer from.

The most forceful argument in defense of oral immunity is that caries is a disease of modern man, uncommon in early man, and rare in any other mammals living on an unrefined diet. It is the highly refined, low-fiber, sucrose-rich diet, which does not result in tooth wear, that renders the oral tissues susceptible to its own commensal flora. The principle of developing vaccines against some oral commensals should therefore be questioned. If we interfere with the long-established hierarchy of organisms in the oral ecosystem, there is a risk that a new and more complex problem would arise. In reducing the population of one species, the population of others will certainly rise to occupy the available habitat. The new hierarchy may not be as easy for the host to control; the fine balance of the ecosystem is lost, and new, and perhaps more aggressive, pathogens may emerge.

A final problem in developing a caries vaccine is that there is already a long list of immunizations for children. There may be resistance among parents and health care personnel to the addition of yet another vaccine to the list for a non–life-threatening disease like dental caries. If dentists are aware of the oral ecosystem and the effective performance of the immune system in maintaining it, they can contribute to its protective capability by offering dietary and oral hygiene advice to the public. It should not be necessary to restore teeth or to develop a caries vaccine, because dental caries is preventable by simple means. When it has occurred and is in progress, the process may be arrested, provided the environment is modified.

Key Notes

The oral and gut microbiota have an essential role in the development and maturation of the immune system. During infancy, the encounter with environmental bacteria and the mother's microbiota provides a window of opportunity to acquire not only a tolerance of symbiotic bacteria but also the appropriate response in later life to pathogens.

Review Questions

1. How does the gut microbiota contribute to the health of the human host?
2. How is the production of the secretory product pIgR controlled?
3. What is the value of oral tolerance if it allows so many organisms to populate the mouth?
4. What possible reason can be suggested for the comparative resistance of farm raised children to pollen allergy?
5. What are the challenges in developing a vaccine for caries?

References

[1] Dominy SS, et al. Porphyromonas gingivalis in Alzheimer's disease brains: Evidence for disease causation and treatment with small-molecule inhibitors. Sci Adv. 2019 Jan; 5(1)

[2] Marsh PD. Microbial ecology of dental plaque and its significance in health and disease. Adv Dent Res 1994; 8(2):263–271

[3] Lertpimonchai A, Rattanasiri S, Arj-Ong Vallibhakara S, Attia J, Thakkinstian A. The association between oral hygiene and periodontitis: a systematic review and meta-analysis. Int Dent J 2017; 67(6):332–343

[4] Reddy J, Africa CW, Parker JR. Darkfield microscopy of subgingival plaque of an urban black population with poor oral hygiene. J Clin Periodontol 1986; 13(6):578–582

[5] Chistiakov DA, Bobryshev YV, Kozarov E, Sobenin IA, Orekhov AN. Intestinal mucosal tolerance and impact of gut microbiota to mucosal tolerance. Front Microbiol 2015; 5:781

[6] Mitselou N, Hallberg J, Stephansson O, Almqvist C, Melén E, Ludvigsson JF. Cesarean delivery, preterm birth, and risk of food allergy: Nationwide Swedish cohort study of more than 1 million children. J Allergy Clin Immunol 2018; 142(5):1510–1514.e2

Suggested Reading

The Oral Environment

Ashby MT. Inorganic chemistry of defensive peroxidases in the human oral cavity. J Dent Res 2008;87(10):900–914

Dale BA, Tao R, Kimball JR, Jurevic RJ. Oral antimicrobial peptides and biological control of caries. BMC Oral Health 2006;6(Suppl 1):S13

Dawes C. Salivary flow patterns and the health of hard and soft oral tissues. J Am Dent Assoc 2008;139(Suppl):18S–24S

Gorr SU, Abdolhosseini M. Antimicrobial peptides and periodontal disease. J Clin Periodontol 2011;38(Suppl 11):126–141

Proctor GB, Carpenter GH. Chewing stimulates secretion of human salivary secretory immunoglobulin A. J Dent Res 2001;80(3):909–913

Siqueira WL, Custodio W, McDonald EE. New insights into the composition and functions of the acquired enamel pellicle. J Dent Res 2012;91(12):1110–1118

The Biofilms of the Oral Environment

Beighton D. Can the ecology of the dental biofilm be beneficially altered? Adv Dent Res 2009;21(1):69–73

Costalonga M, Herzberg MC. The oral microbiome and the immunobiology of periodontal disease and caries. Immunol Lett 2014;162(2 Pt A):22–38

Hajishengallis G. Immunomicrobial pathogenesis of periodontitis: keystones, pathobionts, and host response. Trends Immunol 2014;35(1):3–11

Hajishengallis G, Lamont RJ. Dancing with the stars: how choreographed bacterial interactions dictate nososymbiocity and give rise to keystone pathogens, accessory pathogens, and pathobionts. Trends Microbiol 2016;24(6):477–489

Lamont PJ, Burne R, Lantz M, Leblanc D. Oral Microbiology and Immunology. New Jersey: Wiley-Blackwell; 2006

Listgarten MA. Structure of surface coatings on teeth. A review. J Periodontol. 1976 Mar;47(3):139–147

Listgarten MA. The structure of dental plaque. Periodontol 2000. 1994 Jun;5:52–65

Lovegrove JM. Dental plaque revisited: bacteria associated with periodontal disease. JNZ Soc Periodontol. 2004; 87:7–21

Marsh PD. The role of microbiology in models of dental caries. Adv Dent Res. 1995; 9:244–254

Marsh PD. Contemporary perspective on plaque control. Brit Dent J. 2012;212:601–606

Ruby J. The buccale puzzle; The symbiotic nature of endogenous infections of the oral cavity. Can J Infect Dis 2002;13(1):34–41

Twetman S, Keller MK. Probiotics for caries prevention and control. Adv Dent Res 2012;24(2):98–102

Oral Ecology and Dental Caries

Ainamo J, Holmberg SM. Oral health of dentists' children. Scand J Dent Res 1974;82:547–551

Dodds MW, Chidichimo D, Haas MS. Delivery of active agents from chewing gum for improved remineralization. Adv Dent Res 2012;24(2):58–62

Kidd EAM. The essentials of dental caries. Oxford, United Kingdom: Oxford University Press; 2005

Ramos-Gomez F, Ng MW. Into the future: keeping healthy teeth caries free: pediatric CAMBRA protocols. J Calif Dent Assoc 2011;39(10):723–733

Stephan RM, Miller BF. A quantitative method for evaluating physical and chemical agents which modify production of acids in bacterial plaques on human teeth. J Dent Res 1943;22:45–51

Tellez M, Gomez J, Pretty I, Ellwood R, Ismail A. Evidence on existing caries risk assessment systems: are they predictive of future caries? Community Dent Oral Epidemiol 2013;41(1):67–78

The Influence of Fluorides on the Oral Ecosystem

Breaker RR. New insight on the response of bacteria to fluoride. Caries Res 2012;46(1):78–81

Featherstone JD, Doméjean S. The role of remineralizing and anticaries agents in caries management. Adv Dent Res 2012;24(2):28–31

Lawrence HP, Benn DK, Sheiham A. Digital radiographic measurement of approximal caries progression in fluoridated and non-fluoridated areas of Rio de Janeiro, Brazil. Community Dent Oral Epidemiol 1997;25(6):412–418

Psoter WJ, Reid BC, Katz RV. Malnutrition and dental caries: a review of the literature. Caries Res 2005;39(6):441–447

Mucosal Immunity and Oral Ecology

Challacombe SJ, Sweet SP. Oral mucosal immunity and HIV infection: current status. Oral Dis 2002;8(Suppl 2):55–62

Johansen FE, Kaetzel CS. Regulation of the polymeric immunoglobulin receptor and IgA transport: new advances in environmental factors that stimulate pIgR expression and its role in mucosal immunity. Mucosal Immunol 2011;4(6):598–602

Marsh PD, Martin MV, Lewis MAO, Williams DW. Oral Microbiology. Churchill London: Churchill Livingstone; 2009

Moingeon P, Mascarell L. Induction of tolerance via the sublingual route: mechanisms and applications. Clin Dev Immunol 2012;2012:623474

Smith DJ. Prospects in caries vaccine development. J Dent Res 2012;91(3):225–226

5 Cell Differentiation in Embryology and Repair

Abstract

Cells are the central role players in the study of biology. Everything on our earth, which is organic, has come from cells. This is true for the fossil fuels, oil, coal, and natural gas to the fabrics, wood, leather, feathers, cotton, silk, and wool to bone and the two components of teeth: enamel and dentin. The ability of cells to produce such a wide array of products is a measure of just how specialized they can become, often in the same organism. It is also a measure of the level of ordered and coordinated interaction between cells, which allows complex structures to be made. A chick embryo develops a beating heart only 48 hours after a single cell is fertilized. This chapter will be about how cells in the same body become specialized or differentiated, and then how they interact to form complex structures like teeth. There are many similarities in cell interactions, between embryology and wound healing, so this chapter will also describe the replay of embryology that we find during repair of tissues.

Keywords: cell interactions, cell differentiation, gene regulation, cytokines, neural crest cells, tooth development, morphogenesis, healing, angiogenesis

5.1 Cell Interactions in Differentiation

5.1.1 Cell Differentiation

We can recognize four basic types of tissue in mammals. They are epithelium, muscle, nerve, and connective tissue. Each tissue group has a wide diversity of cell types, for example, among the epithelial types of cells are many subtypes such as skin, salivary gland secretory cells, and ameloblasts, the cells which form tooth enamel. So, there are many more than just four different types of cell; in fact, there are over 250 cell types in humans. The information that determines a cell's type is contained in a manual of genetic instructions, the genome, kept in chromosomes inside the nucleus. Every cell of a single species has the same genome; cell types vary due to the expression of different genes within the genome. This expression is regulated by many moderating factors collectively called epigenetic moderators. Many of these moderators are themselves the products of gene expression from within the cell which enhance or inhibit the expression of other genes. These moderators sometimes act alone but more often operate as a network of influences between different moderators. Other moderators reach the cell from promoters in the surrounding matrix or as messengers from other cells. Some of these cell messengers (*cytokines*) are commonly found during development and in the adult, such as nerve growth factor (NGF) and bone morphogenic protein (BMP). Other cytokines, such as sonic hedgehog (SHH) may be more specifically involved in the differentiation of tooth-forming cells and in determining the morphology of the different tooth types (incisor, canine, and molar).

Cells become differentiated when they express specific genes which will serve a particular cell function. Some of these functions may be quite specialized. For example, when the preodontoblast differentiates to form a functioning odontoblast, it begins to lay down collagen fibers in a specific orientation within an extracellular matrix and then it mineralizes the matrix. Cell differentiation occurs frequently during embryology and healing.

5.1.2 Cell Differentiation during Embryology

The first events during embryology are the division of primitive stem cells, firstly, to form the cells of the endoderm, ectoderm, and mesoderm and then at many subsequent stages of further specialization, as cells follow different pathways to maturity. The 250 cell types can be represented as a branching tree (▶ Fig. 5.1).

The differentiation of cells which will form the pulp–dentin, alveolar bone, cementum, and periodontal ligament all have their origins in the neural crest. During the early development of the embryo, the neural plate folds up and closes to form the neural tube which becomes the brain and spinal cord. Cells from the crest of the neural folds detach from the epithelium and enter the mesoderm layer. They are known from this point on as cells of the ectomesenchyme. They migrate far and wide. The migration includes two types of cells. Some of them are committed to their future identities before their migration starts. Others, who travel with them, remain multipotential. The departure and migration of neural crest cells take place during just a few days. On reaching their destination, they differentiate into a variety of cell types, but primarily, the cells of the peripheral nervous system. These include cells of the sensory, sympathetic and parasympathetic ganglia, and the adrenal medulla. They also become pigment cells of the skin and the cells of the branchial arches (▶ Fig. 5.1). The neural crest cells which migrate to colonize the branchial arches have the

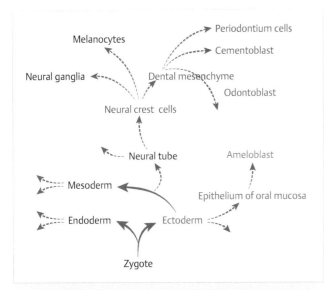

Fig. 5.1 A diagrammatic representation of the pathways of differentiation of some cell lines associated with tooth formation. Each tooth is formed from cells which have taken a different developmental route. The odontoblast has its origins from the neural crest, whereas the ameloblast is derived from the oral epithelium.

capacity to begin tooth germ formation. They are collectively known as dental mesenchymal cells.

On their own, these cells are not capable of forming a tooth. This inability to independently progress toward a fully differentiated cell has been studied in cell cultures. If a clump of identical stem cells is artificially grown in isolation, they do not differentiate, but if they are cultured along with a different cell type, they may progress to a further stage of differentiation. This is the case with the dental mesenchymal cells of the developing tooth germ. They require the proximity of cells from the dental lamina, a downgrowth of the oral epithelium to begin to differentiate into tooth-forming cells.

A similar dynamic applies to the cells of the oral epithelium, which will differentiate into ameloblast. In the case of the ameloblast, these moderators come from cells forming dentin, the odontoblasts. Only when the first dentin has been formed, the cytokines will be released which trigger the ameloblast to differentiate into a cell which is able to form enamel. The process of differentiation of one cell by the cytokines produced by a cell of another type has been called induction. It is a process repeated many times during the various stages of differentiation of the cells of the dental lamina and of the dental mesenchyme as they progress to becoming ameloblasts and odontoblasts. Cytokines are just one of the many epigenetic factors which control the expression of genes (*see Appendix E.1 Epigenetic Modulation*).

5.1.3 Cell and Matrix Interactions in Tooth Development

We have seen the role of gene regulation in bringing forth a new cell line at the right time, but there is less understanding of the mechanism which control tissue shape. What directs a mass of growing cells into the shape of an eye, or tooth, or limb? This process is called morphogenesis, literally the genesis of shape and

structure. In order to fully understand the organization and behavior of cell masses, it is worthwhile being familiar with the types of interactions which occur between a cell, its neighboring cells, and the extracellular matrix (*see Appendix E.2 Morphogenesis*).

The development of the teeth begins with a condensation of epithelial cells of the oral ectoderm, the dental lamina (▶ Fig. 5.2). This forms by a thickening of the epithelium cells along the ridge of both branchial arches which will form the maxilla and mandible. In response, the dental mesenchyme becomes condensed in an area, where the future tooth will develop into a clump of cells which will eventually form the dentin–pulp complex. The initiative for tooth formation then passes to this condensation of cells, and they induce the epithelium to grow downward as a bud, becoming a cap, and eventually a bell-shaped mass of cells. The cells on the inner lining epithelium of the bell are called the inner enamel epithelium (IEE), and they will become the future ameloblasts. The induction continues to pass from one formative tissue to the other in a series of exchanges almost like a verbal dialogue. The preameloblasts do not mature fully and begin to lay down enamel until the odontoblast has formed dentin. Both ameloblasts and odontoblasts retreat from each other as the hard tissues are formed; the ameloblast migrates toward the surface of the future crown and the odontoblast toward the center of the tooth.

The cells of the IEE and the cells lining the outer surface of the bell, the outer enamel epithelium fuse together and form a sheath of cells which define the shape of the tooth root. This sheath of cells carries the name of its discoverer, Hertwig. Not only does Hertwig's sheath define the shape of the root dentin, but it may induce the differentiation of the surrounding mesenchymal cells to form cementoblasts, which lay down cementum against the newly formed root (*see Chapter 3.6.2 Origins of Cementum*). For a complete description of the embryological development of teeth, a text in dental histology should be consulted.

> **Key Notes**
>
> Embryonic cells have the potential to become specialized so as to form any cell from the entire spectrum of adult tissues. The distinctive cell type is determined by the expression of specific genes. Differentiation is the process whereby a particular set of genes is expressed. It is determined by a network of interacting moderating factors, operating both inside and outside the cell.

Review Questions

1. Define cell differentiation in terms of gene expression.
2. What factors determine the differentiation of primitive cells?
3. What are the embryological origins of ameloblasts and odontoblasts?

5.2 Tooth Morphogenesis

5.2.1 Generic Tooth Forms

During the evolution of mammals, the teeth became more specialized than those of their reptile ancestors. Reptiles' teeth were, and still are today, rather similar cone-shaped pegs. In contrast, mammals have developed a recognizable group of

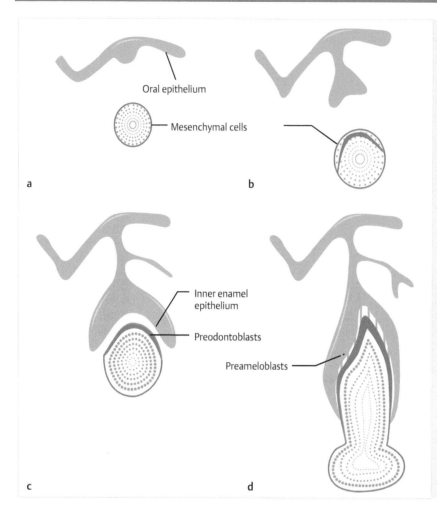

Oral epithelium

Mesenchymal cells

a

b

Inner enamel epithelium

Preodontoblasts

Preameloblasts

c

d

Fig. 5.2 A diagrammatic representation of the early stages in the development of a tooth which illustrate induction at a number of occasions. (a) The oral epithelium induces the mesenchyme to condense in areas of a future tooth. (b) The mesenchyme induces a downgrowth of oral epithelium. (c) The "cap" of epithelium induces differentiation of the nearest mesenchymal cells into preodontoblasts, cells which will later form dentin. (d) Further interactions occur between the preodontoblasts and the inner enamel epithelium, which become preameloblasts.

generic shapes to the teeth. There are some notable variations in the details, but all mammals from the elephant to the armadillo conform to the blueprint for four basic generic tooth shapes. In both these two examples, the elephant and the armadillo, some or all of the tooth types are missing.

Firstly, there are a group of single-rooted teeth in front of both jaws which are usually flat and spade shaped. These are the incisors and they work against the teeth of the opposing jaw like flat pincers. The exceptions are the ruminants whose mandibular incisors work against the tongue; the maxillary incisors are absent. At the corner of the arch of teeth, just below the nostril is the second type of tooth which is spear shaped and often the longest tooth. This is the canine. Then there is often a space in the dentition. This is an important option as in some mammals it separates the process of grazing, browsing, or nibbling, with the process of shredding and grinding. The teeth toward the back of the jaw are larger and have a more complex crown and root system. They are subdivided into premolars of intermediate size and molars which are larger.

It is convenient to describe mammalian dentition using a formula which lists the combination of generic types on one side of the jaw. The convention of the dental formula is to list the number of each tooth type in the maxilla over the number in the mandible (▶ Fig. 5.3). There is a wide range of dentitions, all suited to the dietary and feeding habits of each animal, but they

all are constructed using the same theme of four basic tooth shapes. Note that cows, sheep, and antelope do not have any maxillary incisors. They graze by using their tongue to rasp of grass against the lower teeth.

During tooth development four generic shapes of tooth are formed. These four shapes are characterized by increasing complexity of the crown and root form. Incisors have one sharp edge (or cusp) and a tiny second one, the cingulum, on the lingual side. Canines have a pointed sharp edge and a bit more of a second cusp, which makes the tooth rounder. Premolars have a well-defined second cusp and may have two or three roots. Molars have more cusps and many roots. Some generic shapes have been adapted. For example, the elephant tusk is a very large lateral incisor.

The mammalian teeth, in comparison to reptilian teeth, play a primary role in its survival. There can be few other anatomical structures which so clearly define the life span of an animal as the teeth of a mammal. When the teeth are worn out, it dies of starvation. It is not a process which is usually witnessed, as wild animals go away somewhere private to die, but domestic animals reveal the true crisis of being toothless. The mandibular incisors of sheep are crucial to their ability to graze, but it is not uncommon, in some countries, for them to suffer from a type of periodontal disease called broken mouth. The incisor teeth become so mobile that they cease to function and the animal's life is at an end.

Dogs, wolves, bears, etc.	I	$\frac{3}{3}$	C	$\frac{1}{1}$	Pm	$\frac{4}{4}$	M	$\frac{2}{2}$
Rats, mice, squirrels, beavers	I	$\frac{1}{1}$	C	$\frac{0}{0}$	Pm	$\frac{1}{1}$	M	$\frac{3}{3}$
Lions, tigers, cats, leopards	I	$\frac{3}{3}$	C	$\frac{1}{1}$	Pm	$\frac{2}{2}$	M	$\frac{3}{3}$
Pigs and boars	I	$\frac{3}{3}$	C	$\frac{1}{1}$	Pm	$\frac{2}{2}$	M	$\frac{3}{3}$
Cows, sheep, antelope	I	$\frac{0}{3}$	C	$\frac{1}{1}$	Pm	$\frac{3}{3}$	M	$\frac{2}{3}$
Monkeys, baboons, man	I	$\frac{2}{2}$	C	$\frac{1}{1}$	Pm	$\frac{2}{2}$	M	$\frac{3}{3}$

Fig. 5.3 A diagrammatic representation of the four generic tooth shapes of mammals. Incisors, canines, premolars, and molars are represented by the dental formulas in this selection of mammals. Each dentition has evolved to suit the dietary opportunities and feeding requirements of each mammal.

5.2.2 Cusp Morphology

It has been noted in *Chapter 1* The Origins of Teeth that for the mammalian tooth to perform its vital function, the cusps must wear away to provide a composite tooth surface in order to become an effective working tool. It is also clear from the brief review above that the structural design of the dentition is specific and crucial to the survival of every mammalian type. It can be therefore be inferred that one of the defining characteristics of this structural design is the conformation of the unworn tooth cusps.

In comparison with the dentition of modern humans, whose tooth cusps have not been revealed by reliable evidence to serve a significant function, the cusp design of quadrupedal mammals is of significant importance. It is therefore not surprising to discover that during mammalian tooth development, it is the cusp formation which defines the structure and function of the dentition.

The cusps and roots of teeth are formed during development by folds in the inner enamel epithelium, the layer of cells which will lay down enamel (▶ Fig. A.2). The shape of the inner enamel epithelium and the alignment of the ameloblasts will determine the future shape of the crown (▶ Fig. 5.4). In a review of this process by Simmer and coworkers, it is suggested that the shape of this layer of ameloblasts is determined by several influences, the most significant of which is the gradient of the rate of division of preameloblasts.[1] The rate of division is expressed as the mitotic index, which is the ratio of dividing cells to those cells not dividing. The mitotic index of the inner enamel epithelium (preameloblasts) is more rapid in some areas than others. There is thus a gradient between the fastest and slowest dividing cells. Where the mitotic index is highest, the sheet of cells expands rapidly, and a bulge (cusp slope) appears. Where it is slower, the curve of the cell sheet does not expand as rapidly and remains more tightly curved leading to a relatively pointed cusp tip. The cusp tips are formed at points, where the cell division is slowest. When cell division stops, the ameloblasts start to form enamel and that part of the sheet of ameloblasts becomes rigid.

If the enamel epithelium of the developing tooth has a high mitotic gradient, there will be a marked difference between the rounded curve of a region with a high mitotic index and the pointed curve of a region with a low mitotic index. The result then of a steep mitotic gradient is a tooth with a flat buccal/lingual aspect and a pointed cusp.

These suggestions regarding the control of cusp morphology are mostly speculative, although they do suggest that cusp conformation may be the driving factor in determining crown and root morphology. The progressive increase in cusp folding which occurs from incisor to molar teeth may well be controlled by diffusion through a morphogenic field of a factor which regulates the mitotic index of enamel-forming cells. There are no data at present which provide conclusive evidence for the mechanisms of tooth morphogenesis. It is likely, however, that the patterns generated by developing tooth germs are related to generic forms determined by cusp morphology which is influenced within a morphogenic field.

Key Notes

The mammalian dentition has evolved four distinct tooth forms, each adapted to performing a specific function in mastication. The exact combination of forms is a reflection of each mammal's diet.

Review Questions

1. What relation does cusp design have on the masticatory function of teeth?
2. How does the mitotic rate of the inner enamel epithelium affect cusp morphology?

5.3 Cell Interactions in Repair and Regeneration

5.3.1 Wound Healing

The first stage in wound healing is the formation of a blood clot which fills the wound space. This happens within a few minutes and is an essential first step to control further bleeding. The clot

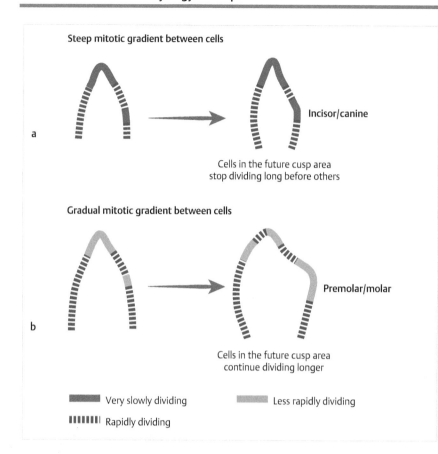

Steep mitotic gradient between cells

a

Cells in the future cusp area
stop dividing long before others

Incisor/canine

Gradual mitotic gradient between cells

b

Cells in the future cusp area
continue dividing longer

Premolar/molar

▬▬ Very slowly dividing   ▭▭ Less rapidly dividing

||||||| Rapidly dividing

Fig. 5.4 A diagrammatic representation of the influence on mitotic gradient of the inner enamel epithelium on cusp morphology. The sheet of enamel-forming cells grows by cell division. A gradient in the rate of division influences the shape of the sheet of cells. **(a)** Where there is a steep mitotic gradient, a pointed cusp shape will form where the division rate is slow and eventually stops. Dentin and enamel formation then begin, and the sheet of cells is held rigidly in place. **(b)** If the mitotic gradient is more gradual and all the cells of the sheet keep dividing, enamel formation is delayed. The tooth bud gets larger and the cusp is less prominent. The final shapes of an incisor, canine, and premolar may be the result of a variation in the mitotic gradient of enamel-forming cells.

also provides some stability to the injury and forms a provisional extracellular matrix into which cells can migrate. The damaged tissues secrete cytokines, which set in motion a series of healing responses. Some of these cytokines attract the influx of cells which are able to control the damage and rebuild the tissue. This mobilization is called *chemotaxis*. Some cells such as fibroblasts migrate in from the surrounding tissue into the wound, providing a more permanent cell matrix of ground substance and collagen fibers. However, the largest influx of cells come from the blood itself. Cell migration from blood vessels is a response to specific cytokines which regulate genes in the endothelial cells of the surrounding blood vessels. These genes code for a protein, P-selectin, which is a cell surface integrin, specific for white blood cells (*see Appendix E.2.3 Integrins*). The integrins on the endothelial cells cause the passing white blood cells to start sticking to the endothelium; they slow down, stop moving, and escape between the endothelium cells. Once out of the blood vessel, they move toward the damaged tissue. White blood cells such as neutrophils and monocytes remove dead tissue and fight infection. These early stages in response to damage may be the onset of inflammation if the level of damage is extensive, or there are bacteria or foreign proteins to be removed. Inflammation is clinically characterized by swelling, heat, redness, and pain and should not be present following limited damage such as a clean cut or tooth extraction. Much depends on the exclusion of harmful bacteria in determining whether healing will be complicated by inflammation. An essential requirement of wound healing is the presence of a stable blood clot. A poor blood supply or the disruption of the blood clot leads to delayed healing

5.3.2 Healing of a Tooth Socket

Stage 1: When a tooth is extracted, the socket should fill with blood which clots to form a natural barrier to infection. This is the first stage of healing. If an extraction socket does not fill with blood clot, it becomes infected and inflammation occurs with pain which may be severe, occurring 2 to 3 days after the extraction. This condition has been named a *dry socket*, though this may be a euphemism for infected socket. The term "dry socket" has been preferred, as the term "infected" is less easily explained to the patient; it might imply a failure to observe a sterile working environment. The fact is that it is an infected socket, though as we now are aware, it has nothing to do with cross-infection control. The infected socket is another example of a noncommunicable disease caused by pathobionts.

This author was trained in an era when boiling water was used to sterilize the forceps to be used for an extraction, and a prophylaxis was performed around the tooth to be extracted. It was also an era before it was routine for dentists to wear gloves. Infected sockets were uncommon, perhaps due to the presurgical prophylaxis. The aim of this procedure was to avoid forcing subgingival plaque down the root surface and into the socket when applying downward pressure on the extraction forceps. While there was little understanding of the endogenous origins of oral infections, at that time, it appears to have been a sensible practice.

The frequency of dry sockets in some studies is as high as 10% of all tooth extractions. One of the associated risk factors is the amount of anesthesia used and the length of time required to extract the tooth. It is usual to employ an anesthetic solution with an added vasoconstrictor in order to reduce the blood supply to the surgical area, therefore prolonging the presence of the anesthetic agent in the tissue. If increased amounts of anesthetic agent are used, there is an increased amount of vasoconstrictor introduced into the surrounding tissue. Bleeding into the socket from the surrounding tissues is therefore restricted. If the extraction takes more than a few minutes, the blood from vessels ruptured during the initial displacements of the tooth, clots before it can fill the socket. When the tooth is eventually removed, there is little further bleeding and the socket remains "dry," though it soon fills with saliva and is contaminated within hours. Within 48 hours, the damaged and necrotic gingival and periodontal tissues have become infected. The poor blood supply to this necrotic tissue does not allow antibiotics to reach the infected tissue and the formation of a biofilm over the damaged tissue is resistant to antiseptic mouth wash.

Stage 2: If a stable blood clot does form, the second stage of healing can begin (▶ Fig. 5.5). This is the development of a blood supply within the clot. It starts with the budding of capillary endothelial cells and new blood vessel formation. This *angiogenesis* is activated by genes whose expression is driven by locally produced cytokines, the most important of which is vascular endothelial growth factor (VEGF). The development of an adequate blood supply is a critical requirement of both healing and the embryological development and growth of fetal tissue. Tissue which has a poor blood supply such as cartilage is unable to heal. The replacement of embryological cartilage of the future long bones begins with the ingrowth of endothelial cells which will form blood vessels. (see *Chapter 7.3.6 Endochondral Bone Formation*).

The differentiation of cells capable of blood capillary formation is followed by both increase in cell numbers and change in their relationship to one another. They become orientated into

tube-like structures which stimulate basement membrane type collagen, on to which finally endothelial cells are able to attach and remain. The growing tubes now branch out and thoroughly extend throughout new tissue, so that no cell is further than a few microns form a capillary. This process of angiogenesis requires wound stability to ensure that the fragile elements of forming blood vessels are not disrupted. This stability is of great importance during the wound healing of bone augmentation of a surgical site planned for implant placement. One technique for augmentation makes use of a rigid titanium mesh which defines the area where new bone formation is required. The mesh is filled with bone or other granules which provide a scaffold for a blood clot and also allow the penetration of new blood vessels between the granules. The formation of a blood clot and its stability within the mesh are of critical importance to allow angiogenesis and eventual differentiation of bone cells. The granules may or may not assist or participate in the growth of new bone in the graft site.

The outcome of this second stage of healing is the production of granulation tissue. This wound tissue is well vascularized and contains mostly fibroblast cells which have produced a loose and not particularly well-organized tissue. The further organization of granulation tissue in the tooth socket involves the secretion by fibroblasts of collagen fibers which strengthen the wound and provide a suitable matrix onto which bone mineral can be laid down. During this second stage of healing of a tooth socket, epithelium cells from the damaged margin of the wound begin to migrate across the wound.

Stage 3: The third stage of healing of a tooth socket involves the transformation of granulation tissue into bone. The cells which form bone are osteoblasts and they emerge by the differentiation of stem cells associated with the new blood vessels. Generally, it takes about 6 weeks to fill the socket with poorly organized bone, which is very similar to the bone first formed during embryology, before it becomes resorbed and reformed as lamellae bone.

5.3.3 Healing of a Pulp Exposure

Traumatic exposures: An exposure of the dental pulp, which has occurred through accidental penetration during cavity preparation, is defined as a traumatic exposure. It implies that the dentin immediately surrounding the exposure is not contaminated by caries organisms. There is mounting evidence that the pulp–dentin is able to repair even large traumatic exposures. The response of a completely healthy pulp to a calcium hydroxide dressing after a traumatic exposure was first described by Schroder.[2] A layer of necrosis is seen within an hour due to the high pH of the calcium hydroxide. After a week, new collagen has formed against the necrotic zone and the beginnings of a calcifying front. Odontoblast-like cells orientate against the calcifying front and develop cellular extensions around which bone-like tissue is deposited after 4 weeks. After 12 weeks, a hard tissue barrier with tubules has formed (▶ Fig. 5.6). This work by Schroder provided early evidence for the capacity of pulp cells to differentiate into odontoblasts and to form new dentin.[2] Subsequent studies have traced the origins of newly differentiated odontoblasts and confirmed the readiness of dental pulp stem cells to differentiate, particularly under the influence of cytokines derived from the extracellular matrix, pulp fibroblasts,

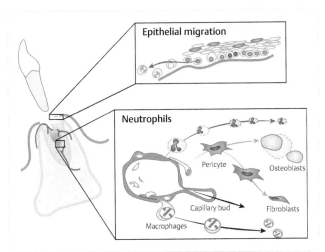

Fig. 5.5 A diagrammatic representation of the events occurring during the first 48 hours after tooth extraction. The first stage of damage control involves hemostasis, the formation of a stable clot and infection control. After 6 hours, repair begins with migration of neutrophils, macrophages, and fibroblasts into the wound. The cells from the surrounding epithelium become less tightly-attached to each other and migrate over the blood clot. Budding of capillaries begins the vascularization of the wound. Perivascular cells differentiate into fibroblasts and osteoblasts.

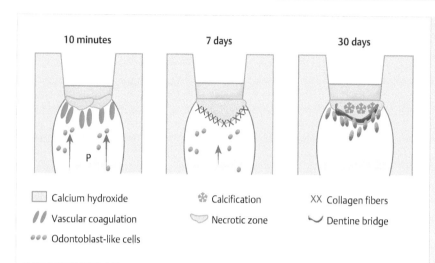

Fig. 5.6 A diagrammatic representation of the stages in the repair of a pulpal exposure using a calcium hydroxide dressing. After 7 hours, a traumatic pupal exposure, sealed with calcium hydroxide, shows a necrotic layer and increase in vascularization. After 7 days, cells which resemble odontoblasts have migrated toward the exposure; collagen has been formed against the necrotic tissue which has begun to calcify. After 30 days, a dentin-like bridge has formed against the calcified necrotic tissue. (Adapted from Schröder 1985.[2])

serum, and odontoblasts adjacent to the exposure. An important condition for the formation of a successful dentin bridge is a low level of inflammatory response of the pulp following the pulpal exposure. Even moderate levels of inflammation appear to be associated with a failure of the pulp to form a dentin bridge.

In addition to calcium hydroxide for managing vital pulp exposures, mineral trioxide aggregate (MTA) and enamel protein derivative (Emdogain) have been found successful.[3] Some workers conclude that it is not what you put over the exposure, but the state of the underlying pulp, which determines whether a dentin bridge will form. In spite of significant advances in the management of traumatic exposures, there is no single technique that can achieve predictable and reliable results in preserving pulp vitality.

Carious exposure: A carious exposure implies that in removing carious dentin the pulp has become exposed. It is likely therefore that there is some degree of existing infection and inflammation of the pulp. The pulp is not uniformly affected by deep carious lesions. A superficial inflammation may be eliminated by the effect of a calcium hydroxide dressing, leaving a pulp tissue capable of healing. On the other hand, a more pronounced and widespread pulpal inflammation may be increased by the irritation of the calcium hydroxide. Schroder writes, "The degree of inflammation, the time of irritation and infection, and the location of the exposure must thus be regarded as decisive factors for the healing of the inflamed pulp rather than the effect of calcium hydroxide as such."[3] This statement indicates that the use of calcium hydroxide or the more recent use of MTA or Emdogain to induce dentin bridge formation in a carious exposure will have to be a carefully considered clinical decision. Unfortunately, there is a poor correlation between signs and symptoms and the histological state of the pulp, so as yet there is no precise definition of an "irreversible pulpitis."

Pulp tissue death with abscess formation is considered to be irreversible, but it is possible that vital pulp remains deep to an abscess. The ability of the pulp tissue to stop bleeding without the presence of a blood clot may provide some indication that a dentin bridge could form under the influence of calcium hydroxide. In view of the considerable time required to perform endodontic treatment on a molar tooth, the possibility of inducing a dentin bridge after removing infected dentin and pulp tissue should be considered.

One of the limiting factors in the ability of the dental pulp to control acute inflammation is its limited blood supply. This is imposed by the narrow constriction of vessels entering and leaving the pulp through the apical foramen. Another limiting factor is the rigid containment of the pulp tissue within the pulp chamber. It is said to have a low compliance. The tissue expansion which normally results from the formation of an inflammatory exudate has nowhere to go, and the tissue pressure within the pulp chamber increases. This further inhibits the vascular supply and increases pulp sensitivity. The prognosis for healing of an infected pulp is improved in young permanent teeth and deciduous teeth, where the apex remains open allowing an increased vascular flow.

5.3.4 Cytokines and Extracellular Matrix in Healing

During the first stage of wound healing, bleeding is controlled by the adhesion of platelets (sticky blood cell fragments) to each other. This adhesion can be encouraged if fibronectin is added to wounds, presumably by encouraging the adhesion of platelets and the migration of fibroblasts and epithelial cells into the wound. The inflammatory process and organization of granulation tissue and tissue repair are processes activated by a variety of cytokines. These include platelet-derived growth factor (PDGF), vascular permeability factor (VPF), and transforming growth factor (TGF). TGF-β regulates numerous cellular functions including the immune response. It is the most powerful chemotactic stimulus to polymorphonuclear leukocytes (PMNs). Epidermal growth factor encourages the formation of new epithelial cells after injury. Bone morphogenic proteins (BMPs) are cytokines which conduct a dialogue between the extracellular matrix and bone-forming cells. They have a short but critical appearance at a bone fracture site and disappear after 72 hours.

The clinical application of cytokines is well illustrated by the ability of BMP extracts to close cranial bone defects, which do not normally repair with bone. BMPs have also been used to stimulate reparative dentin by causing the rapid differentiation of primitive mesenchymal cells of the pulp into odontoblasts.

Cytokine messages create a high degree of complexity due to their varying level of concentration and their interaction with

Legend (Fig. 5.6):

10 minutes   7 days   30 days

☐ Calcium hydroxide   ✳ Calcification   XX Collagen fibers
// Vascular coagulation   ◡ Necrotic zone   ◡ Dentine bridge
••• Odontoblast-like cells

other inhibiting and facilitating cytokines. For example, TGF-β is a cytokine with many different properties, including the ability to increase its own secretion. It does not act in isolation, and therefore the interactions between cytokines may be as complex as the interaction between the gene moderators which regulate their expression.

5.3.5 Comparison between Repair and Embryology

Similarities between embryology and healing: Repair and embryology are both characterized by similar series of stages beginning with chemotaxis, cell migration, attachment, proliferation, and finally differentiation. Both processes are concerned with the formation of new tissue, and in both processes, the shape of the new tissue mass must be controlled. As embryology is an event of the past, its replay during healing may be referred to as recapitulation. There are many ways in which repair may recapitulate embryology, and there are some important differences. We have seen that new tissue, such as dentin, requires a new generation of specialized cells and that these new cells are derived by the differentiation of multipotential or stem cells in the pulp. The process of new cell differentiation is similar in both healing and repair. In both cases, new cell types are formed by the expression of particular genes which initiate and control a new range of cell behavior. As in embryology, two processes are important moderators in the expression of genes, the action of cytokines, and the role of the extracellular matrix. The processes governing embryonic bone development are largely recapitulated during fracture healing.

Angiogenesis, the development of a new blood vessels, is crucial to both embryology and healing. The transformation of embryonic cartilage into bone would not occur without the ingrowth of endothelial cells, which form blood vessels and eventually extend throughout the entire cartilage in a long bone, with the exception of the joint surfaces. The same process of vascularization occurs when an extraction socket heals, or when a free bone graft is used to augment dental alveolar bone in order to support implant fixtures. The cells within a free bone graft die within minutes after harvesting disrupts the grafts blood supply. The bone graft must first become vascularized in order to become receptive to remodeling and to fuse with its surrounding receptive bed. Not infrequently, this vascularization fails to occur, and there is instead a progressive resorption of the bone graft until it disappears.

Angiogenesis requires both the differentiation of stem cells into endothelial cells and their migration into the wound or graft with the support of a matrix onto which the cells can form a capillary. This matrix includes fibronectin, as it provides anchorage for the cells, which provides the traction required for migration. Other matrix proteins form the framework for tube-like formations of cells, which will become capillaries (*see Chapter 6.2.2. Fibronectin*).

In the absence of fibronectin, complete embryological development does not occur. Its role in healing is illustrated by its capacity to increase the rate of wound healing in eye operations.

Differences between embryology and healing: Important differences between embryology and healing are the limited ability of some tissues and all organs to regenerate. In the adult, new nerve cells and muscle cells have been considered incapable of differentiating from more primitive precursors in order to regenerate lost tissue. Even precursor cells during embryological development may have a limited period of competency to become adult-specialized cells. Oral epithelial cells are responsive to differentiate into enamel-forming cells but only during a window of 6 to 12 days. After that period of competency, no new enamel-forming cells can be made, although, as we have noted, the same is not true for the dentin-forming cells which can be replaced throughout life. As a consequence of the inability of some adult cells to be replaced in order to allow damaged tissue to regenerate, it is impossible for a new tooth to be grown or a new nervous tissue to repair damage to the spinal cord. Of course, every cell carries the information in its DNA to become any one of the 250 different cells in the body. It is not therefore impossible that a precursor or stem cell for neurons will be found and the cytokines artificially made, which will induce it to differentiate and regenerate damaged nerve tissue. Stem cell production by inducing alterations in adult cells has been achieved using gene replacement techniques with four transcription factors. The induced pluripotent stem cells of the patient's own genome have promise in regenerative medicine, but at present, there are still difficulties to be overcome.

The limitations of regenerating some tissue types are less overwhelming than the limitations in producing a new organ. Organs not only contain several different types of cells, but they have complicated morphology which developed under the surrounding influence of many other events occurring simultaneously during the growth and development of the embryo. The repair of damage to odontoblasts requires the differentiation of precursors which are capable of laying down reparative dentin. The dentin is not the same as that formed during embryology, as it lacks the morphology of normal tubules. So, repair is a less coordinated process than regeneration.

5.3.6 Nutrition, Embryology, and Healing

In developing nations, and particularly in those where poverty is common, the health risks to the fetus, of malnutrition in the mother, are immediate and obvious. In developed nations, malnutrition of pregnant mothers is less severe, and so its impact on the growing fetus takes longer to emerge. However, there is evidence that even moderate levels of malnutrition, which occur during embryology, have long-term influences on the future health of the adult (*see Chapter 4.5 Nutrition and Oral Ecology*). Birth weight and its relationship to the weight of the placenta are related to the risk, in later life, of heart and lung disease. Adults who, as newborn babies, were heavier, longer, and who had light placentas, are half as likely to suffer from these diseases as adults who were lighter and shorter babies. The nutrition of a growing embryo therefore influences both immediate and long-term prospects of the individual's capacity to resist infections, heal rapidly, and return to health.

Malnutrition in children reduces their immune capacity, and they have an increased risk of suffering from measles, malaria, severe diarrhea, and acute necrotizing ulcerative gingivitis (ANUG). A complication of ANUG is noma, a severe infection of the oral cavity and face which occurs in communities with poor environmental sanitation. It results from complex interactions between malnutrition, infections, and compromised immunity.

Nutrition is an essential factor in both embryology and healing as both these processes require energy. Interactions between cells and their environment are crucial to the ordered processes which occur during embryology and healing.

Key Notes

Repair follows a similar cascade of events as embryology, starting with chemical and neural signaling. The matrix, in healing tissue, into which cells migrate, differentiate and grow, is the blood clot. The formation of a vascular system is as critical in repair and healing as it is during embryology.

Review Questions

1. What is the function of a blood clot in the initial response to tissue damage?
2. What factors might lead to the development of an infected tooth socket?
3. Why is the stability of a blood clot essential to the successful healing of a tooth socket?
4. What factors determine whether the repair of a pulp exposure will be successful?
5. What similarities are there between embryology and healing?
6. What differences are there between embryology and healing?
7. How does nutrition affect embryology and healing?

References

[1] Simmer JP, Papagerakis P, Smith CE, et al. Regulation of dental enamel shape and hardness. J Dent Res 2010;89(10):1024–1038

[2] Schröder U. Effects of calcium hydroxide-containing pulp-capping agents on pulp cell migration, proliferation, and differentiation. J Dent Res 1985;64 (Spec No):541–548

[3] Bollu IP, Velagula LD, Bolla N, Kumar KK, Hari A, Thumu J. Histological evaluation of mineral trioxide aggregate and enamel matrix derivative combination in direct pulp capping: an in vivo study. J Conserv Dent 2016;19 (6):536–540

Suggested Readings

Tooth Morphogenesis

Mark MP, Bloch-Zupan A, Ruch JV. Effects of retinoids on tooth morphogenesis and cytodifferentiations, in vitro. Int J Dev Biol 1992;36(4):517–526

Mina M, Kollar EJ. The induction of odontogenesis in non-dental mesenchyme combined with early murine mandibular arch epithelium. Arch Oral Biol 1987;32(2):123–127

Nusslein-Volhard C. Gradients that organize embryo development. Sc Am 1996;275 (2):54–55; 58–61

Sharpe PT. Neural crest and tooth morphogenesis. Adv Dent Res 2001;15:4–7

Cell Interactions in Repair and Regeneration

Barker DJ. The fetal origins of diseases of old age. Eur J Clin Nutr 1992;46 (Suppl 3):S3–S9

Harichane Y, Hirata A, Dimitrova-Nakov S, et al. Pulpal progenitors and dentin repair. Adv Dent Res 2011;23(3):307–312

Kidd EAM. The Essentials of Dental Caries. Oxford, United Kingdom: Oxford University Press; 2005

Maes C, Kobayashi T, Selig MK, et al. Osteoblast precursors, but not mature osteo blasts, move into developing and fractured bones along with invading blood vessels. Dev Cell 2010;19(2):329–344

Quain AM, Khardori NM. Nutrition in wound care management: a comprehensive overview. Wounds 2015;27(12):327–335

Seux D, Couble ML, Hartmann DJ, Gauthier JP, Magloire H. Odontoblast-like cytodif ferentiation of human dental pulp cells in vitro in the presence of a calcium hydroxide-containing cement. Arch Oral Biol 1991;36(2):117–128

6 The Extracellular Matrix

Abstract

Connective tissues are composed of cells and their surrounding extracellular matrix. They are derived from the mesenchymal component of the embryonic mesoderm. In spite of this common origin, there are some noticeably different structural types (e.g., blood and bone). Each type, however, is made up of the same components, namely tissue-forming cells, which are not usually in contact with one another, and an extracellular matrix (ECM). The ECM provides a physical scaffold around the connective tissue cells which may attach to the matrix for support. The nonfibrous components of the ECM include glycosaminoglycans (GAGs) and glycoproteins (GPs). The fibers of the ECM include collagen, elastic, and reticulin fibers. All matrix molecules also play some additional bioactive role in the differentiation of precursor connective tissue cells and the regulation of their activity. Some of these bioactive components have been called matricellular proteins, describing their dual function.

Keywords: connective tissue, extracellular matrix, glycosaminoglycans, glycoproteins, collagen, matricellular, bone glycoproteins, fibronectin, laminin

6.1 Glycosaminoglycans

The extracellular spaces of all vertebrates are taken up by water and very large molecules called glycosaminoglycans, previously referred to as mucopolysaccharides. As the name suggest, these molecules are polymers of a variety of polysaccharides (*Greek* glykis = sweet). The polymer unit is a disaccharide made up of a glucosamine (amino sugar) and either a glycan (uronic sugar) or galactose. Some GAGs are covalently linked to a protein core in an arrangement like a bottle brush (▸ Fig. 6.1).

6.1.1 Types of Glycosaminoglycans

Hyaluronic acid: This molecule has been called the "goo" that holds tissue together. It has important properties which make it particularly suitable as a lubricant in synovial fluid. It is viscoelastic, which means that it may respond to loads with both elastic rebound and viscous resistance. When a joint is suddenly loaded, it induces an elastic response from the synovial fluid, which protects the joint from damage. Loads which are less rapidly applied allow the synovial fluid to flow and the joint to move freely. Hyaluronic acid also surrounds and protects cartilage cells from compression.

This GAG is one of the few which is nonsulfated and not linked to a protein core. Hyaluronic acid may be a huge molecule of molecular weight 100,000 to 10 million. It is in the form of a long loosely tangled chain (▸ Fig. 6.1). It occurs in most connective tissue but is a vital component of synovial fluid.

Chondroitin sulfate: This GAG is found in bone, cartilage, the periodontal ligament and the dental pulp. It is a smaller molecule than hyaluronic acid, though as with other GAGs, the molecular weight varies depending on the source and the stresses being applied to it.

Dermatan sulfate: This GAG is found in skin, cardiovascular structures, and tendons.

Heparin sulfate: It is found in and released by mast cells and found in skin and lung tissue. *Keratan sulfate.* This GAG is found in cartilage and the cornea.

6.1.2 Properties of Glycosaminoglycans

The biological role of GAGs is related to their very large size and extremely large numbers of charged sites.

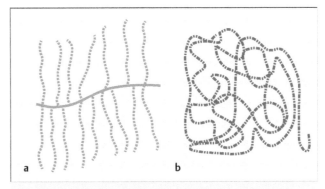

Fig. 6.1 Diagrammatic representation of the structure of glycosaminoglycans (GAGSs). (a) Some GAGs have a core of protein to which are attached GAG side chains. **(b)** Hyaluronic acid is a single chain of GAGs which is long and coiled.

Space occupancy: The space occupied or "domain" of a molecule is more important than its weight. Hyaluronic acid has a domain so large that a single molecule occupies a sphere of 1 μm.

Osmotic pressure: Each GAG molecule exerts a high osmotic pressure, as though it was composed of several separate molecules.

Water retention: The most important property of GAGs is to bind or trap relatively large amounts of water, about 60% of the total content of water in soft tissue structures. This maintains the turgidity of skin and other structures. Water retention also accounts for the ability of GAGs to resist compression as the water molecules are unable to be squeezed out of the entangled meshwork that characterizes GAGs.

Resist compression: While the fibrous component of connective tissue resists tensile forces, GAGs resist compressive forces. This together with their slipperiness makes them an important component of synovial fluid and contributes along with collagen to the load-bearing capacities of cartilage.

Concentrated ions: GAGs have the ability to concentrate calcium ions, many times more than the surrounding tissue, because of the large number of charged particles within the meshwork of the molecule. The role of GAGs in the pulp may be to assist calcification of secondary dentin and to protect the pulp from vibration. Inflammatory exudate in the pulp may be absorbed by GAGs and so prevent build-up of pressure.

6.2 Glycoproteins

GPs are polymers consisting of long chains of covalently linked polypeptides (amino acid residues). Short carbohydrate (CHO) side chains of about 7 to 10 sugars are linked to the peptide. The side strings of sugar usually end with sialic acid, giving the carbohydrate side chain a negative charge (▶ Fig. 6.2). Neighboring ends of sialic acid repel each other, and this tends to

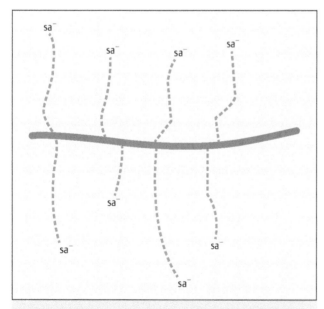

Fig. 6.2 Diagrammatic representation of the structure of a glycoprotein. A central core of polypeptides is linked to carbohydrate side chains of different lengths but all ending with a sialic acid residue.

keep the whole molecule straightened out and away from adjacent GP molecules. The large molecules are therefore long and slippery like buttered spaghetti. The amount of CHO side chain varies. It may be as little as 5% and as much as 50% in salivary GPs. This high CHO content in salivary GPs is important in providing the ionic bonds with enamel which form pellicle. GPs in saliva provide good lubrication and a source of sugars, which bacteria can utilize. GPs have a wide range of other functions apart from their importance in saliva.

They are the markers on the cell membranes of red blood cells. These markers confer the four major types of blood, A, B, AB, and O. They also form part of the cell wall of bacteria to which antibiotics can attach. While GPs do not form a large component of the extracellular matrix like GAGs do, they are of great importance as they interact with cells to regulate their differentiation and activity.

6.2.1 Bone Glycoproteins

Osteocalcin is a GP which makes up 20% of the noncollagen proteins of bone. One of its amino acid residues gives osteocalcin its strong calcium-binding properties.

Bone sialoprotein (BSP) has, as the name suggest, a large proportion of sialic acid. It appears in osteoid of embryonic (woven) bone and may be important with the other noncollagen bone proteins in initiating mineralization.

Osteonectin is a strongly acidic glycoprotein, which is readily phosphated and binds strongly to hydroxyapatite. Synthetically produced osteonectin increases the rate of bone regenerating properties when applied to healing bone.

6.2.2 Fibronectin

During embryonic development, and during wound healing, cells do not keep their place but migrate in an organized way. In order to move they need something to hold onto. Once they are anchored, a local extension of the cell membrane is squeezed out by a contraction in the cytoplasm. The extruded foot now attaches itself and provides an anchorage for the rest of the cell to move by further contractions within the cytoplasm brought about by the shortening of actin fibers. Fibronectin is a GP which provides anchorage, so it makes a convenient pathway for migrating cells. A trail, made by smearing a pathway of fibronectin on a cell culture dish, stimulates neural crest cells to start moving along the trail. If some of the fibronectin on the path ahead is inactivated with a specific antibody, the cells lose their way. They recover their direction after some random movements when they find the path again. Fibronectin-rich spaces in the embryo suggest that many kinds of cells may migrate along these routes. Absence of fibronectin has been noticed in tissue cultures of cancer cells. These cells do not adhere well to a substrate or to each other. They also have a poorly organized internal structure which gives them a variety of shapes. Fibronectin added to tumor cells in culture restores a more contained shape and improves their adhesion.

6.2.3 Laminin

All epithelial cells are either attached directly or via other epithelial cells to a basement membrane. This membrane is held together by a web of type IV collagen but contains other proteins. One that is biologically active is a GP called laminin, which has a powerful inductive effect on cells. Laminin plays a crucial role in bringing about cell differentiation, which can be demonstrated by studying the behavior of cells in tissue culture. If mammary gland cells are removed from mice and grown in tissue culture, they quickly lose their regular cuboidal shape and their ability to make milk proteins. If they are grown in the presence of laminin, they regain their form and produce milk. Basement membrane also provides the necessary structural support for new tissue formation.

Endothelial cells will not form into capillaries unless basement membrane is present. This process, angiogenesis, is essential for developing and healing tissues. Salivary gland cells in tissue culture also require basement membrane extract, before they will form into branching glands. Types I and II collagens also provide the framework around which new blood vessels form.

6.2.4 Metalloproteins

There are a group of matrix proteins which bind copper and calcium, the so-called metalloproteins. One of these, osteonectin, which has been mentioned as a bone GP, has a powerful influence on cell shape. It also influences cell behavior, inhibiting cell migration but enhancing angiogenesis. Metalloproteins, like many other matrix proteins, provide a framework for tissue organization and the trigger which starts off cell differentiation and morphogenesis. The opposite process, that of breaking down matrix proteins, is an equally important process in tissue repair and remodeling of tissue during growth. A group of enzymes called metalloproteinases (collagenase and stromelysin) are responsible for breaking down metalloproteins.

6.2.5 Periostin

Periostin is a recently designated matricellular protein concerned with cell development, repair, and disease, particularly in tissues rich in collagen. In repair, it may be involved in the recruitment of preosteoblasts to form a bone callus and also stimulate the production of collagen from fibroblasts (*see Chapter 6.4 Matricellular Proteins*).

> **Key Notes**
>
> GAGs are the "goo" that holds together the extracellular matrix. Their properties provide resistance to compression of synovial fluid and protect the dental pulp and periodontal ligament from being disrupted by impact forces. GPs provide support for cell messengers and cell movement. They are the "sign posts, control points, and highways" for connective tissue cells.

6.3 Fibrous Matrix Proteins

6.3.1 Collagen

Collagen is the most abundant protein in the body comprising about 20% of the body weight. It is an extracellular fibrous protein produced by fibroblasts. Collagen is a long fibrous polymer, and this structure gives to it the ability to resist tension. It is, however, quite flexible (in the young) and insoluble. If heated with water (hydrolyzed), it eventually becomes a soluble gelatin which has been used, in the past, as glue (*Greek* kolla = glue). It is of great interest to dentists, as the destruction of dentin and periodontium both involve the breakdown of collagen. Other more important diseases of collagen occur when enzymes (collagenases) produced by the body break down collagen in the cartilage of joints (rheumatoid arthritis). Failure to produce normal collagen causes a variety of genetic diseases (Marfan's syndrome, scleroderma). The loss of the flexibility of collagen, which occurs in the elderly, accounts for many of the tissue changes which accompany old age.

Collagen structure: Common to all collagen fibers is a basic structural unit, a long, thin macromolecule, about 1.5-nm wide and 300-nm long. It is called tropocollagen and is made up of three polypeptide chains wound around each other in a right-handed twist, like rope. The structure of a three-strand rope is revealed when the end unravels. The strands have clearly been twisted to hold them together but cannot be simply twisted back into a rope, unless each strand is itself twisted in the opposite direction to the major strands of the rope. The tropocollagen molecule is twisted in a left-handed direction, but the three polypeptide chains are twisted in a right-hand direction.

Each chain is joined with others at each end, lined up and stacked parallel to others. Microfibrils are aligned together to form fibrils, which in turn are joined to form individual collagen fibers (*see Appendix H.3 The Heritage of Fibrous Polymers*).

There are some interesting features of the individual polypeptide chains. The most common amino acid is glycine, followed by proline, hydroxyproline, and alanine. The amino acids are held together by peptide bonds, which are normally quite rigid and allow no twisting of the chain. However, glycine does allow rotation to occur and the chain to be twisted. The whole proline molecule becomes part of the peptide backbone giving the chain a twist to the left, which determines a fixed distance separating the coils of the chain. Every third residue comes to lie vertically above the other. From the glycine residues, interpeptide hydrogen bonds keep each chain coiled together to form a superhelix. The three chains are also held together by strong covalent bonds between the lysine residues. This pattern is repeated for 95% of the length of the molecule. At one end, there is a region which lacks the triple sequence; this is called the *telopeptide* region, and it confers specific species antigenicity (▶ Fig. 6.3).

Slight variation in structure of collagen have led to 28 types being recognized, mostly based on the structures in which they are found. The collagen found in bone, teeth, skin, and tendon has two chains that are identical, (type α_1 chains) and one (type α_2 chain) which is slightly different. These collagen type I fibers are arranged in longitudinal bundles whose purpose appears to be to resist tension. The collagen found in cartilage (type II) has three type α_2 chains. The fibrils are arranged in a network which holds together the large GAG molecules of chondroitin sulfate. Two other collagen types, III and IV are found in the aorta and basement membrane, respectively. The types III and IV fibrils are arranged like a coarsely woven fabric and in fact provide a sheet-like structure underneath epithelia and around the aorta (▶ Fig. 6.4).

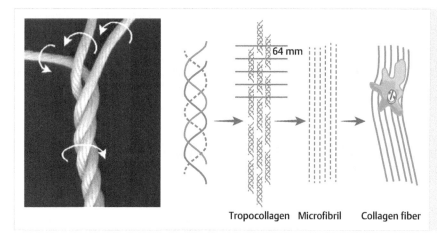

Fig. 6.3 Diagrammatic representation of the structure of tropocollagen. A rope is formed by twisting each strand one way (anticlockwise), and then twisting all three in the other direction (clockwise). The rope illustrates the three helical molecular chains of amino acids which coiled in the opposite direction, make up the basic molecular unit of tropocollagen.

64 mm

Tropocollagen Microfibril Collagen fiber

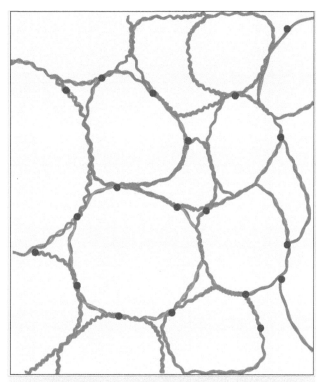

Fig. 6.4 Diagrammatic representation of the structure of type IV collagen. Type IV collagen forms a fine network of fibrils which support other proteins such as fibronectin and laminin in basement membranes.

Collagen synthesis takes place in two stages. Firstly, it is intracellular and then follows an extracellular stage. The polypeptide chain is first assembled on the ribosomes, and the completed chain released into the endoplasmic reticulum. The hydroxylation of the proline and lysine residues then occurs with the help of a hydroxylase enzyme, oxygen, ferrous ion, and ascorbic acid (vitamin C). Hence, a dietary lack of ascorbic acid prevents complete hydroxylation. Scurvy is a condition caused by reduced cross-linkages required to strengthen the collagen fiber.

The *proto*collagen chains come together to form a triple helix. At this stage further modification occurs, in that a carbohydrate component, galactose is linked onto the chain in certain places. Having been hydroxylated and glycosylated, the chain is now called *pro*collagen and is ready for secretion. The telopeptide regions are removed outside the cell, and the *tropo*collagen thus formed is ready to form fibrils.

The tropocollagen molecules are laid head to tail, but the joins of a fibril are not in the same place as its neighbor. The tropocollagen molecule junctions are staggered a quarter of the neighbor's length giving a banded appearance due to the regular appearance of small gaps (about 67 nm) in between each molecule. Cross-links occur within the tropocollagen molecules (intramolecular) and between the molecules (intermolecular). Both types of cross-linkages involve lysine and hydroxylysine residues.

The cross-linkages increase with age making the collagen molecule tougher and less soluble. Collagen fibers may be orientated parallel to the long axis of a tendon. Their orientation also contributes to the structure of lamellar bone and dentin. It is likely that the orientation is controlled by some environmental factor, which may be an electrical polarity of the tissue, or the presence of strains resulting from stresses.

Collagen turnover: Collagen is broken down and replaced in most tissues, though the rate of turnover varies considerably. In tendons, the rate would be slow, but in the periodontal ligament it would be rapid (24 hours in the mouse). The process of breakdown is initiated by partial phagocytosis of a fibril into a lysosomal vacuole in the fibroblast. Collagenase enzymes split the bonds holding the chains together, and proteolytic enzymes attack the polypeptide chains. Collagen turnover is an essential process in bone remodeling which occurs throughout life.

In periodontal disease, there is breakdown of collagen which may be the result of both bacterial collagenases and endogenous collagenases from polymorphonuclear leukocytes.

6.3.2 Elastin

Elastin fibers are thin branching elastic fibers. They can stretch up to 1.5 times their original length without breaking, but this elasticity decreases with age. They are found in arteries, lungs, and skin. Elastin differs from collagen in composition, in that there are more nonpolar amino acids (e.g., valine and alanine). The molecule structure tends to be globular until straightened out.

6.3.3 Keratin

In contrast to both elastin and collagen, keratin is an intracellular fiber. Also, unlike collagen the molecule is a single α-helix chain. The chains are twisted together to form a cable, and a number of cables form a microfibril (7-μm diameter). The process of keratinization of epithelial cells involves the progressive dehydration of the microfibrils and cross-linkage with sulfide bridges. The result is a highly insoluble fiber with great mechanical strength.

6.4 Matricellular Proteins

All matrix molecules play some additional bioactive role in the differentiation of precursor connective tissue cells and the regulation of their activity. Some of these bioactive components have been called matricellular proteins, describing their dual function. They include the structural proteins such as collagen, fibronectin, laminins, and periostin, as well as proteoglycans, glycoproteins, and metalloproteins. They provide molecular signals to resident cell populations that are essential for maintenance of normal connective tissue structure and function. They are most active during development of connective tissues but return to activity once more during repair and disease. They can thus be quite transient, their regulatory activity short lived. The interaction and regulation which occur between these proteins and connective tissue cells include functions such as cell differentiation, migration, morphology, mineralization, apoptosis, and collagen synthesis. The route of interaction involves the attachment between specific binding sites of the matrix protein (*ligands*) with *integrins* on the surface of connective tissue cells. The integrin goes right through the cell membrane and attaches to actin filaments held together in a sack-like aggregate of molecules, called focal adhesions. In this way, the integrin provides a robust connection between the cell and the extracellular matrix. Apart from providing matrix adhesion, integrins have a second powerful function. They are capable of initiating changes in cell shape, intracellular signaling, and differentiation. They activate gene expression through a series of signals, which start at the cell membrane and move in toward the nucleus causing transcription of specific genes (*see Appendix E.2.3 Integrins*).

Key Notes

Collagen and keratin are large fibrous polymers which have essential structural and protective roles. Collagen along with other structural and supportive matricellular proteins of the connective tissue plays an active role as part of the network of signaling molecules which control cell activity, particularly during healing.

Review Questions

1. What are the main properties of GAGs?
2. How does the viscoelasticity of hyaluronic acid contribute to the properties of synovial fluid?
3. How do salivary PGs influence the oral environment?
4. Explain the effects of scurvy in terms of altered collagen synthesis.
5. What is conveyed by the term matricellular proteins?

Suggested Readings

Darnel J, Lodish H, Baltimore D. Molecular cell biology scientific American books. New York: WH Freeman and Co Ltd; 1990

Goodsell DS. Our molecular nature; the bodies motors machines and messages. New York, NY: Springer-Verlag; 1996

Hamilton DW. Functional role of periostin in development and wound repair: implications for connective tissue disease. J Cell Commun Signal 2008; 2(1–2):9–17

Young MF. Bone matrix proteins: more than markers. Calcif Tissue Int 2003; 72(1):2–4

7 The Physiology of Bone

Abstract

Bone has three main functions. Its earliest function, on an evolutionary scale, was to protect the brains of the first bony fish. It later developed in these bony fish as a flexible skeleton of rigid components against which swimming muscles could work with great efficiency. Finally, it provided a store and source of calcium, whose homeostasis was important. There is little further that can be added to the role of bone in mammals and man. Teeth and bones share a common property. They are both hard and are resistant to dissolution by acids. This is because part of their structure is made of apatite crystals, which are only slightly soluble. The bones and teeth of a mammal may remain intact for hundreds of years after it has died. When we handle such old relics, it is hard to realize that they were once dynamic, reactive, and constantly changing components of a living body. Living bone is constantly being turned over, resorbed, and remodeled in response to changing demands. One of the challenges to astronauts, who spend any prolonged period in the zero gravity of space, is the rapid resorption of bone which is no longer weight bearing. Maintaining the bone around teeth and preventing its resorption if the teeth are lost provide one of the great challenges of dentistry. The more we understand of the dynamics of bone resorption and remodeling, the better we will manage the clinical problem of bone loss.

Keywords: mineralization, apatites, solubility product, matrix vesicles, epitaxy, intramembranous, cartilage, growth, development, functional matrix, remodeling, stress

7.1 The Mineralization Process

7.1.1 Composition of Biological Apatites

Calcium and phosphate have a strong affinity for each other and therefore form stable compounds, which have structural and physiological importance in many living organisms. Collectively, they are referred to as biological apatites. The name is derived from the Greek "apatite" to deceive. Apatite is a very hard salt and almost insoluble in water. Crystals of apatite form the bulk of the mineralized part of hard tissues in bones and teeth. The crystals are not pure apatite; they include carbonate, citrate, sodium, and magnesium, in amounts of about 1% each. There are small amounts of fluoride and traces of heavy metals.

The proportions of calcium and phosphates in the crystals of apatite are not consistent; the most common form, however, is hydroxyapatite ($Ca_{10}(PO_4)_6 OH_2$), but there are other apatites in which the calcium and phosphate parts are in different ratios. The ratio of Ca: PO_4 in hydroxyapatite is 1.67, the highest of all the apatites and the most insoluble.

7.1.2 Solubility of Apatites

When crystals of an almost insoluble salt like apatite are placed in water, both calcium and phosphate ions enter the water. The process continues until the solution around the crystals is saturated and can hold no more ions. At this point, the salt and the solution are in equilibrium. If, at this point, either Ca^+ or PO_4^- is added to the solution, the reaction would go into reverse, and ions would precipitate onto the crystal. So, the reaction may move in either direction, dissolution or precipitation. The principles of saturated solutions may be summarized by the following relationship:

$Ca_3 PO_4$	→Dissolves	$3Ca^{++} + 2 PO_4^-$
Apatite crystal	←Precipitates	Saturated solution

The concentration of ions in such a saturated solution will be depend on the solubility of the apatite and will have a constant value known as the solubility product (K^{sp}). The K^{sp} will be highest for the most soluble apatites.

$$K^{sp} = [Ca^{++}]^3 \times [PO_4^-]^2$$

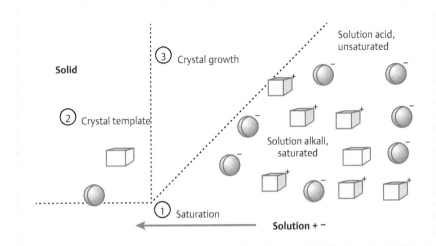

Fig. 7.1 A diagrammatic representation of the stages in the production of hydroxyapatite crystals. 1. The first stage in crystal formation is the increase is salt concentration until the solution is saturated. Saturation is reached sooner in an alkali medium. 2. Crystals begin to form in a specific pattern determined by the template offered by existing crystals. 3. Once the crystals first form, they grow rapidly provided the solution remains saturated.

Before precipitation of ions can occur, their concentrations must reach certain levels for a given set of conditions. The different ions, calcium, and phosphate, in this case, do not have to be in the same proportions, but the product of their concentrations, $[Ca^+] \times [HPO_4^-]$, must reach the solubility product (K^{sp}). In test tube experiments (in vitro), this product must reach $4.3 \, mmol^2$ before nuclei of hydroxyapatite will form. If the pH does not change, this solubility product is constant. The solubility for any apatite is decreased if the solution is alkali. Hence, precipitation of salt would be assisted in an alkaline medium.

7.1.3 Production of Apatite Crystals

There are three recognizable stages in the production of hydroxyapatite crystals (▶ Fig. 7.1). Firstly, Ca^+ and PO_4^- must accumulate in such concentration as to exceed the solubility of an apatite salt and to precipitate. Secondly, the ions must precipitate in a specific pattern which will allow other ions to spontaneously arrange themselves in the proper orientation for the third stage, which is crystal growth.

The presence of existing crystal nuclei alters the conditions very significantly. Existing crystals reduce the concentrations required for precipitation to as low as $0.83 \, mmol^2$, compared to the concentration of salts required to allow precipitation in a test tube of $4.3 \, mmol^2$. The concentration product of $[Ca^+] \times [HPO_4^-]$ ions in tissue fluid is around $1.76 \, mmol^2$. This means that hydroxyapatite cannot precipitate without a local catalyst or template, but once nucleation has occurred, crystals can grow rapidly in body fluids.

In newly formed bone, about 70% of the mineral is amorphous calcium phosphate (ACP), but in older bone, the proportions of ACP and hydroxyapatite are reversed. ACP may form first and then become crystallized into hydroxyapatite as this has been observed in in vitro studies. In vivo, a local increase in pH would encourage this change from ACP to hydroxyapatite.

7.2 Mechanisms of Mineralization

Mineralization is the deposition of apatites and other salts in an extracellular matrix of fibers and ground substance. As calcium is not the only mineral involved, it is incorrect to refer to the process as calcification. Mineralization goes on throughout life as bone is continually being deposited and removed from the skeleton. The mineralization of the teeth is for the most part confined to their period of development. There is no completely satisfactory explanation for the apparent control of the process of mineralization. It is not clear how it is initiated in embryonic development, and it is not certain how the process, once started, is restrained. There are at least two possible processes which could be involved in the control of mineralization. The first results directly from cellular activity via the production of vesicles high in calcium content; the second depends on the presence of matricellular proteins including collagen.

7.2.1 Control of Mineralization by Organic Components

The matrix in which mineralization takes place contains collagen, proteoglycans, citrates, lipids, and plasma constituents. The cells concerned in the mineralization process all contain large quantities of the enzyme alkaline phosphatase. There is some evidence for the involvement of each of these organic components in mineralization.

Crystal growth may be initiated by the presence of a nucleus in a saturated solution. This nucleus may be an impurity or a previously formed crystal introduced into the solution, which acts like a template against which ions can form up in order. This process is referred to as *epitaxy*. Support for the epitaxy theory has come from electron microscope studies which have shown that hydroxyapatite crystals are initiated first at the light bands of 64.0-nm repeating collagen, and that the crystals orientate along the long axis of the collagen fiber. It is also suggested that for crystal formation to occur within the fiber, the phosphate and calcium ions must pass through the gaps between the tropocollagen molecules. For type I collagen, the gap is 0.6 nm (large enough for the phosphate molecule), but for the type II collagen, (soft tissue) the gap (0.3 nm) is too small, and the collagen does not calcify.

A calcium-*phospholipid*-phosphate complex has been isolated from young bone and found to induce crystallization. Acidic phospholipids from dentin have also been found to have the same potential. Phospholipids are also associated with the matrix vesicles (*see Chapter 7.2.2 Control of Mineralization by Cells*) in calcifying cartilage. Glycosaminoglycans (GAGs) in cartilage seem to have an inhibitory effect on mineral nucleation.

Their removal may be necessary to make room for mineral crystals.

7.2.2 Control of Mineralization by Cells

All the components of supportive connective tissue, including the matrix of fibers and ground substance and its mineralization with apatite, are formed as a result of bone-forming (osteoblast) and bone-removing (osteoclast) cells. The activity of osteoblast and osteoclast is influenced by systemic hormones such estrogen, parathyroid, calcitonin, and growth hormone. At a local level, the activity of these cells is also influenced by a wide range of local chemical mediators, and the matrix molecules around the cells, which are both supportive and inductive. The provision of high concentrations of calcium at levels which are highly toxic to cells would seem to require mechanisms which take place outside the cell, although it is possible that mineralizing cells could accumulate and store high levels of calcium safely in their mitochondria.

The final concentration, however, is not achieved in the cell but in an extracellular vesicle. Membrane-bound vesicles about $100 \mu m$ in diameter have been found within the organic matrix destined to become bone, and within predentin, and in the pre-calcifying zone of cartilage. The contents of these *matrix vesicles* are rich in acid phospholipids, which have a strong affinity for calcium. One of these, phosphatidylserine, not only binds calcium but also inorganic phosphate as well. Matrix vesicles also contain high concentrations of phosphatases, enzymes which generate phosphates. Matrix vesicles are able to concentrate both phosphate and calcium ions until the threshold for the precipitation of hydroxyapatite is reached.

> **Key Notes**
>
> Hydroxyapatite is an almost insoluble salt. In solution, a small number of ions dissolve until the solution is saturated. When apatite crystals are formed, the solution not only has to be saturated, but crystallization must be assisted by cellular and matrix factors.

Review Questions

1. What is the salt which forms the mineral part of bone?
2. Why is it that the concentration of apatite ions in tissue fluid would allow continual crystal growth yet be insufficient to initiate mineralization?
3. What role do cells have in mineralization?
4. What role does the cell matrix have in mineralization?

7.3 Methods of Bone Formation

7.3.1 Origins of Bone

The tissues which form the skeleton of vertebrates are cartilage and bone. The early fish all had cartilaginous skeletons, and some, like sharks and rays still have not progressed beyond using cartilage for their backbones and fins. Many millions of years ago, some fish developed a modification to cartilage. These first truly bony fish actually still had a backbone of cartilage, but they grew protective sheets of bone under the skin around the head, improving the protection of the brain and eyes. These bony plates are still part of our skeletons and are known as the dermal (skin) bones of the skull. Bone had many other advantages over cartilage, particularly where a rigid thin structure was required. The flesh of fishes-like mackerel and trout is well supported with "bones" to support the action of strong swimming muscles. Land animals do not have the support water gives to the body and require the skeleton to prevent them from collapsing under their weight. Cartilage would not support the weight of a horse, but bone, with its mineral crystals, toughened by a network of collagen fibers is able to withstand heavy compression. Bone is, however, brittle; it does not withstand tension well. If the horse should fall badly, a leg bone might snap under the tension. Parts of the mammal skeleton which must be flexible, like the ears, respiratory passages, and the ends of long bones, are made of cartilage.

7.3.2 Structure of Cartilage

Cartilage has a very simple structure when viewed under a microscope. The only cells visible in mature cartilage are chondrocytes. The matrix surrounding the cells usually has a glassy appearance and is given the name *hyaline cartilage* (*Greek* hyalos = glass). Hyaline cartilage can be found keeping the airway open, from the nose to the bronchi and covering the articular surface of joint surfaces. The matrix is not in fact featureless, as it contains a fine network of collagen fibers embedded in an extracellular matrix. In some cartilage, such as that found between the intervertebral disks, the fibers are visible, as they are more densely packed. This, so-called *fibrous cartilage*, is stronger but less flexible than hyaline cartilage. When prepared for histological section, the matrix of cartilage takes up basic dies (basophilic) because it contains acid GAGs. These GAGs are huge molecules which account for some of the important physical properties of cartilage (*see Chapter 6.1 Glycosaminoglycans*). GAGs retain large amount of water which is attracted to the molecule and trapped within its large domain. It is difficult to squeeze this water out of the GAG molecule, so cartilage is resistant and to compression. One of its great disadvantages is that if it is torn or damaged, it has little ability to repair itself because it does not have a blood supply. Nutrients reach the cartilage cells by diffusion from the perichondrium, a surrounding layer of dense connective tissue. Cartilage is not a biologically active tissue.

7.3.3 Cartilage as a Skeletal Material

Cartilage is a useful skeletal material in the developing embryo. At this time and during infancy, the skeleton needs to grow fast. Cartilage is flexible and can grow by expansion from within (interstitial growth) and so increase in size rapidly. Bone, being rigid, cannot grow except by addition of new bone to the surface, so expansion is gradual. With the exception of the dermal bones of the skull, the bones of the skeleton develop first in cartilage, which is later replaced with bone. Cartilage also has a crucial role in the interface between skeletal elements. Not only it is a growth zone in young bones, but also it later remains to provide the joint surfaces. The combination of GAGs and a network of collagen gives it a high resistance to compression, flexibility, and a slippery surface. This makes it an ideal material for joint surfaces which have to sustain high impact, such as those of the lower limbs. There are some exceptions, however. The temporomandibular joint surfaces and the disk in between are not cartilage but dense fibrous tissue. The reason for this may be that cartilage provides a suitable surface in a joint as long as it is stable and well fitting when loaded (like the knee joint). The temporomandibular joint rotates and slides while under load in a grinding manner, and the joint surfaces are not well fitting. If the lining surface were incompressible cartilage, there would be concentrations of pressure to the supporting bone. Fibrous tissue, on the other hand, allows for some distortion under load thereby conforming to the constantly changing points of contact between the joint surfaces. The intervening disk, also of dense fibrous tissue, ensures smooth movement of the joint under load (*see Chapter 9.2 The Structure of the Temporomandibular Joint*).

7.3.4 Intramembranous Bone Formation

The first bones to form in the embryo are those which surround the brain. These skull bones form in between the outer membrane of the brain and the skin, hence the name, intramembranous. The cells which form bone are osteoblasts. These are specialized cells which are differentiated from stem cells in bone marrow and the periosteum. The osteoblasts secrete a matrix around themselves which is rich in collagen fibers and ground substance known as *osteoid*. The ground substance consists of the GAG chondroitin sulphate and osteocalcin. The osteoblasts then start depositing calcium and other mineral salts into the osteoid, where the salts precipitate as crystals. These first spicules of bone appear as an ossification center, which grows progressively in size to fuse with other ossification centers (▶ Fig. 7.2). This first formed bone is called embryonic,

or woven bone, because it is not well organized. Bone which first forms during repair of fractures, or in tooth sockets after extraction, is also irregular, woven bone.

The organization of this bone soon begins by its removal by osteoclasts. These are multinucleated giant cells, whose origins are from monocytes. Osteocytes emerge from blood vessels and remove a tunnel of bone around the blood vessel, which in the two dimensions of a histological section appear as a circular ring of bone removal (▶ Fig. 7.3). The osteoclasts's work is done. Osteoblasts begin to form bone against the inner walls of the tunnel in layers of concentric plates called *lamellae*. The layers are distinguished by the regular orientation of collagen fibers. The tunnel is not completely filled up, as a central bundle of blood vessels remains. As the lamellae are formed, some osteoblasts remain trapped in between them. They are in this situation, called osteocytes, as they no longer form bone. They retain contact via long cellular projections, with osteoblasts, and contribute greatly to control bone metabolism from their inner caverns.

The concentric lamellae of bone and central blood vessels have been called a haversian system. The haversian system in three dimensions forms the basic structural unit of bone and is called an *osteon*. The concentric tubes of plated bone resemble the stem of a leek, but of course they are microscopic in size. The process of cutting a tunnel and lining it again is in order to align the collagen fibers, before they are surrounded by crystals of bone salts. This alignment gives the osteon great strength, as not only are the fibers arranged in a number of useful directions, but their direction is reversed in each adjacent layer of the osteon. Fibers in each osteon are formed as either long spirals, transverse circles, or longitudinal rods (▶ Fig. 7.4). Osteons have greater density than embryonic bone and are the reason this bone has a compact appearance, even when it is not magnified. If the leg bone of any mammal is sectioned through the shaft, it will be seen to consist of a thick dense tube called the cortex and an inner softer center called the medulla. The medulla in the center of long bones may be filled with red bone

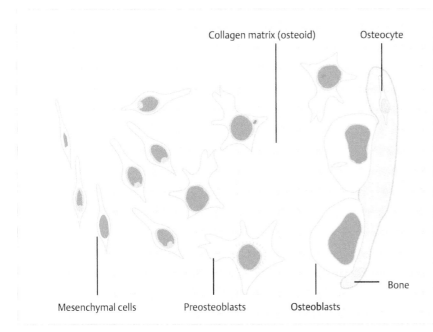

Collagen matrix (osteoid)   Osteocyte

Mesenchymal cells   Preosteoblasts   Osteoblasts   Bone

Fig. 7.2 A diagrammatic representation of the stages of embryonic or woven bone formation. Mesenchymal stem cells differentiate into pre-osteoblasts, which further differentiate into osteoblasts. Osteoblasts lay down a matrix of osteoid, which contains collagen fibers in a ground substance of the glycosaminoglycan, chondroitin sulfate. Mature osteoblasts secrete calcium and phosphate salts, which form crystals of hydroxyapatite around the collagen fibers. The bone formed may trap osteoblasts, which become osteocytes.

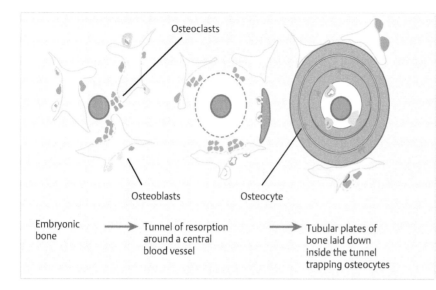

Fig. 7.3 A diagrammatic representation of the formation of lamella (compact) bone. Embryonic bone surrounding a blood vessel is remodeled, forming a tunnel. Against the walls of the tunnel, new osteoid, containing ordered collagen fibers, is laid down then mineralized forming concentric plates of lamella bone. The blood vessel and surrounding plates of lamella bone are called an osteon.

Osteoclasts

Osteoblasts Osteocyte

Embryonic bone → Tunnel of resorption around a central blood vessel → Tubular plates of bone laid down inside the tunnel trapping osteocytes

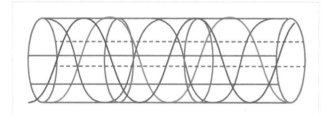

Fig. 7.4 A diagrammatic representation of the arrangement of collagen fibers in an osteon. There are circular, longitudinal, and spiral fibers, which provide resistance to fracture when bone is deformed under strain.

marrow in the young and fatty tissue in older subjects. If the bone is sectioned at either end of the shaft, the medulla is seen to be filled with spongy-looking bone.

The dense bone of the cortex is compact lamella bone, and this can be confirmed by examining a section using a microscope. The spongy inner core appears to lack any pattern of arrangement. When a section is examined microscopically, it appears even less structured, as all that can be detected is isolated spicules of bone. However, if a radiograph is made, a distinct orientation of spicules may be seen. These spicules have been called trabeculae, and so the bone is called trabecular bone (▸ Fig. 7.5) (*see Appendix F.1 Stress and Trabecular Orientation*).

7.3.5 Growth of Intramembranous Bone

We have noted that intramembranous bone formation occurs in the skull bone to protect the brain. It is clear that as soon as some bone has formed, it cannot increase in size from within, but only by the apposition of new layers of bone on the surface. The shape may be controlled by both appositional growth on the outside and resorption on the inside. Where two cranial bone surfaces meet, for example, the parietal and frontal bones, a fibrous suture separates the two membranous bones until

growth ceases (▸ Fig. 7.6). Bone growth by apposition and resorption is a relatively slow process; it serves well enough for the bones of the skull which are in infancy, disproportionately large, but grow slowly, and must at all times provide a rigid protective shield for the brain.

Growth of the axial skeleton must be more rapid in order to achieve adult size during the years of childhood. The axial skeleton also has to grow while bearing the weight of the child. Bone-forming cells at sutures would have to be capable of withstanding considerable compression due to weight and at the same time provide a high growth rate. Subperiosteal appositional bone formation would not meet the demands made for growth of the axial skeleton.

7.3.6 Endochondral Bone Formation

The axial skeleton of the embryo is therefore first formed in cartilage. Cells forming cartilage (chondrocytes) are flattened parallel to the surface and several layers deep. The rubbery consistency of the cartilage surrounding each chondrocyte protects it from compression due to the weight of the child. It has been noted that the matrix of chondroitin sulfate and type II collagen fibers provide cartilage with resistance to compression and a slippery joint surface. Nests of chondrocytes are able to form cartilage rapidly. Unlike the rigid matrix surrounding bone cells, cartilage can increase in size by expansion from within, that is, by interstitial growth. The chondrocytes increase in size and their extracellular matrix increases in mass. Then they begin to calcify their surrounding matrix with hydroxyapatite crystals. Their mission is suicidal. As soon as they have completed this task of growth and calcification, they die by a process known as *apoptosis* (programmed cell death). The calcified matrix becomes the framework against which osteoblasts start to form bone (▸ Fig. 7.7).

Before new bone can replace the calcifying cartilage, a blood supply (*angiogenesis*) must be established. Blood vessels penetrate the cartilage in the center of the shaft, the diaphysis and at each end, the epiphysis. The new blood vessels move into the

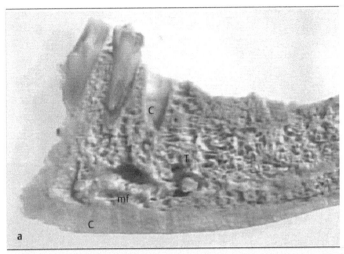
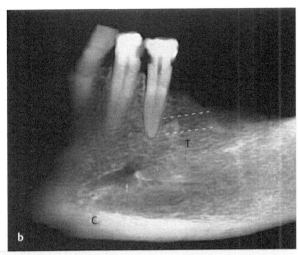

Fig. 7.5 The structural appearance of compact and trabecular bone. (a) A sagittal section through the mandible, with a few remaining anterior teeth, shows the compact cortical bone (C), thickest at the lower border of the mandible. Most of the posterior teeth have been lost for some time before death. Note, the absence of any cortical bone on the residual alveolar ridge. One of the premolar teeth has been removed postmortem, and the cortical bone lining the tooth socket is visible. The mental foramen is visible (mf). The central spongy bone has supportive trabeculae (T) which are not readily recognizable. **(b)** The radiograph of the same sample reveals the direction of trabeculae, which are more radiopaque, and therefore slightly lighter than the surrounding spongy bone.

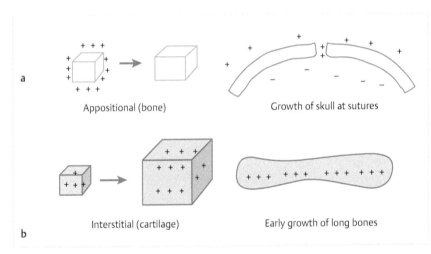

Appositional (bone)

Growth of skull at sutures

Interstitial (cartilage)

Early growth of long bones

Fig. 7.6 A diagrammatic representation of the difference between interstitial and appositional bone growth. (a) A growing skull bone increases in size slowly by apposition (++) and changes shape by a balance of apposition (++) and resorption (– –). **(b)** Long bones increase in length rapidly, as growth occurs first, by interstitial growth of cartilage before bone formation occurs.

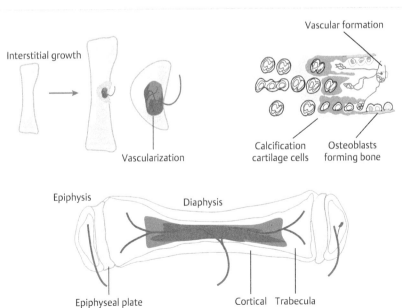

Interstitial growth

Vascularization

Vascular formation

Calcification cartilage cells

Osteoblasts forming bone

Epiphysis

Diaphysis

Epiphyseal plate of cartilage

Cortical bone

Trabecula bone

Fig. 7.7 A diagrammatic representation of the conversion of a cartilaginous limb into bone. Blood vessels invade the cartilage and begin to vascularize it. As this occurs, some cartilage cells calcify their surrounding matrix and die, leaving channels for blood vessels to follow. Osteoblast lays down bone against the calcified cartilage and gradually replaces it, except for two plates, which remaining at the epiphysis, and allows continued growth of cartilage until adulthood.

spaces created by the dying cartilage cells and establish a highly active connective tissue capable of supporting the principal bone-forming cells the osteoblasts. Having a calcified matrix to work against the replacement of the calcified cartilage by bone proceeds swiftly. This type of bone formation by replacement of cartilage is called *endochondral* ossification. Bone is also being formed on the outside of the cartilage in the perichondrium. This periosteal bone contributes to thickening the long bones, but the major growth in length is still achieved by cartilage growth. The cartilage is gradually replaced with bone along the shaft of the long bones and at the ends (*epiphysis*) of the bone where it forms a joint. In between the shaft and the epiphysis is a plate of cartilage which remains the active growing site until the adult dimensions of the bone are reached. The *epiphyseal plate* then ossifies, fusing the shaft and epiphysis, and growth in length of the bone stops. The time of fusion of the epiphyseal plate of bones of the wrist is a useful indicator of the biological age of an adolescent (*see Chapter 7.5.2.1 Measuring Growth*).

7.3.7 Summary of Differences between Cartilage and Bone

As we have seen, cartilage may become calcified, so mineralization is not always a useful distinction between cartilage and bone. There are, however, some essential differences between bone and calcified cartilage, which are related to their internal structure.

- Firstly, in bone, the collagen fibers are arranged in layers and organized into longitudinal, circular, and spiral patterns, which are all united into a macroscopic structural unit, the osteon. This orientation gives bone structural strength which cartilage lacks. The fibers in cartilage are arranged in an interlocking mesh, and there is no macroscopic structural unit.
- Secondly, bone is well vascularized, and this has a number of consequences:
  - It interacts with the physiology of the entire body in providing a reservoir of calcium. This reservoir ensures that a constant blood and tissue calcium level can be maintained.
  - Bone is capable of repair as inflammatory cells can be brought to damaged sights and eventually new bone laid down.
  - Bone is always being remodeled and is therefore capable of responding to changing patterns of stress, which the body experiences.

7.4 Development of the Skull and Jaws

7.4.1 Development of the Mandible

After 6 weeks of development, there is a "J-shaped" core of cartilage within the first branchial arch called Meckel's cartilage. The hooks of the "J" almost meet in front at the midline. Mandibular bone forms around the lateral aspect of Meckel's cartilage. An ossification center first appears in the region of the bifurcation of the inferior alveolar nerve. From this point, a wave of ossification spreads forward and backward forming a gutter around the inferior alveolar nerve. At this time, the tooth germs lie above the developing mandible, but as they grow in size, they will begin to lie in the same trough of bone as the nerve. The cartilage eventually disappears as the mandible develops around and mainly outside Meckel's cartilage. In spite of the proximity of the cartilage, the mandible does not begin formation by endochondral ossification. It is primarily formed, like other bones of the face, by intramembranous ossification. The mandibular bone develops two processes as it grows backward: the coronoid and the condylar processes. During the 10th week, a condensation of mesenchyme develops in the future ramus region. Cartilage develops and migrates down in a cone shape toward the lingula. The cells are replaced by bone (endochondral ossification) except those at the head of the condyle, where cartilage may remain up to the age of 20 years. Two other sites of secondary cartilage are formed at the coronoid process and in the midline. The part of Meckel's cartilage, which is not resorbed, forms the malleus and the sphenomandibular ligament.

7.4.2 Development of the Temporomandibular Joint

The disk of the temporomandibular joint is formed by a condensation of mesenchyme between the condyle and the articular surface of the temporal bone. This mesenchyme becomes organized into dense fibrous tissue, continuous with the future lateral pterygoid muscle. At 12 weeks, clefts in the fibrous tissue appear, and these form two cavities leaving a layer between which will become the interarticular disk. Thus, the surfaces of the condyle, the disk, and the surface of the temporal bone are covered with dense fibrous tissue during development and throughout life.

7.4.3 Synchondrosis of the Cranial Base

The base of the fetal cranium begins as a cartilaginous plate. Within this plate centers of ossification appear which will become the occipital, sphenoid, and ethmoid bones. At birth, these bones are still separated by cartilage from the original plate, which is now called a synchondrosis (*Greek* Syn = together). Growth occurs at the synchondrosis by endochondral bone formation, which is similar to the growth at the epiphysis of the long bones, except that ossification occurs on both sides of the cartilage (▶ Fig. 7.8). The last to fuse is the spheno-occipital synchondrosis, which closes at about 15 years for males, and 13 for females.

Key Notes

Bone formation requires osteoblasts to lay down a matrix of osteoid before mineralizing the matrix with bone salts. The first formed woven bone is remodeled by repeated resorption and deposition. The lamellar bone which results is densely organized and orientated so as to provide the greatest strength to weight ratio possible.

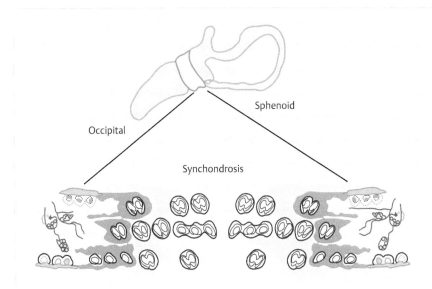

Fig. 7.8 A diagrammatic representation of the growth of the base of the cranium. The cranial base grows due to the fusion of two epiphyseal plates of cartilage which form a synchondrosis.

Occipital

Sphenoid

Synchondrosis

Review Questions

1. What were advantages of bone to early fish and later land reptiles and mammals?
2. What makes cartilage resistant to compression?
3. Why is the first formed bone called woven bone?
4. What is an osteon?
5. What is the difference between cortical and medullary bone?
6. What are trabeculae?
7. What are the limitations of appositional bone growth?
8. What are the events which must precede endochondral bone formation?
9. What are the essential differences between calcified cartilage and bone?

7.5 General Features of Growth

The essential feature of growth is change in size, proportion, or function of cells and tissues. There is a limit to the size cells can grow to. This limit is dictated by the relationship between volume and surface area; the larger the cell gets, the less is the surface area relative to the volume. Thus, surface area available for transport becomes progressively reduced as the cell gets bigger. The margins of large cells, like ameloblasts, become folded to increase the membrane area. The membrane area of nuclei also may become extended by folding (e.g., polymorphonuclear leukocytes) or by combining several nuclei within one cell (e.g., osteoclasts).

The changes in cell function are usually toward greater specialization. They become progressively differentiated from a stem cell (e.g., odontoblasts and cementoblasts both originate from mesenchymal cells of the dental papilla).

Tissues grow in size, both by an increase in *cell mass* and an increase in the *tissue matrix*, produced by the cell. Increase in the size of some growing tissue, like dentin or cartilage, is mostly due to an increase in cell secretions and not brought about by an increase in cell mass.

Cell mass increases due to an increase in number of cells known as *hyperplasia* or an increase in the size of each cell known as *hypertrophy*. Cell hyperplasia accounts for the vigorous growth of an embryo. Cell hypertrophy accounts for the increase in muscle mass and brain size. The shape of organs and bones is controlled by differential rates of growth.

7.5.1 Phases of Growth

The timing of cell division, differentiation, secretion, or movement accounts for the specific shapes of tissues and organs. The overall growth pattern is thus the result of a meticulously orchestrated series of growth phases. Only 48 hours after fertilization, a chick embryo's heart is beating. Each growth phase occurs within the environment of other growth events and may be dependent on them. Development of the secondary sex characteristic in puberty depends on the growth of the gonads and the production of sex hormones. While these events are controlled by timing devices, controlling the genetic expression of traits, the final growth rate, is affected by environmental factors such as diet and general health. A plot of increases in stature up to the age of 24 months gives an indication of growth phases and spurts. The plot of height against time shows a gradual increment with a slightly varying gradient. However, the plot of actual increments shows how irregular the growth rate is (▶ Fig. 7.9). Growth in height is not uniform but occurs in spurts. Most increase in height occurs before and just after birth, with a second peak at puberty. In the first year after birth, the body height increases by 50%, but the body weight usually triples. It is difficult to predict the mature dimensions from infant and child growth rates, but the later the growth spurts occur, the smaller in stature the adult is likely to be. If normal growth is retarded by disease (e.g., lack of thyroid hormone), and the disease is later cured, a spurt of "catch-up growth" occurs, which may leave the adult individual with no sign that there was ever deficient growth. Growth is not uniform over time nor does it occur at the same rate all over the body. The infant skull is

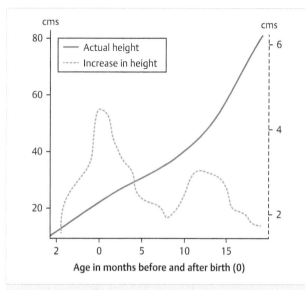

Fig. 7.9 A chart showing increments in growth plotted against actual increase in height during the first 24 months. Actual height (cumulative) is shown by the solid line, plotted against the y-axis on the left, and the x-axis, age. Increments of growth are plotted against the y-axis on the right, and age, showing that growth occurs in spurts.

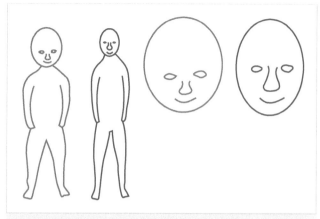

Fig. 7.10 Growth spurts of the axial skeleton and face are illustrated by the proportions of the long bones to the skull and the face to the cranium. The ratio of the skull height to total body height in the child is about 1:5. The ratio of the skull height to total body height in the adult is about 1:8. This illustrates the relatively rapid growth rate of the skeleton as the child matures. The ratio of the face height of the child to its cranium is about 1:2, whereas the ratio of the adult face to cranium is about 2:3. This illustrates the relatively rapid growth rate of the face as the child matures. In comparison to the rest of the skeleton, the cranium grows little throughout development.

proportionately large in comparison with the body, a ratio of about 1 to 5, whereas the adult skull is relatively small; the proportions of skull to body ratio are 1 to 8. The cranium of the infant is relatively large in comparison to the face; growth after birth is slow. The growth of the face and eyes during childhood is noticeable and accounts for the emerging proportions of the adult face (▸ Fig. 7.10).

7.5.2 Measuring Growth

The appearance of the epiphysis occurs at different times and is a useful diagnostic guide to the skeletal age of a growing child. For example, the appearance of the sesamoid bones of the thumb is a useful guide to the onset of puberty. As epiphysis appears at different times, so they fuse at different times after the growth spurt. The sequence in which this happens is quite predictable, but it does not always occur at the same chronological age for every individual. Orthodontists need to be able to predict the onset and end of the adolescent growth spurt in order to time their treatment. The pattern of epiphyseal fusion of the wrist bones provides them with a more useful estimate of skeletal age than the actual (chronological) age does.

The relative importance of different regions of bone growth has been discovered by a variety of experiments. If the condyles of a rat are removed, there is little change in the eventual proportions of the mandible. Tissue cultures of condylar cartilage do not grow vigorously; further evidence that there is no intrinsic capacity for condylar growth. Cultures of fibrous sutures, and even synchondrosis, also show little intrinsic growth activity. In contrast, tissue cultures of epiphyseal cartilage grow vigorously on their own. While the growth of long bones may be explained by the intrinsic activity of the growing epiphysis, the factors responsible for cranial and facial growth are less obvious.

7.5.3 Soft Tissue (Functional) Matrices

The pressures and tensions generated by soft tissues may be the driving force behind the growth of bone cavities, such as the cranium and eye socket. Melvin Moss believed that it was the *function* associated with a soft tissue matrix, which was the origin of the growth force.[1] As the head is a complex of growing sites, Moss divided the head into a few capsular matrices. The cranium was one matrix, which was driven by the space requirement of a growing brain. The eye socket was another matrix, which grew in response to the growing eye. The space required by the growing face was the result of the functional requirements of breathing. Moss's theories have been mostly upheld by recent research.[2] It has been confirmed that the primary inherent determinant of growth is soft tissue. Bone and cartilage are secondary sites, which react to the soft tissue growth. The implications of the soft tissue matrix theory are that by altering the level of soft tissue function in a matrix, the growth activity of the surrounding bones could be controlled. Hence, an underdeveloped mandible may be responsive to orthodontic treatment that consists of an appliance, which alters the functional activity of the matrix and encourages normal growth.

7.6 Growth of the Skull and Jaws

7.6.1 Growth of the Cranium and Face

We have noted that the synchondrosis at the base of the skull does not appear to be a major growth force, but that the growth may be encouraged by a functional matrix. Thus, the increase in size of the frontal lobes causes expansion at the sutures between the frontal, parietal, sphenoidal, and temporal bones. The expanding anterior cranial fossa carries the bones of the

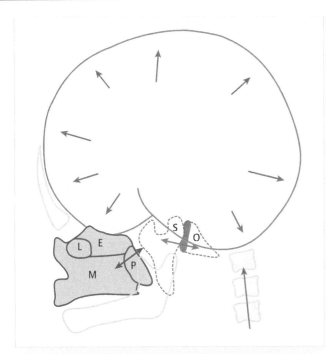

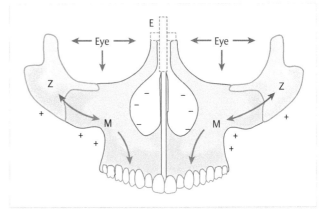

Fig. 7.12 A diagrammatic representation of the growth of the face. The eyes contribute to growth at the sutures, between the maxilla (M) and the zygoma (Z). The expanding dentition contributes to the downward growths of the maxilla. Resorption inside the maxillary sinuses increases their volume.

Fig. 7.11 A diagrammatic representation of the growth response of the face and cranium to soft tissue growth. Growth of the brain carries the maxilla, mandible, and vertebral column apart and creates tensions causing expansion of the cranium. The cranial base, also expands due to growth of the spheno-occipital synchondrosis (S, sphenoid; O, occipital). The lower face develops downward and forward by growth of the ethmoid (E), lacrimal (L), maxilla (M), palatine (P) bones. The growth of the eyes and frontal lobes also displaces the lower face downward and forward.

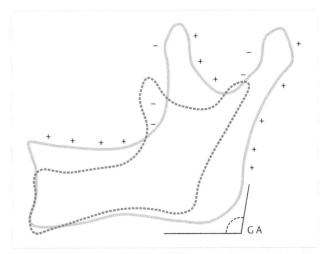

Fig. 7.13 A diagrammatic representation of the growth of the mandible by apposition and resorption. Tracing of the newborn (*dotted line*) are superimposed on the growing mandible. The gonial angle (GA) becomes reduced as the child grows, by appositional growth of the posterior border.

upper face away from the pterygoid plates and the mandible. Posterior growth of the maxilla retains the contact with the pterygoid plates (▶ Fig. 7.11). Growth of the eyes places tension on the sutures between the ethmoid and lacrimal bones and the adjacent superior surfaces of maxillary bones. The maxilla is displaced downward and the zygomatic arch outward. However, the size of the maxilla increases at the same time due to the developing dentition. The teeth account at least for the vertical growth of the maxilla. The vault of the palate would become extremely deep were it not for the deposition of bone over the palatal surfaces of the maxilla and palatine bones. The palate does not thicken because at the same time bone resorption takes place on the floor of the nose and maxillary sinuses. The face becomes wider with age due to lateral tension on the maxillary zygomatic sutures, as a result of eye growth, brain growth, and the development of molar teeth and the widening dental arch (▶ Fig. 7.12).

7.6.2 Growth of the Mandible

The mandible is held in a sling by the muscles of mastication, both elevators and openers. If the growth force of the condylar cartilage is minimal, it is not clear what force carries the mandible away from the temporal fossa and thereby encourages it to grow. One possibility is that the cranium and upper face are being pushed away from the mandible by the elongation of the cervical vertebrae (▶ Fig. 7.11). The growing and active tongue

may also push the mandible downward and forward. The following description does not imply any understanding of the dynamics but merely traces events.

Implanted metal markers on the growing mandible have shown that the condyle grows upward and backward (▶ Fig. 7.13). The extension of the condyle is assisted by subperiosteal apposition on the posterior border of the ramus and resorption on the anterior surface of the ramus and sigmoid notch. Growth of bone on the posterior surface of the angle decreases the gonial angle from about 135 degrees in the newborn to about 100 degrees in the adult. The main increase in the depth of the body is due to the development of the alveolar bone. The mandible widens due to cartilage growth at the midline symphysis. The posterior growth of the condyle and ramus also contributes to increase in the intercondylar distance.

Bone growth occurs by subperiosteal apposition onto the surface of existing bone or by bone formation within the epiphysis of long bones. The main stimulus for appositional growth is pressure caused by the growth of soft tissue. Growth at the epiphysis of long bones is controlled by local growth factors and hormones.

Review Questions

1. Why do we not find cells the size of chickens?
2. What are the limitations of bone growth by subperiosteal apposition?
3. What processes maybe responsible for the increase in size of a tissue?
4. How is growth of the face and cranium explained by Moss's proposal?
5. Which sutures are involved in the growth of the maxilla downward and forward?
6. What are the differences between growth at an epiphyseal plate and at a synchondrosis?

7.7 Bone Remodeling

One of the main functions of bone is as a structural element of the skeleton serving the functions of locomotion and protection. Bone may be subject to quite substantial forces during function, but it has limited structural strength. In order to understand the principles of bone remodeling, it is useful to take an engineer's view point of bone as a structural support of the skeleton. The design and mass of a bone must provide the required structural support without high risk of fracture or being unnecessarily heavy. The extreme challenges of bone as a structural material is well illustrated in birds, whose bone must be strong enough not to break but light enough to allow the bird to fly. Bird bones exploit the strength and lightness of tubular structures and the benefits of bracing under arch forms (*see Appendix F.2 Remodeling to Achieve Optimal Stress*).

The components of bone, matrix, and mineral are continually being resorbed and redeposited. This process is called remodeling, and it continues from the very earliest fetal bone formation until death. If the rates of these two processes are balanced, there is no net gain or loss in bone mass. The factors which initiate and control bone remodeling are local cytokines, hormones, and mechanical stress.

7.7.1 Mechanical Loads and Bone Remodeling

Stress (force per unit area), when applied to a weight-bearing bone, causes bone strain (deformation), which, if excessive, could cause microfractures to develop. Like other man-made structural elements, repeated microfracture may lead eventually to total rupture (*see Appendix H.1 Cracks, Composites, and Teeth*). Before this happens, there are adaptive changes in architecture or mass (or both) which are brought about by remodeling so as to increase the capacity of bone to resist stress and strains. Bone remodeling may be directed so as to increase bone mass. Increased resistance to fracture may also be achieved by modifying the bone shape so as to reduce stress concentrations. For example, if a carpenter needs to strengthen roof timbers, in order to support a change to heavier roof tiles, he or she might either use more or thicker roof timbers or reposition the old ones with an increase in roof pitch. The internal architecture in bone may be similarly modified. Bone becomes stronger if the trabeculae become thicker and also if they are orientated at right angles to stress lines.

The relationship between stress and trabecula orientation was described by Wolff and subsequently by Frost.[3,4] In a study on sheep mandibles the degree of trabecula orientation was found to predict the resistance of the mandible to fracture.[5] Modifications to trabeculae orientation and size may still be insufficient to reduce stress down to sustainable levels, and so cortical thickness and total bone mass may be increased. The racket arm of professional tennis players gradually becomes heavier than the non-racket arm; the leg bones of long-distance runners also become heavier as their training program begins to involve marathon distances. In both these examples, this increase in bone mass takes several months. Newly enthusiastic road runners may suffer from microfractures, so-called stress fractures if they do not allow time for this restructuring and increase in bone mass to develop.

The response of bone to an increase in strain may therefore be via two mechanisms: increase in bone mass and altered arrangement of trabeculae. In contrast, a reduction in stress applied to bone may cause a shift in the balance of bone turnover leading to a net loss of bone mass. This reduction in stress occurs as a result of prolonged immobility, for example, during a long illness or during immobilization to allow healing of a bone fracture. One of the challenges of space medicine is to prevent the loss of bone mass which occurs when astronauts spend long periods in a zero-gravity environment.

An experimental model used by Rubin and Lanyon consisted of a turkey's wing bone, which was detached from all forms of loading but still had its vascular supply intact.[6] Loss of bone weight occurred immediately but could be prevented by very slight and brief periods of loading, provided that the frequency was low (15 Hz). Bone loss was also prevented by surrounding the isolated fragment with a low-frequency electromagnetic field. These experiments leave us in no doubt that certain levels of bone strain stimulate an increase in bone mass and that total absence of strain causes bone loss (*see Appendix F.2 Remodeling to Achieve Optimal Stress*).

7.7.2 Cellular Process of Bone Remodeling

The removal of bone by osteoclasts, and laying down of new bone by osteoblasts, takes place isolated from the bone marrow in what has been called a bone multicellular unit (BMU). This is a specialized vascular tunnel confined by a covering of bone cells. The essential structures within the BMU are new capillaries and bone cells. The levels of the cytokine vascular endothelial growth factor (VEGF) are raised. This factor stimulates the formation of new blood vessels and is an essential requirement of bone formation and remodeling whether during development, bone remodeling in the adult, or healing. It is known that the presence and concentration of other powerful cytokines need to be confined in this microenvironment. They are the factors which contribute to regulating the activity of osteoblasts and osteoclasts. At a cellular level, the process of remodeling is achieved by osteoclasts and osteoblasts. Osteoblasts secrete the organic as well as the calcium and phosphate salts which precipitate to form the inorganic component.

Osteoclasts are multinucleated cells which differentiate from monocytes under the influence of osteoblasts. Osteoblasts carry on their cell membranes, a ligand called receptor activator of NF-kB ligand (RANKL). This ligand binds onto a matching receptor RANK on the cell membrane of precursor osteoclasts and promotes their differentiation into mature osteoclasts. The expression of this receptor RANK on the osteoclast is stimulated by colony-stimulating factor 1 (CSF-1). CSF-1 also has a chemotactic effect on stimulating the migration of precursor osteoblasts from the blood (▸ Fig. 7.14). The receptor RANK may be blocked by a tissue cytokine called osteoprotegerin (OPG) thus preventing the activity of bone removal. OPG is increased in the presence of estrogen. This means that when estrogen levels are low, as in menopause, the blocking effect of OPG on osteoclast differentiation is removed, and there is more osteoclast activity.

The osteoclasts attach to the bone surface and secrete powerful enzymes, which dissolve bone salts and the organic components of the matrix. The acids (carbonic anhydrase) and enzymes (collagenase) used to accomplish this are toxic, and so the process is kept well isolated by a brush border, which acts as a skirt around the contact area of the cell membrane with

bone. Calcium and phosphate ions are released from the dissolved bone, and the osteoclast moves onto a new patch of bone. Bone morphogenic proteins (BMPs), which were sequestered by the osteoblast during bone formation, are also released, and they activate adjacent osteoblasts to lay down bone. The process of bone resorption and deposition thus goes on simultaneously. Resorption may balance deposition.

In summary, the differentiation and activity of osteoclasts are under the regulation of osteoblasts. Osteoclasts do not have the same reciprocal influence on osteoblasts. It has been found that osteoblasts can function even if osteoclasts have been knocked out.

7.7.3 Transformation of Stress to Bone Cells

As we have noted above, bone remodeling may be influenced by changes in the strain environment of bone which result from functional loads. The mechanism by which bone strains are transformed into chemical signals is not clear, although it is thought to be via osteocytes. Osteocytes have long cellular processes which are sensitive to deformation. They are surrounded by a fluid which is confined to channels around the osteocyte processes. Osteocytes have cilia on their cell membranes which are sensitive to fluid flowing past them. As the bone was deformed, this fluid would flow back and forth, and this movement might be detected by the osteocyte.

The deformation of bone crystals would also generate piezoelectric charges, which have been shown to influence bone remodeling. Osteocytes are all connected to each other by *gap junctions* which would transmit electrical signals between them.

Microfractures of bone cause osteocyte death which is followed by a cycle of remodeling which prevents further damage. Osteocyte death would be at the extreme upper end of a signaling process, which has to have a wide enough range to respond to both high and low levels of bone strain. When the strain falls below a certain level, the osteocyte would need to respond by downregulating bone formation to reduce bone mass, a process which would occur in prolonged states of weightlessness.

7.7.4 Tooth Repositioning

During the preeruptive phase, the tooth is repositioned from within the alveolar bone until it emerges into the oral cavity. During the next phase of eruption and posteruption, it makes contact with its opposing tooth. Further repositioning occurs as the tooth continues to erupt to compensate for occlusal wear. It is not clear what generates this posteruptive force, but as discussed in *Chapter 8 Eruption, Occlusion, and Wear*, the periodontal ligament (PDL) is probably partly responsible.

Erupted teeth are not rigidly held in their socket but can be displaced during chewing by as much as 20 μm in a lateral direction, though much less in an axial direction. This movement is partly due to the resilience of the PDL, but it is also due to deformation of the bone around the tooth socket. During tooth displacement, therefore, some compression of the PDL and alveolar bone occurs, where the pressure is greatest. If tooth displacement is sustained or frequent, the tooth may

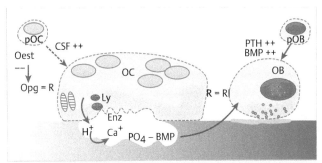

Fig. 7.14 A diagrammatic representation of the interaction between preosteoclasts and osteoblasts during bone remodeling. Preosteoblasts (pOB) are stimulated to differentiate into mature osteoblasts by parathyroid hormone (PTH) and bone morphogenic protein (BMP). Preosteoclasts (pOC) are induced to migrate from blood vessels under the influence of colony-stimulating factor (CSF), which also activates the expression of the ligand RANK (R), on the membrane of pOC. When this ligand binds onto RANKL (Rl) on the cell membrane of the osteoblast (OB), the induction of the preosteoclast to differentiate is completed. Osteoclast lysosomes (Ly) produce enzymes (Enz) and acids (H⁺) which dissolve bone salts (Ca⁺ and PO₄⁻) and remove bone matrix in a safely contained area. Released from the dissolving bone, BMP acts as a positive feedback loop by stimulating new bone formation by the odontoblast (*shaded blue*). The receptor RANK on the osteoclast cell membrane is blocked by the cytokine osteoprotegerin (Opg), which therefore inhibits the maturation of pro-osteoclasts, and bone resorption is reduced. The secretion of Opg is inhibited by estrogen (Oest). During menopause, when estrogen levels drop, Opg levels rise, as does the activity of osteoclasts which leads to osteoporosis, a loss of bone mass.

reposition permanently in the socket. The new position is created by resorption of bone on the side of the tooth socket to which the tooth is being displaced and deposition of bone on the opposite side of the socket.

Teeth may be repositioned using an orthodontic appliance which produces a light sustained force, usually in a lateral direction. If the PDL on the resorption side is examined a number of characteristic features are found. There is increased osteoclast activity on the bone lining the socket, and the blood vessels appear to be compressed. Analysis of the oxygen tension in the tissue shows hypoxia on the resorption side. An increase in a number of cytokines is found on the resorption side, predominant among them are two derivatives of arachidonic acid, prostaglandins, and leukotrienes. Another prominent cytokine istumor necrosis factor (TNF). These substances are normally associated with the inflammatory reaction, and the concentration of other cytokines mediating inflammation is also increased. On the deposition side, there is greater osteoblast activity and the blood vessels are dilated.

There is some uncertainty about the nature of the signals which are transmitted to bone cells, which control the remodeling of the tooth socket.

7.7.5 Remodeling of the Tooth Socket

There is more than one possible explanation for the remodeling of a tooth socket by an orthodontic appliance. The assumptions are that there is some displacement of the tooth and some degree of compression of the soft tissue. This compression may be responsible for the anoxia, and release of cytokines which stimulate inflammation such as prostaglandins, interleukin-1 (IL-1), and TNF-α.

- *Cells signaling compression:* Compression causes an increase in the rate of differentiation of osteoclasts brought about by changes in RANKL and OPG levels. The activity of osteoclasts is raised for about 5 days after the force is applied, after which time the numbers of osteoclasts decrease due to apoptosis (programed cell death) (▶ Fig. 7.15). The conclusion is that the compression of the tissue causes via a pathway of cell messengers, the resorption of bone.

There are at least two problems with this conclusion. Firstly, it assumes that tissue compression remains sufficiently constant to trigger the cascade of events necessary to invoke osteoclast activity. In view of the rich collateral blood supply of the PDL, it seems likely that an initial rise in tissue pressure would be reduced by escape of tissue fluids through the collateral network of vessels and by absorption of water by the large matrix molecules of the connective tissue. Secondly, it is important to note that the compression generated under experimental conditions is of soft tissues, not bone. There is no proposed link between soft tissue compression and the control system, which induces skeletal bone remodeling, namely input from sensors of bone strain. It is known that the control system of skeletal bone responds to increased levels of compression by increased bone formation. Weight-supporting bones of the axial skeleton are under constant compression, yet resorption does not occur.

It is important to close the distance between a view that bone cells and their molecular environment are the key to bone remodeling and the engineer's view that bone is a

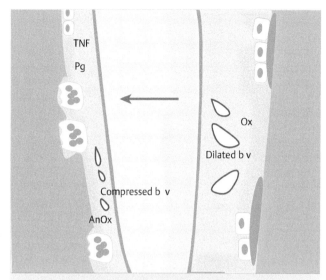

Fig. 7.15 A diagrammatic representation of the events in the periodontal ligament (PDL) following tooth displacement. Pressure on the side of the PDL to which the tooth is displaced causes compression of blood vessels (bv), hypoxia (AnOx), an increase in prostaglandins (Pg) and tumor necrosis factor (TNF). These factors, and others, account for the activation of osteoclasts and resorption of bone. The side of the PDL opposite to that which is compressed shows increased vascularity (Ox) and bone formation.

structural element and as such its structural design will be influenced primarily by patterns of bone strain during loading, which brings us to the possibility that there is another explanation for the process of tooth repositioning following tooth displacement.

- *Protective reaction:* The bone resorption observed as a result of soft tissue compression may be a protective reaction driven by cell messengers to relieve the compression and ischemia, which may cause damage and possible necrosis to soft tissues. The bone resorption which occurs in the socket of a tooth under a constant orthodontic force and that which occurs on the residual alveolar ridge under the functional loads of a removable appliance may be protective of soft tissues, rather than the result of a requirement for structural remodeling.

7.7.6 Tooth Displacement and Cell Rests of Malassez

It is possible that factors other than soft tissue compression and a protective reaction could operate during the repositioning of a tooth due to orthodontic forces. The first factor to consider is that a tooth repositions not due to the force applied but due to its *displacement* in the tooth socket. The distinction is of course only slight, as one causes the other, but it has to be noted that very light forces, not sufficient to cause compression, may cause displacement.

For example, tooth repositioning occurs quite naturally as a result of approximal wear and the gradual *mesial drift* of the dentition. The relatively light forces responsible for this wear and subsequent drift do not have to be high enough to compress the PDL but just enough to displace the tooth, perhaps only microns.

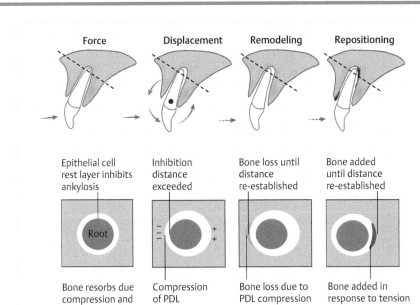

Fig. 7.16 A diagrammatic representation of two possible mechanisms for the remodeling of the tooth socket. A force is shown causing tooth displacement, remodeling, and finally repositioning. The epithelial cell rests (ECR) prevent ankylosis by creating an inhibiting zone, preventing bone formation. If a tooth is permanently displaced, and the periodontal space is reduced, the inhibitory zone of the ECRs comes into effect and causes bone resorption. Where the periodontal space increases the inhibitory zone is removed and bone formation occurs. The tissue compression caused when a tooth is displaced causes the releases of cytokines from periodontal fibroblasts which activates osteoclast activity resulting in bone resorption.

The epithelial cell rests of Malassez, which surround the root, are known to regulate periodontal repair. These cells have been shown to have an inhibitory influence on bone formation but a positive influence on cementum formation. They also influence osteoclasts by producing a cytokine which increases osteoclast activity.[7] Thus, if a tooth is displaced in a lateral direction, the root and its cell rests come close enough to the bone on the side to which the displacement occurs for the cell rests to initiate osteoclastic activity.[8] A negative balance of bone would occur with loss of bone on the displaced side of the socket. Tooth repositioning occurs naturally during eruption and drift, without conspicuous force being applied, though sufficient clearly, to induce tooth repositioning (▶ Fig. 7.16).

7.7.7 Response of Alveolar Bone to Dentures

When the teeth are removed, the bone around the tooth resorbs, leaving a residual alveolar ridge of bone on which dentures may be placed. In the mandible, this resorption occurs more rapidly than it does in the maxilla. Resorption of the mandibular residual alveolar ridge may continue until there is so little left of the body of the mandible that there is danger of fracture. It is customary to assume that dentures contribute to this bone loss, and this does seem to be the case in most patients. However, there are edentulous patients from very poor communities, who have never worn dentures but yet have lost most of their alveolar bone. The actual cause of bone loss in these cases is not clear, but the influence of a reduction of normal bone strains may be responsible. If bone strain stimulates bone formation, dentures might be expected to maintain alveolar bone, although in the usual course of events, bone resorbs in spite, or perhaps because, of wearing dentures.

There are important differences between loading the alveolar bone via teeth and via a denture. With the teeth present, the transmission of a bite force to bone is via the PDL. This ligament is rich in collagen and large matrix molecules. It is thus well

designed to resist compression, provided that the entire ligament area is recruited for support. This occurs when the bite force is predominantly directed down the long axis of the tooth. The force is thus safely transmitted to bone without soft tissue damage. However, the denture transmits its load through a single layer of oral mucosa, the total area of which, perhaps 12 cm^2 for a mandibular denture, is far less than the estimated 200 cm^2 of PDL. So, the pressure on oral mucosa under a mandibular denture is considerably greater than on the PDL. The periosteum is a membrane of bone cells covering the outer surfaces of bone. This membrane is trapped, and pinched, like the mucosa superficial to it, between the denture and the underlying bone. It would not be surprising, though there are no data, if it were found that cells in the periosteum were compressed as much by a denture as cells in the PDL are compressed by an orthodontic appliance. If bite forces could be transmitted direct to the bone, resorption should not occur, in fact, the bone should respond well to compressive strains. This direct transmission is achieved by dental implants.

7.7.8 Response of Bone to Implants

Dental implants are placed in bone, and in orthodox techniques left completely unloaded for 3 months. This period of rest is to allow an intimate attachment of bone to the fixture surface, known as osseous integration. It may be possible at placement of the implant to achieve primary fixation. This requires that a threaded fixture can be screwed into an identically sized osteotomy site, with sufficient torque to be stable enough to support light loads immediately.

The stable fixation of the implant within bone is as important as the stable fixation of the two sections of a fractured bone, which may be achieved with a plaster cast, or metal pins. Even microscopic motion during this phase of reunion may cause later failure.

A recent development in bone research is the use of BMPs, harvested from primate bone, to encourage bone repair of surgical defects. BMP for clinical use is available and is the only bone cytokine to have been licensed. A readily available stimulus to healing around an implant is to use the patient's own platelets. Platelet-rich plasma is harvested from the patient and placed into the prepared implant site.

Once union between the implant and bone has occurred, the implant may be safely loaded. The bite force is now directly transmitted to the bone and restores stimulating levels of bone strain. The trabeculae start to becomes denser around the implant, and further bone loss is halted.[9,10] The shape of an implant may alter the distribution of bone strain, and therefore design is an important factor in maintaining bone around the implant.

7.7.9 Systemic Factors and Bone Turnover

There are systemic factors which contribute to bone remodeling such as the levels of parathyroid hormone, thyroxine, growth hormone, and estrogen. One of the vital functions of bone is to participate in calcium homeostasis. This is maintained by endocrine activity, causing the release or removal of calcium from the blood. There is a reduction in both intake and absorption of calcium with ageing. Muscle activity is also reduced which further contributes to a negative bone balance. The loss of bone mass in the elderly can be reduced by a well-balanced diet, physical activity, and the avoidance of bone toxins such as smoking, alcohol, high-protein, and caffeine intake.

Bone loss may begin early in middle-aged women, as a result of a reduction in estrogen associated with menopause. Estrogen inhibits the activity of osteoclasts by suppressing osteoprotegerin synthesis, so when levels diminish, activity of osteoclasts increases (▶ Fig. 7.14). Thus, loss of bone mass with age or menopause is not due to reduction in osteoblast activity (bone healing is not impaired) but due to increased activity of osteoclasts. When there is a widespread and sustained negative balance in bone turnover, it causes a progressive loss of total bone mass, a condition known as *osteoporosis*. This condition may result in such weakening of the bones that they fracture readily, a common site being the vertebrae and the hip. Osteoporosis may be managed by the patient taking the drug bisphosphonate. This drug inhibits the increase in osteoclast activity and reduces the bone resorption. Unfortunately, there may be complications from high levels of this drug, which may affect the healing of an extraction socket and cause an uncontrollable necrosis of alveolar bone.

Osteoporosis is less common in people of African than of Caucasoid origin. This may account for the observation that loss of alveolar bone following tooth extraction appears to be less noticeable in African patients. Osteoporosis appears to occur more frequently within the same family.

Key Notes

Bone remodels in response to levels of strain, which either exceed or fail to reach optimum levels. Levels of bone strain are perceived by changes in fluid flow around osteocyte cell processes and by piezoelectric currents, generated in bone crystal. Bone surfaces may be resorbed, in response to compression, in order to prevent damage to cells of the periodontal ligament or periosteum.

Review Questions

1. What is the possible origin of bone inhibiting factors in the periodontal ligament?
2. What evidence is there that bone mass is lost after long periods of inactivity?
3. What is the link between estrogen levels and osteoclast activity?
4. What is the difference between strain developing in soft tissue such as the periodontal ligament and strain developing in bone?
5. What role could the cell rests of Malassez have in the remodeling of the tooth socket?
6. Why is bone loss inevitable in the elderly and how can it be minimized?

References

[1] Moss ML, Salentijn L. The primary role of functional matrices in facial growth. Am J Orthod 1969;55(6):566–577
[2] Richards GD, Jabbour RS. Foramen magnum ontogeny in Homo sapiens: a functional matrix perspective. Anat Rec (Hoboken) 2011;294(2):199–216
[3] Wolff J, Maquet PGJ, Furlong R. The law of bone remodeling. New York, NY: Springer-Verlag; 1986:126
[4] Frost HMA. A 2003 update of bone physiology and Wolff's Law for clinicians. Angle Orthod 2004;74(1):3–15
[5] Wilding RJC, Ferguson MM, Farr N, McKellar G. Changes in bone strength during fracture repair predicted by fractal analysis of radiographs. Proceedings of the 2nd International Meeting of Fractals in Biology and Medicine. Ascona, Switzerland: Kargar; 1997
[6] Rubin CT, Lanyon LE. Regulation of bone formation by applied dynamic loads. Calcif Tissue Int 1985;37:411–417
[7] Talic N, Evans CA, Daniel JC, George A, Zaki AM. Immunohistochemical localization of alphavbeta3 integrin receptor during experimental tooth movement. Am J Orthod Dentofacial Orthop 2004;125(2):178–184
[8] Lindskog S, Blomlöf L, Hammarström L. Evidence for a role of odontogenic epithelium in maintaining the periodontal space. J Clin Periodontol 1988;15(6):371–373
[9] Wilding RJC, Slabbert JGC, Kathree H, Delport P, Owen CP, Crombie K. The use of fractal analysis to reveal remodeling in alveolar bone following the placement of dental implants. Arch Oral Biol 1995;40:61–72
[10] Suer BT, Yaman Z, Buyuksarac B. Correlation of fractal dimension values with implant insertion torque and resonance frequency values at implant recipient sites. Int J Oral Maxillofac Implants 2016;31(1):55–62

Suggested Readings

Mechanisms of Mineralization

Cui L, Houston DA, Farquharson C, MacRae VE. Characterisation of matrix vesicles in skeletal and soft tissue mineralisation. Bone 2016;87:147–158

Development of the Skull and Jaws

Berkowitz BWK, Moxham BJ, Linden RWA, Sloan AJ. Oral Biology; Oral Anatomy Histology, Physiology and Biochemistry. London: Churchill Livingstone; 2010.

Growth of the Skull and Jaws

Atkinson PJ. Patterns of bone growth. In: Poole DFG, Stack MV, eds. The Eruption and Occlusion of Teeth. Colston Papers No 27. Boston, MA: Butterworths; 1976
Björk A, Skieller V. Facial development and tooth eruption. An implant study at the age of puberty. Am J Orthod 1972;62(4):339–383

Enlow DH. Childhood Facial Growth and Development in Oral Histology by Ten Cate. Mosby; 1989.

Hoyte DAN. Growth of the face and jaws compared with the rest of the skeleton. In: Poole DFG, Stack MV, eds. The Eruption and Occlusion of Teeth. Colston Papers No. 27. Boston, MA: Butterworths; 1976

Lavelle CLB, Osborn JW. Growth of the skull and jaws. In: Osborn JW, ed. Dental Anatomy and Embryology. Oxford, United Kingdom: Blackwell Scientific Publications; 1981

Standerwick RG, Roberts WE. The aponeurotic tension model of craniofacial growth in man. Open Dent J 2009;3:100–113

Bone Remodeling

Eriksen EF. Cellular mechanisms of bone remodeling. Rev Endocr Metab Disord 2010;11(4):219–227

Feng X. Chemical and biochemical basis of cell-bone matrix interaction in health and disease. Curr Chem Biol 2009;3(2):189–196

Fujiyama K, Yamashiro T, Fukunaga T, Balam TA, Zheng L, Takano-Yamamoto T. Denervation resulting in dento-alveolar ankylosis associated with decreased Malassez epithelium. J Dent Res 2004;83(8):625–629

Georgiadis M, Guizar-Sicairos M, Gschwend O, et al. Ultrastructure organization of human trabeculae assessed by 3D sSAXS and relation to bone microarchitecture. PLoS One 2016;11(8):e0159838

Maes C, Kobayashi T, Selig MK, et al. Osteoblast precursors, but not mature osteoblasts, move into developing and fractured bones along with invading blood vessels. Dev Cell 2010;19(2):329–344

Mackie EJ. Osteoblasts: novel roles in orchestration of skeletal architecture. Int J Biochem Cell Biol 2003;35(9):1301–1305

Robling AG, Castillo AB, Turner CH. Biomechanical and molecular regulation of bone remodeling. Annu Rev Biomed Eng 2006;8:455–498

Sandy JR. Tooth eruption and orthodontic movement. Br Dent J 1992;172(4):141–149

Seeman E. Structural basis of growth-related gain and age-related loss of bone strength. Rheumatology (Oxford) 2008;47(Suppl 4):iv2–iv8

Talic NF, Evans CA, Daniel JC, Zaki AE. Proliferation of epithelial rests of Malassez during experimental tooth movement. Am J Orthod Dentofacial Orthop 2003;123(5):527–533

Wang Y, Jia L, Zheng Y. Bone remodeling induced by mechanical forces is regulated by miRNAs. Biosci Rep 2018;38(4)

Xiong J, Mrozik K, Gronthos S, Bartold PM. Epithelial cell rests of Malassez contain unique stem cell populations capable of undergoing epithelial-mesenchymal transition. Stem Cells Dev 2012;21(11):2012–2025

8 Eruption, Occlusion, and Wear

Abstract

Eruption is a lifelong activity, which begins with the emergence of a tooth from the alveolar bone, and then proceeds to the more gradual process, which keeps the tooth in contact with its opponent in order to compensate for tooth wear. The stability of the dentition is influenced by the nature of forces transmitted to teeth. The effect these forces have is partly determined by the direction, magnitude, and frequency of the force and also the angles of the occlusal surfaces of opposing teeth. Forces generated by the tongue are also of great influence to the stability of the dentition. There is considerable variation in the size, and relationship, between the maxillary and mandibular dental arches, which, while they may not be considered ideal, are nevertheless quite normal and functional. Tooth wear is also normal, in fact a requirement of efficient masticatory function, though it is seen by many clinicians as undesirable and requiring repair or reconstruction.

Keywords: eruption, stability, arch form, normal occlusion, ideal, tooth wear

8.1 Eruption

8.1.1 Phases of Eruption

Eruption is a lifelong process, but it can be conveniently described in three main phases (▶ Fig. 8.1).

- The preeruptive phase describes the passage of a tooth from its crypt in the alveolar bone, through the bone between it and the oral cavity, through the oral mucosa and into the oral cavity. The tooth takes with it the remains of the enamel epithelium which becomes the future epithelial attachment.
- The eruptive phase describes the migration of the tooth into the oral cavity until it makes contact with the tooth in the opposing arch. The deciduous teeth make this journey uninterrupted, but some of the permanent teeth which succeed a deciduous tooth are only able to erupt after the roots of the deciduous tooth have been resorbed by osteoclasts.
- The posteruptive phase describes the continued eruption of the tooth as wear occurs. Movement of the tooth is considerably slower in this phase of eruption than the preceding two.

A permanent tooth may take 2 to 4 years to move through the alveolar bone and into occlusion. Its most rapid progress is seen just after breaking through the oral mucosa, when its root would be two-thirds complete. The maxillary incisors show the most rapid movement, about 1 mm/mo. Molar teeth achieve only half this rate, and if crowded move at 1 mm/6 mo.

8.1.2 Formation of the Epithelial Attachment

When enamel formation is complete, the internal and external enamel epithelium fuse to form the reduced enamel epithelium

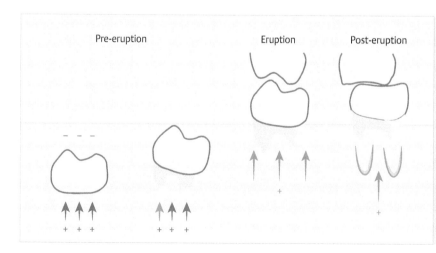

Fig. 8.1 A diagrammatic representation of the three phases of tooth eruption. During the preeruptive phase, bone deposition at the base of the follicle and resorption of the overlying alveolar bone cause the tooth bud to migrate toward the surface. During the eruptive stage, root growth and continued bone deposition at the base of the root allow the tooth to emerge into the oral cavity. During the posteruptive stage, periodontal ligament tension provides the continued eruption against the opposing tooth as wear occurs. The slow apposition of cementum and further alveolar bone growth compensate for tooth wear.

Pre-eruption   Eruption   Post-eruption

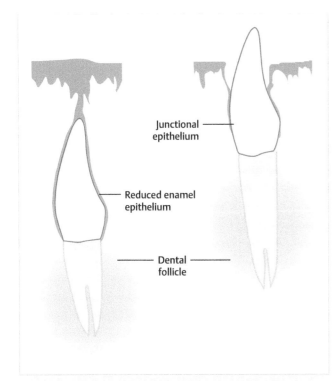

Fig. 8.2 A diagrammatic representation of the formation of the epithelial attachment and the gingival sulcus. The reduced enamel epithelium fuses with the oral epithelium before the tooth erupts. The tooth moves through a core of epithelium, so that connective tissue and the dental follicle are never exposed to the oral cavity. The is converted to the epithelium of the gingival sulcus, but where it remains attached to enamel it becomes the junctional epithelium.

Junctional epithelium

Reduced enamel epithelium

Dental follicle

(REE). The cells still in contact with the enamel develop hemidesmosome, which attaches to the enamel surface. As the tooth erupts, the REE cells mingle with the oral epithelium and hence form a "junction" between the tooth and the future gingiva (► Fig. 8.2). At no time during eruption, there is a break in this epithelium, and hence there is no bleeding or risk of infection as the tooth emerges through the oral mucosa. During eruption of the first teeth, they may provoke a mild immune response comprising swelling around the erupting tooth and a slight fever. After the first few teeth have erupted, the process generally occurs without the child noticing that a new tooth has arrived. The erupting permanent tooth passes through a band of fibrous connective tissue, the gubernaculum, which connects the tooth germ with the oral mucosa. So, like the deciduous tooth, the permanent tooth does not cause a break in the epithelium as it erupts into the mouth.

8.1.3 Eruptive Mechanisms

For the unerupted tooth to emerge from its bony surrounds, it is clear that two processes have to occur. The first is the removal of bone above the tooth to create a pathway for the tooth to emerge. The second is the deposition of bone under the developing root of the tooth to help move the unerupted tooth out of the alveolar bone. These two processes are achieved by bone

remodeling, which we have noted is an event which is controlled by osteoblasts, which mediate the removal of bone over the tooth by osteoclasts. Osteoblasts lay down new bone under the growing root. The molecular events which control bone deposition and removal around the erupting tooth and its follicle are similar to those described in bone remodeling (*see Chapter 7.7 Bone Remodeling*). Just before eruption begins, there is a burst of osteoclast activity above the follicle. This is initiated by the protein colony-stimulating factor 1 (CSF-1). This factor attracts monocytes from the blood and also blocks osteoprotegerin (OPG), an inhibitor of the differentiation of monocytes into osteoclasts. The influences of CSF-1 are augmented by raised levels of vascular endothelial growth factor (VEGF). VEGF initiates angiogenesis (new blood vessel formation), and receptor activator of nuclear factor kappa-B ligand (RANKL), which stimulates the differentiation of osteoclasts. At the same time, bone is being deposited at the base of the follicle which is reflected by raised levels of the bone morphogenic protein (BMP). The importance of the osteoclasts and osteoblasts in eruption is confirmed by several studies which show that a tooth will not erupt if the dental follicle is removed. These two mechanisms, bone deposition and bone removal, explain the preeruptive phase of eruption in which the tooth emerges from the alveolar bone. There have, however, been some alternative explanations which have been popular:

- Tissue fluid pressure within the pulpal tissue was thought to help push the tooth out. The evidence, however, is contradictory, so this explanation has not stood up to scrutiny.
- Root elongation occurs as the tooth emerges until the root is fully formed. There is no evidence that root growth is an eruptive force in the preeruptive phase as rootless teeth can erupt, and teeth may fail to erupt, though they have fully developed roots.

During the eruptive and posteruptive phase, alveolar bone growth continues although once the preeruptive phase is over, there is no bone to impede the tooth's progress and no further need for any osteoclastic activity. If bone growth at the base of the tooth continued at the preeruptive rate, it would soon exfoliate the tooth. Bone deposition around the emerging root is, however, essential in providing the full development of the tooth socket. Periodontal ligament tension was thought to be able to pull the tooth out of its socket. This does not seem possible during the preeruptive phases, as inert replicas are able to erupt without any ligament.

There is evidence that the periodontal ligament fibroblasts may exert some tensional force on the tooth during its eruptive and posteruptive phases. During the posteruptive phase, both continued active eruption and bone growth may be mechanisms of compensating for tooth wear. No theory of tooth eruption mechanism can claim to account for all aspects of eruption. A view has emerged that eruption might be brought about by different mechanisms at different stages, which at the present state of our knowledge is probably the best explanation. Deposition and removal of alveolar bone may be the driving mechanism at the preeruptive stage while periodontal ligament forces may be mostly responsible for posteruptive and continued eruption.

8.1.4 Tooth Position after Eruption

The final position of a tooth which has erupted into the mouth is thought to be determined by a balance of all the forces acting on it. The forces include the following:
- An eruptive force directed coronally.
- A biting force directed down the long axis of a tooth toward the root apex, which would balance the eruptive force. If the bite force were directed at an angle to the long axis of a tooth, it would cause the tooth to rotate, and reposition laterally. When a cusp articulates well into the opposing tooth fossa, such laterally displacing forces are reduced. Cusps may serve to guide the erupting tooth into a stable position within the dental arch.
- The lateral forces of the tongue and lips. The forces of the tongue are especially powerful during swallowing.
- The lateral forces encountered by adjacent teeth (*see Chapter 1.2.3 Tooth Wear in Man*).

The magnitude, direction, duration, and frequency of all these forces make impossible any simple equation which might determine the equilibrium position of a tooth. However, when one of the above components is completely absent from the equation, the consequences may be predictable. If there is no opposing tooth (most commonly due to extraction), the eruptive force of a tooth is unopposed, and it may continue to erupt. If this does happen, the tooth appears to bring its gingival attachment and the alveolar bone with it at first. This has been termed periodontal growth, and may occur quite naturally in subjects whose teeth have been worn by a course diet (*see Chapter 8.3.2 Consequences of Tooth Wear*). If the tooth continues to erupt without the alveolar bone, the distance from the cementoenamel junction (CEJ) to the alveolar bone crest increases. This process has been termed *active eruption*. Later, the gingival and periodontal attachment may move apically and the root surface may be exposed. This process is termed *passive eruption*. These observations suggest that continued eruption occurs both due to alveolar bone growth and the active eruption of the tooth.

Overeruption due to loss of opposing teeth may destabilize the entire arch of teeth and in order to prevent this, especially in young children, appliances may be fabricated which exert a light but sufficient force to prevent overeruption.

8.1.5 Incomplete Eruption

The complete eruption of a tooth may be blocked by other teeth whose eruption is more advance, and already have occupied a place in the dental arch. One of the most common sights for this incomplete eruption is the mandibular third molar. The bud of this tooth may be orientated in a mesial direction, and unless there is sufficient space for it to erupt mesially and coronally, its eruption is blocked by the second molar. Less common is for the maxillary canine tooth bud to be orientated in a horizontal direction, and this position may make eruption impossible. More commonly, the maxillary canine does erupt into the oral cavity, but there is insufficient space, and it is blocked out of the arch in a labial position. This problem occurs as the maxillary canine is the last tooth to erupt, and there may not be sufficient space after all the other teeth have erupted.

Overcrowding is a common problem in the modern human dentition. Human teeth vary considerably in size; the teeth of males are slightly larger than the teeth of females. Anthropological studies reveal a *normal distribution* of tooth sizes throughout a population. A normal distribution means that if the frequency of the data is plotted on a curve, it is evenly distributed and the curve looks like a bell. there will be a similar proportion of individuals at one end of the curve, who have unusually small teeth, and an equally similar number of individuals at the opposite end of the curve, who have unusually large teeth. One of our ancestors (or cousins), Australopithecus *robustus*, had huge teeth and an unusually large jaws to accommodate them. If we should inherit a tendency for larger teeth and a smaller face, the problems of overcrowding are likely.

It is common to assume that the contact of a tooth in the opposing arch is required to prevent continued or overeruption. An uncommon growth disorder causes a failure in alignment of the maxillary and mandibular dental arch. The result is called an anterior open bite. It can be so severe that only the third molars meet when the jaw is closed. It is surprising therefore to find that the teeth do not overerupt. This condition may require surgical repositioning of entire sections of the teeth and alveolar bone. It is not certain what would be the long-term stability of the dentition if it were not treated.

8.1.6 Deciduous Dentition

The deciduous dentition consists of five teeth in each quadrant, two incisors (1 and 2), a canine (3), and two molars (4 and 5). The purpose of the deciduous dentition is to provide the growing child with effective chewing ability consistent with the size of the jaws. It allows time for the development and growth of larger and more durable teeth. The first deciduous teeth begin to calcify in the fourth month of pregnancy and erupt 6 months after birth (▶ Fig. 8.3). The mandibular incisors are the first to erupt, followed by the maxillary incisors. The next teeth are not the canines but the first deciduous molars. Then come the canines and lastly the second molar. In most cases, the mandibular teeth erupt before their maxillary counterparts. Root formation continues to occur from 12 to 18 months after a tooth has erupted. By the age of 2 to 4 years, the entire deciduous dentition has erupted (▶ Fig. 8.4).

No permanent teeth will erupt until the age of 6 or 7, but the formation of the permanent teeth is already advanced. The permanent incisors and first molars begin to calcify at birth. At the age of 4, the crowns are fully formed.

8.1.7 Differences between Deciduous and Permanent Teeth

Size: The deciduous teeth are smaller than the permanent teeth.

Enamel: The enamel of deciduous teeth is whiter and opaquer. It is also softer and so wears more rapidly.

Crown: The crown shape of anterior deciduous teeth is more bulbous than permanent teeth.

Root: The roots of deciduous teeth are shorter and narrower than those of permanent teeth.

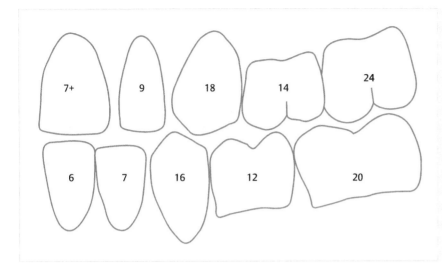

Fig. 8.3 A chart of the age in months, when each tooth of the deciduous dentition erupts.

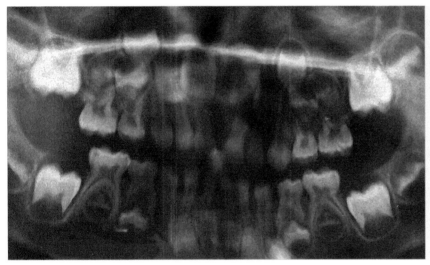

Fig. 8.4 A panoramic radiograph of the dentition of a 4-year-old boy. All the deciduous teeth have erupted. Note that the crown formations of the first permanent molars are complete.

Dental pulp: The pulp chambers in deciduous teeth are larger, but the pulp canals are narrower than permanent teeth. In deciduous teeth, there is no clear distinction between the pulp chamber and the root canal, whereas in permanent teeth, there tend to be clearly defined entrances to the root canal. This is particularly true of multirooted teeth where there is a well-defined floor of the pulp chamber with separate openings for each root canal.

8.1.8 Mixed Dentition

The changeover period between the deciduous and permanent dentition happens gradually, so that there is a period, the mixed dentition, when there are both deciduous and permanent teeth. This stage begins with the eruption of the permanent maxillary incisors at 6 years and ends with the loss of the last deciduous tooth, the canines. During the mixed dentition period, the permanent teeth erupt in a fairly predictable order although there is some variation seen (▶ Fig. 8.5). Eruption of the permanent teeth may be earlier than normal if the overlying deciduous tooth is extracted early. If the deciduous second molar is lost early due to caries, the permanent first molar may drift forward

as it erupts, thereby reducing the space for the second premolar which may then be crowded out.

Key Notes

As a tooth erupts into the oral cavity, it becomes subject to a variety of forces. The final position occupied by the tooth is not just dependent on the magnitude of these forces, but also the duration, frequency, and direction of these forces. Light continuous forces may have a greater impact than infrequent, short-acting, high forces.

Review Questions

1. What is to be gained by dividing eruption into different phases?
2. What forces in the ligament could generate tension?
3. When do the first deciduous teeth begin to calcify?
4. Tetracycline antibiotics have a side effect of staining developing teeth gray. If a child was given tetracycline at the age of 6 months, which teeth would you expect to show staining?

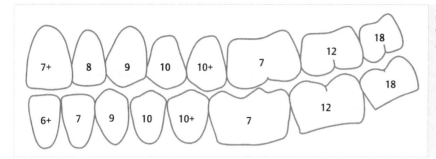

Fig. 8.5 A chart of the age in years, when each tooth of the permanent dentition erupts. The ages are approximate and for females.

5. What are the possible causes of incomplete eruption in permanent teeth?
6. When do the first permanent teeth begin to calcify?
7. What is meant by the mixed dentition?
8. What is the difference in age between the eruption of the permanent maxillary and mandibular incisors?
9. What situations may cause failure of a tooth to erupt?

8.2 Occlusion

Occlusion is a topic which has exercised the minds of dentists for the last 100 years. There have been entire schools of occlusal philosophy, most of which have been directed toward the anatomy of occlusion or a mechanical interpretation of how the teeth work. The solution to a reliable, evidence-based understanding of occlusion is to focus on the basic physiology, with a little help from comparative evolution. This process should provide some stable ground, on which to choose from the many prescribed clinical practices in occlusion, with some expectation that the choices are based on sound evidence and not on dogma.

8.2.1 Stability of the Dentition

Mammals experience relatively little trouble from their teeth. Their gnawing/nibbling/crushing food processors last lifelong without needing repair. If we look at a mammalian skull, the teeth appear to be indestructible pegs fixed into the jaw bone, but of course they are not static. They are responsive to change, such as physical wear and demineralization, and they are not fixed permanently in one position. In comparison, dental implants are completely static. The long life of mammalian teeth is partly due to characteristics acquired over millions of years of evolutionary selection and also due to their interaction with other teeth which bring stability to the whole and its parts. Modern human dentitions are not as stable as those of our ancient human relatives. We experience caries and periodontal disease which reduce the life of individual teeth and eventually the entire dentition. Loss of even one or more teeth may cause instability in the teeth remaining. This instability may be due to over-eruption when an opposing tooth is lost, or tilting and drifting into a space left by the loss of a neighboring tooth in the arch.

As the dentition is reduced by tooth loss, the load on the remaining teeth becomes excessive, and they become even more unstable and collapse. With dental treatment we try to reduce the disease processes and to restore the stability of individual teeth and the dentition as a unit. It is useful to understand the factors which maintain the stability of the dentition, so as to ensure our restorations contribute to long-term occlusal stability.

8.2.2 Arch Stability

It has been noted above that after eruption teeth stabilize in a position where forces acting on them are in equilibrium. Thus, a tooth would occupy a position in the arch, where the pressures of the tongue and lips were equalized. This theory is supported by the observation that tongue-thrusting habits in children tend to create a longer arch and splay the anterior teeth forward. However, Proffit has shown that even in children without a thrusting tongue, the forward/outward pressures of the tongue during swallowing are considerably greater than the inward forces of lips and cheeks.[1] He therefore doubts that a position of equilibrium exists due to a balance of soft tissue pressures alone. There are other factors which determine the stability of the arch and these include the way the teeth meet each other, occlusion. We have seen that teeth are able to reposition in the bony socket as a result of forces acting on them. For example, teeth drift in a mesial direction as a result of approximal tooth wear and a mesial component of the bite force. This mesial component might be quite a small force. What about the much larger bite forces which would tend to intrude the teeth? When cracking a nut, we may be able to exert a bite force on a single tooth of up to 100 kg. Why does this tooth not become intruded by remodeling of the socket? Proffit reminds us that the magnitude of the force is not the only factor which could cause the tooth to reposition. Duration, frequency, and direction of the force are as important as magnitude in determining how living tissue will respond to force. When cracking a nut, let us consider these other factors:

- The duration of the force is very short—it is all over in less than a second.
- The frequency is very low; we do not crack nuts all day.
- The direction of the bite force is more or less down the long axis of the tooth, so we are spreading the load over the entire periodontal ligament. In spite of the high magnitude of force used in cracking a nut, the supporting tissues are not damaged and do not remodel.

Let us now return to explain the apparent paradox of Proffit's findings. During swallowing, the tongue pushes harder against the mandibular teeth than the lip does. However, the duration of the swallow is short, and the frequency is relatively low. The lip, on the other hand, exerts a light force against the teeth, but its duration is very long and the frequency is continuous. It is the light continual forces which orthodontists find move teeth most effectively, not intermittent high forces. So, continual light muscle forces of the lip may well balance out the infrequent high forces of the tongue, leaving the tooth at the end of the day, balanced by the influences of the lip and the tongue. If the duration and forces generated by the tongue are abnormally high or the lip muscles are flaccid and incompetent, the balance may be disturbed and the teeth may become displaced.

We have noted that there is a mesial direction of force generated during biting which tends to push the teeth forward, keeping the teeth together and the arch intact. If a tooth is lost and the support it gave to its neighbors reduced, the neighboring teeth may rotate into the space it occupied. If the posterior sections of the arch are lost, the maxillary anterior teeth may splay out labially, as they are readily rotated, by having to withstand the full impact of the bite forces which are not directed down the long axis of the tooth (▶ Fig. 8.6). These are the factors which tend to destabilize the arch:

- Loss of one or several teeth causes loss of approximal contact, drifting and tipping; overeruption of an opposing tooth; loss of posterior support; abnormal distribution on remaining teeth.
- Abnormally high-frequency tongue activity which is not necessary for function (parafunctional).
- Absence of adequate muscle tone of the lips (incompetence or mouth breathing).

8.2.3 Tooth Stability

We have reviewed some of the factors which may determine the stability of the dental arch. Let us now consider the factors which may determine the stability of individual teeth. During eruption, teeth are at their most responsive to external forces. One important factor determining the position of an erupting tooth is the stability provided by a balance of muscle forces on the arch. For example, sometimes an incisor erupts slightly out of alignment. However, after a few months it regains its alignment with other teeth. This alignment may be due to the tooth

taking up a position of equilibrium in the arch between lingual and labial forces, but there is another equilibrium and that is between opposing cusps and fossae. As the erupting tooth makes contact with its opposing teeth, the forces generated during biting come into play. We have noted above that cusps may help to align some teeth into a stable relationship, but this early alignment may be abnormal. For example, the emerging maxillary incisor may get trapped behind the mandibular incisor (▶ Fig. 8.7). It is stabilized by the "cusp" of the mandibular incisor and may remain there, in crossbite. This stability is due to the absence of any dislodging force. During chewing and swallowing the maxillary incisor is not subjected to any destabilizing forces. With a little intervention though, using an appliance which holds the teeth apart for a period, and at the same time pushes the incisor forwards, the offending tooth "jumps-the-bite." The appliance may then be removed, as stability is

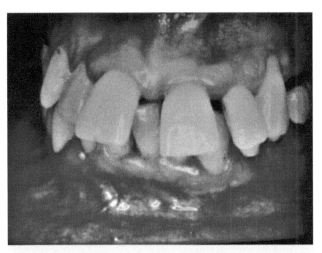

Fig. 8.6 A clinical example showing the collapse of the anterior teeth due to loss of posterior support. Loss of posterior teeth may place excessive loads on the anterior teeth. The inclined contacts are unstable and cause the maxillary anterior teeth to splay outward. Occlusal vertical height is reduced.

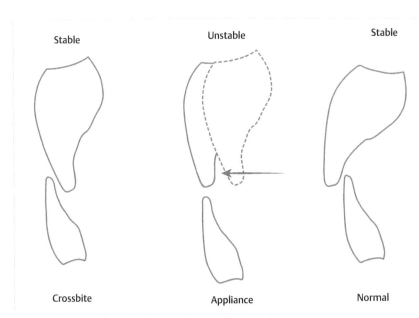

Stable | Unstable | Stable

Crossbite | Appliance | Normal

Fig. 8.7 A diagrammatic representation of an incisor crossbite, which is corrected by a removable appliance. The maxillary incisor is stable in a crossbite relationship. Instability is achieved with a removable appliance which increases the vertical dimension, sufficiently to allow the maxillary incisor to be repositioned. Once stabilized again, there is no further need for the appliance.

restored and the tooth does not jump back to its original position. It is likely that the same sort of stability is achieved once the cusps of posterior teeth have found an opposing fossa. Once positioned into the arch, they are quite stable, and only repositioned as a result of tooth wear. If posterior teeth erupt into a crossbite, they may remain there until corrected by orthodontic treatment.

This role of cusps holds true for herbivores. However, the high single cusps of some teeth serve a different purpose. The canines of carnivores are used to pierce and tear at prey, and they also serve to guide the carnassial (premolar) teeth past each other when cutting through skin, tendons, and bone. Carnassial teeth themselves are high-cusped teeth and vulnerable to fracture, especially during the high bite forces exerted by carnivores. They would impact together and break down without the guidance offered by the canines. Carnassial teeth also must be worn to remain sharp and to reposition constantly in order to remain in contact with the opposite tooth during function. The term *canine guidance* has been used to describe the protection and guidance canines provide in the human dentition as high-cusped premolar posterior teeth are brought together in a scissor-like action.

Orthodontic treatment, which involves repositioning of individual teeth, or the entire dental arch may require some form of retention to secure the dental alterations against relapse when the appliance is removed. Some clinicians have implied that retention may have to be for an indefinite period. The challenge in maintaining a stable occlusion after orthodontic treatment highlights the complex nature of tooth and arch stability.[2]

8.2.4 The Distribution of Bite Forces on Teeth

The most powerful forces which teeth have to resist are those generated by the masticatory muscles. The magnitudes of these forces vary considerably. Within the same individual, they are highest in the first molar region when directed more or less at right angles to the occlusal plane. The position and direction of chewing forces can be estimated by a mechanical analysis of the jaw as a lever and the size and directions of the various chewing muscles (*see Chapter 9.1.2 Variable Forces at the Teeth*).

A comparison of chewing forces between individuals produces no surprises. Males are able to generate greater bite force than females, the young greater than old, the athlete (raised on a hard diet) greater than those on a soft diet, and dentate greater than edentate. These comparisons are all about magnitude. Let us look at those other factors we have identified which influence the response of living tissue to force. Forces which are frequently generated, such as those arising out of repeated habitual activity, have a far greater destabilizing affect than infrequent short-acting forces. These continuous forces may be due to habitual grinding, clenching, or finger sucking.

Given that one or more teeth may be subjected to these frequent forces, what will determine just how disrupting they may be? This will depend on how well the forces are dissipated by the supporting structures. For example, a multi-root molar is better able to resist an abnormally frequent force than a mandibular incisor, purely because it has a larger area of periodontal ligament to support the force. So, root surface area would be

the first factor which would determine the long-term effect of abnormally high or frequent biting force.

The next factor is related to the effective root surface area. If the biting force is applied down the long axis of a tooth, it is resisted by the entire periodontal ligament. If, however, a force is applied to a tooth in a lateral direction to its root, there will be a smaller area of support provided by the ligament. Orthodontists will confirm that a tooth will displace more readily by applying a lateral force than if an intrusive force is applied (▶ Fig. 8.8).

If the tooth subjected to abnormal forces has already lost periodontal support due to bone loss, it is vulnerable to even light, normal chewing forces and may be readily destabilized. Lastly, a tooth which stands out proud of its neighbors is likely to receive an unequal share of the chewing forces. This situation is described by clinicians as an *occlusal interference*. It may result from the overeruption of a tooth due to the loss of its opposing tooth. It may also occur because the tooth has been restored and the restoration overcontoured.

The important possible consequences of occlusal interference are as follows:
- Microdamage to the periodontium with vascular congestion and sensitivity to pressure.
- Pulp hypersensitivity which may develop due to inflammation around the apical nerve bundle. There may be slight extrusion of the tooth and increased mobility.
- Fracture of cusps, particularly when weakened by large intracoronal restorations.
- It has been widely claimed that occlusal interferences may cause temporomandibular dysfunction.

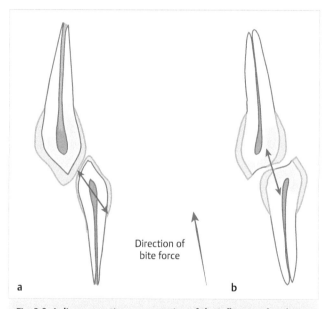

Direction of bite force

Fig. 8.8 A diagrammatic representation of the influence of occlusion contact on tooth stability. (a) When the occlusal contact is inclined to the long axis of the tooth, the reaction (*red arrows*) to the bite force is at an angle to the long axis of the roots and both teeth may be destabilized and rotate. **(b)** When contact with an opposing tooth is made on a flat plane, the reaction (*red arrows*) to the bite force is down the long axis of both teeth, and maximum periodontal support provides stability.

8.2.5 Summary

The factors which tend to destabilize individual teeth are as follows:
- Bite forces of unusually long duration and high frequency.
- A reduced root area.
- Inclined tooth contact.
- Existing periodontal disease.
- Occlusal interference.

8.2.6 Purpose of Cusps

It is important to recognize that pointed cusps which slide past each other like scissors are features of a carnivore's dentition. They have evolved for cutting and tearing. The dentition of man and his ancestors do not have carnivores' features. Our diet is probably somewhat closer to that of a herbivore, but it is not quite that either. Just where, along a line between these two classes of dentition we belong is of interest. Our modern diets, in contrast to those of our ancestors, are so soft and refined that they hardly require teeth at all. Judging from the dentitions of ancestral man, and even Stone Age man, our dentitions appear to have been used for shredding and grinding rather than cutting. They appear to have been well adapted for this work, because they have been found to be in a fair condition at the time of death. If then, our dentition evolved to suit primarily a herbivores diet, our cusps are a liability and will not last long. In fact, a case has been made in *Chapter 1 The Origins of Teeth* that the contribution of cusps to the herbivore's dentition is only fully expressed after some dentin is exposed. The purpose of cusps is to provide, when worn, a suitable pattern of composite surfaces for a particular type of chewing function. The study of occlusion in man has been sidetracked by an assumption that the ideal occlusion was one which was unworn. If a tooth was described as exhibiting wear, it was as good as saying it was "worn out."

It was thought that in the ideal occlusion the teeth should fit exactly together, each cusp in its proper fossa. It has been claimed, as noted above, that errors in cusp relationships, so-called occlusal interferences, may be also defined as "traumatic," that is they would cause or aggravate periodontal disease with loss of bone support. Occlusal interferences were also thought to be responsible for generating tensions in the muscles of mastication, a cause of chronic facial pain (*see Chapter 9.4 Temporomandibular Dysfunction*). Occlusion was therefore carefully studied, frequently on articulators, mechanical devices used to reproduce the geometry of the dentition. These studies led to narrow, but varied definitions of ideal occlusion. They were based more on ideology, of what "should" be correct anatomy and mechanism, rather than intended to reveal the diversity which was both functional and long lasting. The anatomical dogma of the ideal occlusion became the driving philosophy of a large following of dentists and even the formation of an equilibration society which promoted the elective adjustment of occlusions until ideals were met (*see Appendix H.4 Anecdotal Evidence, a Poor Substitute for Science*).

As more physiological and epidemiological methods have been applied to the study of occlusion, a different picture has emerged.

- There is a wide variation in the way teeth come together, which is functional and does not shorten the life span of the dentition.
- Criteria for the ideal occlusion need to broaden from anatomical to physiological criteria. For example, the chewing performance of an individual may tell us more about his or her oral health status, than an analysis of cusp–fossa relationships.
- The prime cause of periodontal disease is a group of motile, anaerobic, gram-negative bacteria and the host's reduced resistance to them.
- In many studies, no association has been found between chronic facial pain and abnormalities in occlusion, although the relationship between occlusion and some types of chromic facial pain, has for many years, been claimed.[3]

8.2.7 Arch and Tooth Relationships

The maxillary incisors and canines are wider than their mandibular counterparts. For this reason, the arch of the maxillary teeth is slightly wider and longer than the mandibular arch (▶ Fig. 8.9). The effect of the longer maxillary arch is to allow the maxillary teeth to meet the mandibular partner and part of the tooth distal to it. So, each tooth meets it opposite partner, and one other tooth, a so-called tooth-to-two-tooth arrangement. This allows the supporting cusps of the maxillary teeth to *intercuspate* with the fossae of the mandibular teeth, and vice versa. This arrangement contributes to stability by spreading the bite force to more than just one tooth and by allowing the cusps to pass between each other when grinding from side to side. The larger maxillary arch also provides stability by allowing the buccal cusps of the mandibular teeth to rest, supported in the central fossa of the maxillary teeth. For this reason, this mandibular buccal cusp is called a *supporting cusp*. Similarly, there is support for the maxillary palatal cusp in the central fossa of the mandibular tooth. Supporting cusps are important to preserve when making adjustments to cusps on restorations.

These supporting cusps appear as though they will provide good stability as long as the teeth are brought together directly into occlusion. However, we know that the posture and movements of the mandible are complex. The mandibular movements bring the teeth together from a variety of anterior and lateral positions. The term *maximal intercuspation* is used to describe the relationship of the teeth when they all in closest possible contact. It used to be common for dentists to believe that this good tight fit should ideally occur when the jaw was in the posture known as *centric relation*. This is when the condyles are in a retruded, unstrained position in the glenoid fossa.

This coincidence of centric relation and maximal intercuspation is not a routine finding in healthy dentitions. A simple exercise will illustrate this point. Sit upright and tuck your tongue back toward the posterior part of your palate (this will encourage a centric relation posture). Now, close your jaw slowly until the teeth meet. Do your teeth close directly into maximal intercuspation? Most likely, the posterior teeth will meet first, and in order to get all your teeth to meet, your jaw will slide slightly forward or even to one side. So, in health, maximal intercuspation does not routinely coincide with centric relation. Nevertheless, the centric relation posture is of great importance when restoring the complete dentition, as

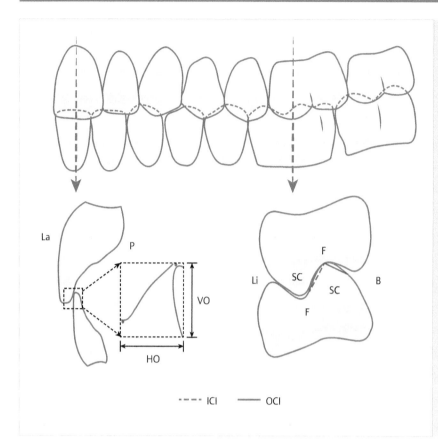

Fig. 8.9 Diagrammatic representation of arch and tooth relationships. At the top of the diagram the dentition is drawn from a lateral viewpoint to illustrate the "tooth-to-two-tooth" relationship between maxillary and mandibular teeth. Note that the maxillary teeth are usually one cusp posterior to their respective mandibular teeth. The diagrams below left illustrate labial (La) to palatal (P) sections (sagittal) through the anterior teeth. The maxillary anterior teeth are related to the mandibular teeth with a vertical overlap (VO), and a horizontal overlap (HO). The diagrams on the right illustrates a buccal (B) to lingual (Li) section (frontal) through the posterior teeth. The supporting cusps (SC) fit into opposing fossae (F). Note that the mandibular molar is tilted slightly lingually and the maxillary molar slightly buccally. This tilt causes the outer cups incline (OCI) to be slightly less steep than the inner cusp incline (ICI).

this postural position provides the operator with a reference point for setting the teeth into maximal intercuspation.

8.2.8 Curves of Occlusion

The mandibular molar teeth are tilted inward and the maxillary teeth slightly outward. This means that the sides of the cusp or "cusp inclines" are altered. The outer cusp incline (OCI) of the mandibular tooth has become less steep due to this tilting. The inner cusp incline (ICI) of the same tooth is steeper (▶ Fig. 8.9). These differences are going to have important consequences as the teeth move against each other. Before we move on, we need to step back from the individual tooth and look at the effect of these tilted positions on the whole arch. Both left and right mandibular molar teeth are tilted inward, so the tips of the cusps fit an imaginary curve, not a flat plane. Such an occlusal curve was described by Spee in 1880 and later by Monson, who described the plane as part of a sphere, which included the lateral component of the curve (▶ Fig. 8.10a).

8.2.9 Tooth Contacts during Function

When we want to grind up hard food, we need to move our jaws from side to side as we bite into the food. If we place the food on the right side and move our jaw to the right in order to start a grinding movement, the condyle on the left will move inward and downward. You can confirm this by putting a finger in each ear or over the condyles and moving the jaw as if to grind toward

the right side. You will feel the condyle on the left, slide forward. The teeth of the left side will probably separate. We will call this left side the balancing side. The condyle on the right side where we are going to be "working" will just rotate, but the teeth will stay close together and grind the food. What effect will occlusal curves have on these working contacts? Recall that the OCI was effectively reduced by the inward tilt of the mandibular teeth (▶ Fig. 8.9). And it is the OCI which guides the opposing teeth over each other on the working side. The ICI have no influence on this working side. However, they do approach close to one another on the balancing side as they are steeper than the working inclines (▶ Fig. 8.10b). If the condylar path was any flatter, they would make contact. In ▶ Fig. 8.10c, if the working incline is reduced by wear, the steeper ICI inclines on the balancing side will indeed come together. So, the difference in inclines between the OCI on the working side and the ICI on the balancing side will, eventually, *compensate* for the tendency of the teeth to separate on the balancing side. This compensation is a consequence of the occlusal curves and so these curves are called *compensating curve*. When the teeth on the balancing side are making contact, we can no longer use the term nonworking, because these teeth are now working. We will have to use a new set of terms.

When the jaw works laterally to chew, we could use the term *buccal phase* of working, and when the jaw moves back inward to chew, what was a buccal phase becomes this *lingual phase* of working. Each tooth may thus function firstly in a buccal phase and then as the jaw moves in the opposite direction, in a lingual phase. During the buccal phase, outer working inclines of the mandibular teeth are in contact. During the

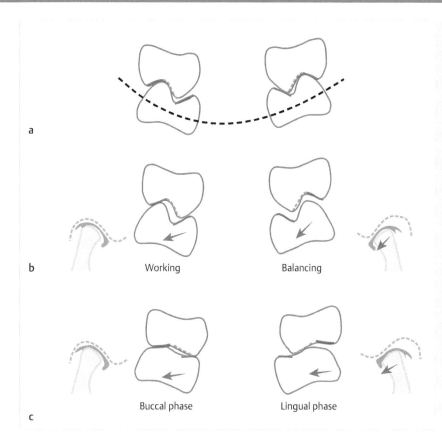

Fig. 8.10 A diagrammatic representation of the influence of occlusal curves in a frontal plane, on functional occlusal contacts. (a) The curves of occlusion are formed by the lingual rotation of the mandibular teeth and the buccal rotation of the maxillary teeth. Note that this tilting reduces the inclination of the working outer cusp inclines (OCIs) which are drawn as *solid red lines*. The inclination of the balancing inner cusp inclines (ICIs) are increased. ICIs are drawn as *broken blue lines*. (b) When the jaw works to one side, the condyle on the opposite (balancing) side moves downward and forward, which tends to disengage the teeth on the balancing side. The increased ICIs (which result from the occlusal curve) of the balancing side brings the teeth on the balancing side closer together. The occlusal curve therefore is said to *compensate* for the separation of the teeth on the balancing side of the jaw during lateral functional movements. (c) Wear of the working side teeth reduces the OCIs which contributes to the continued engagement of teeth on the balancing (opposite) side of the jaw. In the worn dentition, masticatory function occurs on both sides of the jaw during both buccal and lingual phases of movement.

lingual phase, the inner working inclines contact. So, tooth wear is evenly shared by all surfaces of the tooth. We cannot therefore assume that our jaws are adapted to work only on one side at a time unless we treat the human jaw as if we had a carnivore's dentition.

8.2.10 Anterior Tooth Contact

Canine Guidance

We have studied tooth contacts of posterior teeth when chewing on one side and noted that the mandibular supporting cusps move laterally along the outer working incline of the maxillary molars. The steepness of this incline is related to the height of the buccal cusps of both maxillary and mandibular teeth. The buccal cusps of molars are not as high as premolars, and premolar cusps are not as high as canines. So, as the jaw slides laterally, first the molar cusps and then even the premolar cusps become separated by the canines. If the canines are pointed and prominent, as they are in dogs or cats, they may cause almost immediate disocclusion of the posterior teeth when the jaw begins to work to one side. We have noted that canine guidance might contribute to the stability of posterior and anterior teeth (▶ Fig. 8.11).

In humans, we only find a canine guidance in individuals whose teeth have not worn. That includes most of us, who live on a soft diet. It is as if we have been held fast in an immature stage of our dentition before age and a rough diet had worn our teeth. However, given this is the case, how important is this canine guidance? It is instructive to look at those unfortunate people whose permanent canine does not erupt. They retain

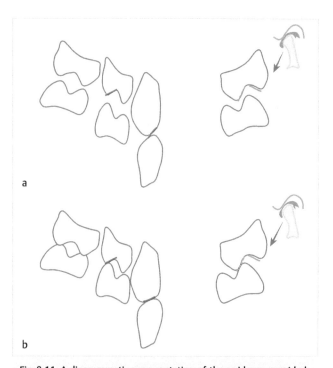

Fig. 8.11 A diagrammatic representation of the guidance provided by the canines during lateral masticatory movements of the jaw. (a) In unworn teeth, the canine guidance is steep and protects the posterior teeth from potentially damaging forces. (b) In slightly worn teeth, the canine guidance is reduced which allows the posterior teeth on the working side to come together simultaneously as in group function. The compensating curve allows the balancing side teeth to contact during function; they are now working in a lingual phase.

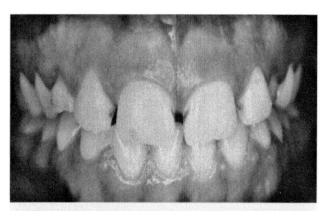

Fig. 8.12 A clinical illustration of the consequence of failure of the permanent canines to erupt. This individual is 21 years old, and the permanent canines have still not erupted. The deciduous canines have worn rapidly, leaving the permanent incisors unprotected. They have splayed and drifted, possibly due to excessive lateral loads, but in addition, there is a loss of arch support due to the reduced width of the deciduous canines.

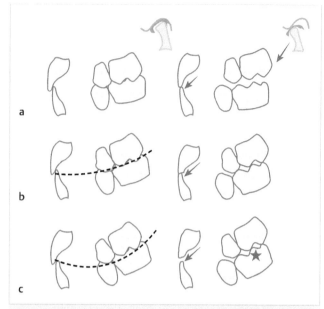

Fig. 8.13 A diagrammatic representation of the guidance provided by the incisors during protrusive masticatory movements of the jaw. (a) In the unworn dentition, there is some degree of horizontal and vertical overlap of the incisors which causes a steep incisal guidance. When the mandible slides forward to incise, the posterior teeth separate. (b) After moderate wear, the overlap is reduced, the incisal guidance is less steep, and the posterior teeth are more inclined to work simultaneously with the incisors, provided there is a sagittal occlusal curve (*broken line*). (c) If the occlusal curve is steep, which may be caused by mesial tilting of molars into a space, a protrusive movement fails to keep the incisor teeth together due to a posterior occlusal interference (*star*).

the deciduous canine for a while, but it is clear that the dentition is not stable. The incisor teeth are likely to become spaced and slightly splayed, and the buccal cusps of one or more posterior teeth may be damaged (▶ Fig. 8.12). The maxillary canine usually has a large, long root which is well designed to take frequent and high lateral forces during chewing. So, canines do protect and stabilize the dentition with high cusps.

In humans, eating a rougher diet, the canine and other buccal cusps wear down, so the lateral loads are shared by all the teeth on that side (▶ Fig. 8.11b). This reduced role of the canine allows *group function* of the teeth on that side. We also see the effect of a compensating curve which allows the teeth on the balancing side to work in unison with the working side teeth.

Incisal Guidance

When we want to cut through food, we use our incisors like rodents do, working the chisel-like mandibular teeth against the maxillary teeth. We need to protrude the mandible, so as to bring the mandibular incisors into an edge-to-edge position with the maxillary incisors (▶ Fig. 8.13). Some vertical and horizontal overlap is usual, which causes the posterior teeth to separate when the jaw is protruded in order to incise. This is just as well as we would find it difficult to exert any working force on our incisors if the posterior teeth interfered. Note, though, that the mandibular molars are slightly tilted forward, and the maxillary molar slightly tilt backward, so we have a curve of occlusion in an anterior–posterior direction (sagittal) as well as the lateral (frontal) curve we have already discussed. This is consistent with Monson's theory of the teeth fitting onto a sphere. This curve reduces the separation of the posterior teeth during protrusion, because the effective cusp inclines become progressively steeper the more the teeth are tilted forward. So, if the curve is steep, the third molars may be quite close to contact as the jaw protrudes. If a mandibular first molar is extracted early in life, the second molar may drift and rotate forward into the space. The effective cusp inclines of the second

molar may be so steep that it interferes with the opposing tooth when the mandible protrudes in order to incise. The rotated tooth then becomes a *protrusive interference*. As the teeth wear, the incisal guidance is reduced, and the posterior teeth may meet during protrusion. This does not cause a problem provided the contact is simultaneous.

8.2.11 Summary of Arch and Tooth Relationships

We have noted that the relationships of the maxillary and mandibular arches and their curves of occlusion have the potential to confer some stability to the arch and to individual teeth. While the teeth are unworn, the canines protect the posterior cusps from damage and ensure that the teeth on the balancing side do not interfere. When there has been moderate wear of the teeth, the potential for stability is fully realized in the following ways:

- Group function occurs on the working side, and in addition, the teeth on the balancing side start to contact and work as well. The workloads are shared over the entire arch.
- The bite forces tend to be more apically directed when the cusps have worn. However, we can also appreciate the importance of a canine-protected occlusion in situations where the cusps are high and pointed.

We have identified some features of the occlusion of natural teeth which tend to stabilize the dentition. We need to review some variations in arch and tooth relationships.

8.2.12 Class II Arch and Tooth Relationships

The essential features of arch and tooth relationships, which are most common, have been described. However, the arch form and tooth relationships of a significant proportion of the population do not conform to these patterns. Variation in arch and tooth relationship does not necessarily imply that they are abnormal or in need of correction. Many individuals who are of Caucasoid ancestry have a smaller mandible and a more prominent maxilla than is usual. When this discrepancy is slight, it makes little difference to the facial profile, but as it becomes more pronounced, we recognize what the laymen may term an undershot jaw. Dentists use the term Class II derived from an early classification of dental malocclusions by Angle. We should note that all classifications are made by man, and not by nature, so there is always a continuum with no clearly defined border between the classes we artificially construct.

We must be wary of adopting definitions of normal, which are so narrow that they exclude variations which are quite healthy. Unfortunately, the prefix "mal" to occlusion conveys something bad or undesirable. However natural variation means that although relationships and patterns may not be usual (average), they are by no means bad or abnormal. There is no evidence to suggest that a dentition which might be described as a malocclusion has a reduced functional capacity or a shorter functional life span.[4] An Angle Class II dentition appears to work as well and lasts as long as a class I dentition.

The criteria for defining a malocclusion, and therefore identifying individuals who may require orthodontic treatment, vary considerably. There are more than 25 indices which may be used. They include a range from those which are based mostly on perceived aesthetic requirement and include patient demands, to those which include an assessment of functional need. These latter classifications, based on functional need, tend to have more restrictive inclusion criteria, and fewer treatments are performed than those based on perceived aesthetic need. There have been few studies to investigate the possibility that orthodontic treatment improves masticatory function.[4]

It is not uncommon to encounter research studies on the epidemiology of malocclusion, which employ some of the more widely inclusive indexes of treatment need, in which the authors categorize only 25% of a sample of individuals to possess ideal tooth relationships. This implies that more than half the children or young adults surveyed may benefit from treatment. One of the unfortunate consequences of taxonomy and classification is the tendency to suspect that there is some intrinsic virtue in that which is most usual. The specimen occupying the popular slot has the true essence. The less common, are seen somehow to be less ideal.

Variations in arch form and tooth position are also subject to the public's determinants of youth and beauty. The widely accepted gold standards are ideal facial profiles and regular white teeth. The public's desire to acquire these standards of perfection drives a significant demand for cosmetic dentistry and orthodontic treatment.

8.2.13 Occlusion and Wear

When the human dentition has worn, it is recognizable as that of an herbivore, and it becomes possible to give a more considered description of tooth contacts during function. The side-to-side grinding may be described in simple terms. We have encountered the concept of a buccal phase of chewing on one side of the jaws and simultaneously a lingual phase on the opposite side. Each tooth may thus function firstly in a buccal phase, and then as the jaw moves in the opposite direction, it functions in a lingual phase. During the buccal phase, outer working inclines of the mandibular teeth are in contact. During the lingual phase, the inner working inclines contact. So, tooth wear is evenly shared by all surfaces of the tooth. It is becoming less clear how to interpret the term "intercuspation." The teeth now fit together well over a wide area of contact. There is no longer a fixed and stable intercuspal position. A new set of criteria for a normal occlusion based on the tooth relationships in the natural worn dentition may be useful. Dentists work with unworn dentitions, but we do not have to assume that they are ideal, or that we should restore them into what may be an unusual condition brought about by our modern diet. This short review of tooth contacts during function should be read together with *Chapter 1 The Origins of Teeth*, on the evolution of mastication, and the section on chewing in *Chapter 10.9 Mastication*.

> **Key Notes**
>
> The dental arch of humans exhibits a variety of shapes, sizes, and relationships with the opposing arch and the face of the individual. The occlusion of the individual teeth is also highly variable. Few of these variants limit the functions of speech and mastication or the stability of the dentition. The greatest threat to the stability of the dentition is tooth loss.

Review Questions

1. What is meant by an occlusal curve?
2. Why is the maxillary arch wider and longer than the mandibular arch of teeth?
3. What is meant by a tooth-to-two-tooth relationship?
4. What are the differences between deciduous and permanent teeth?
5. What factors contribute to the stability of the dental arch?
6. What determines the influence of a premature tooth contact?
7. What do you understand by the term *canine guidance*?
8. What are the possible consequences of occlusal interference?
9. What events may contribute to causing a protrusive interference?
10. What are the consequences of adopting narrow criteria for defining normal when as much as 25% of a sample does not meet the criteria used to define normal?

8.3 Tooth Wear

8.3.1 Types of Tooth Wear

Abrasion refers to tooth wear caused by a course, fibrous, or grit-containing diet. It is a universal feature of mammalian teeth but virtually absent in the dentition of modern humans. Until comparatively recently, grains were milled using stone crushers which contaminated the flour with fine grit. Thus, until the 19th century, the teeth of humans would have shown abrasion. Estimates of tooth wear on skeletal remains from archaeological sites can give some insight into the possible dietary habits of the individuals and the use of teeth as tools.

Attrition refers to wear of the teeth caused by tooth-to-tooth contact. This is most pronounced in the approximal surfaces of the teeth. Attrition would also be found on the opposing surfaces of the canines of carnivores, which act as guides for the cutting edges of the carnassial teeth.

Attrition is seen in patients who grind their teeth, a condition termed *bruxism*. The forces applied to the teeth during bruxism may be so high that a grinding sound can be heard. The cusp surfaces are typically shiny and faceted with microscopic evidence of fine striations running in a recognizable direction. In contrast, abrasion produces a roughened tooth surface without any particular pattern.

Erosion refers to loss of enamel due to exposure to strong acids. Contrary to the process of caries, where acids are produced by plaque and cause a pit or cavity, erosion removes material from the exposed surface of the tooth, leaving a smooth surface. Regurgitated stomach acids are the most common cause of erosion. In the eating disorder, bulimia, the palatal aspect of the maxillary incisors are the worst affected by erosion. A similar pattern of erosion is found in wine tasters, who may sip hundreds of glasses a day during the blending season.

8.3.2 Consequences of Tooth Wear

The benefits which tooth wear confers are that it enables the tooth to remain sharp throughout its life. Prisms of enamel break away leaving a sharp edge which is proud of the supporting dentin. Being softer, the dentin wears faster than the enamel. Wear also reduces the pits and fissures which would otherwise provide shelter for plaque organisms. Approximal wear allows the teeth to drift forward providing space for the third molars to erupt.

Wear would, however, also bring with it several unwanted side effects. The first would be shortening of the working surfaces and loss of contact between the tooth and its opponent in the arch rendering it useless as a tool. The second problem would be sensitivity due to the reduction in thickness of protective layers of enamel and dentin around the pulp. Fortunately, there are two mechanisms, which reduce these undesirable aspects of wear. The first is continued eruption of the tooth. Eruption is a lifelong process, and provided that wear is not too rapid, the continued eruption of the tooth keeps it in contact with its opponent, so there is no loss of function.

We have noted that continued eruption may be brought about by active eruption of the tooth from its socket. This appears to be a function of the periodontal ligament. If an opposing tooth is extracted, the unopposed tooth may continue to erupt and become so extruded that it loses bone support and becomes mobile. This overeruption occurs less frequently in adult and elderly individuals.

An additional process of compensation for tooth wear is continued alveolar bone growth. The supporting socket of the tooth keeps growing and brings the worn tooth back into occlusion. The two processes, alveolar bone growth and continued active eruption, combine to compensate for tooth wear.

Evidence of active eruption would be an increase in the distance between the CEJ and the crest of the alveolar bone. Evidence of alveolar bone growth would be an increase in the height of the alveolar bone. This might be measurable between a static reference point such as the lower border of the mandible or the mental foramen and the crest of the alveolar ridge. A skull of a hunter–gatherer with moderate tooth wear suggests that both active eruption and alveolar bone growth have compensated for tooth wear (▶ Fig. 8.14).

We do not have the same abrasive diet of our hunter–gatherer ancestors, but nevertheless, our teeth continue to erupt throughout life. At least, that is the evidence of a study by Tallgren.[5] She measured the lower facial height of a sample of Norwegian women using lateral skull radiographs. Eleven years later she made the same measurements and found that the facial height had increased. Her conclusion was that continued eruption had occurred, and without tooth wear had increased the vertical dimension in occlusion.

The compensation for wear which secondary dentin provides is effective provided that wear is not too rapid. Wear may be rapid and exceed these compensatory mechanisms if the dentition is not complete due to tooth loss. The few remaining teeth are providing all the masticatory function and wearing faster than normal (▶ Fig. 8.15).

8.3.3 Other Compensatory Mechanisms for Continued Eruption

The thickness of cementum increases throughout life and is a good indicator of age. Forensic scientists use cementum thickness as a guide to determine the age of an unidentified corpse. This increased thickness contributes to the extrusion of the tooth, albeit a small amount. Tooth wear is a stimulus for the formation of secondary dentin around the roof of the pulp chamber. This secondary dentin may obliterate the original pulp chamber and is often seen as a dark patch on the incisal edge of mandibular incisors which have experienced advanced wear. Dentin may be formed inside the tubule thereby reducing the size of the lumen and eventually obliterating it. This process reduces the permeability of dentin thereby protecting the deeper vital tissues. Peritubular dentin is also found in older teeth even if not worn and is another aid to forensic aging.

> **Key Notes**
>
> Tooth wear is an essential process in all mammalian dentitions. It produces a composite surface which is nonclogging and self-sharpening. There are compensating mechanisms which have evolved along with variations in cusp form which allow the teeth to serve as efficient, lifelong food processors.

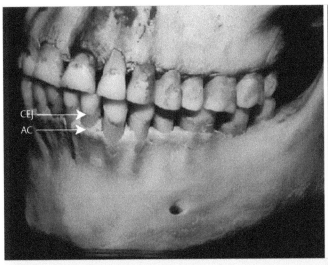
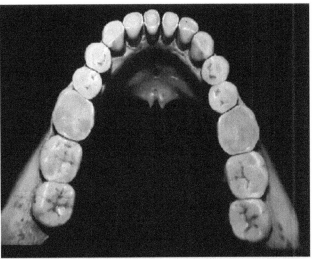

Fig. 8.14 A clinical illustration of the processes of active eruption and continued alveolar bone growth. The skull of a hunter–gatherer estimated to be a young adult, with moderate tooth wear. The separate occlusal view of the same dentition (right) reveals the difference in wear between the first and second molar. This is an indication of the rate of wear, as it represents the amount of wear which took place before the second molar erupted. It appears that the distance of the cementoenamel junction (CEJ) to the alveolar crest (AC) is more than normal (2 mm), and the height of alveolar bone appears to have increased (the roots of mandibular premolars are well coronal of the mental foramen). Continued eruption and alveolar growth compensate for tooth wear and maintain the lower facial height.

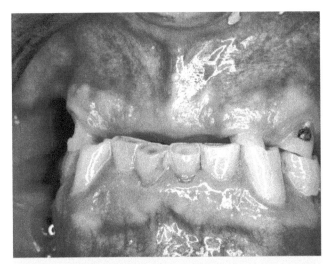

Fig. 8.15 A clinical image of excessive wear caused by tooth loss. The mechanisms of compensation for tooth wear have not kept pace, and a loss of occlusal vertical height has occurred.

Review Questions

1. What mechanisms compensate for tooth wear?
2. What possible advantages to the dentition are derived from tooth wear?
3. Why is there a need for continued repositioning of the teeth once they have erupted?

References

[1] Proffit WR. Equilibrium theory revisited: factors influencing position of the teeth. Angle Orthod 1978;48(3):175–186
[2] O'Neill J. Long-term stability after orthodontic treatment remains inconclusive. Evid Based Dent 2007;8(3):81–82
[3] Woda A, Vigneron P, Kay D. Nonfunctional and functional occlusal contacts: a review of the literature. J Prosthet Dent 1979;42(3):335–341
[4] Henrikson T, Ekberg E, Nilner M. Can orthodontic treatment improve mastication? A controlled, prospective and longitudinal study. Swed Dent J 2009;33(2):59–65
[5] Tallgren A. Changes in adult face height due to ageing, wear and loss of teeth and prosthetic treatment. Acta Odontol Scand 1957;15(Suppl 4):73

Suggested Readings

Eruption

Brook AH, Jernvall J, Smith RN, Hughes TE, Townsend GC. The dentition: the out comes of morphogenesis leading to variations of tooth number, size and shape. Aust Dent J 2014;59(Suppl 1):131–142
Craddock HL, Youngson CC. Eruptive tooth movement—the current state of knowl edge. Br Dent J 2004;197(7):385–391
Kondo Y, Sawada T, Shibayama K, Inoue S. Elastic system fibers in rat incisor perio dontal ligament—immunohistochemical study using sections of fresh-frozen un-demineralized tissues. Acta Histochem 2011;113(2):125–130
Tallgren A. Changes in adult face height due to ageing, wear and loss of teeth and prosthetic treatment. Acta Odont Scand 1957;15(suppl 24):1–112
Wise GE. Cellular and molecular basis of tooth eruption. Orthod Craniofac Res 2009;12(2):67–73

Tooth Wear

Kaifu Y, Kasai K, Townsend GC, Richards LC. Tooth wear and the "design" of the human dentition: a perspective from evolutionary medicine. Am J Phys Anthropol 2003;(Suppl 37):47–61
Kaplan P. Drifting, tipping, supraeruption, and segmental alveolar bone growth. J Prosthet Dent 1985;54(2):280–283
Levers BG, Darling AI. Continuous eruption of some adult human teeth of ancient populations. Arch Oral Biol 1983;28(5):401–408
Lombardi AV. The adaptive value of dental crowding: a consideration of the biologic basis of malocclusion. Am J Orthod 1982;81(1):38–42
Varrela TM, Paunio K, Wouters FR, Tiekso J, Söder PO. The relation between tooth eruption and alveolar crest height in a human skeletal sample. Arch Oral Biol 1995;40(3):175–180

9 The Temporomandibular Joint

Abstract

During mastication, the temporomandibular joint (TMJ) transmits forces to the base of the skull similar in magnitude to those generated by the biting force. For this reason, the disk is fibrous; cartilage would not be tough enough to take the load without breaking up. During incision the reaction force at the joint is higher than it is on the incisors. A bite force at the molars, which is the location where the maximum bite force is possible, causes a reaction on the joint components which are slightly less than during incision. The joint surfaces have a low coefficient of friction. In order to prevent the condyle, sliding out of control during function, a group of muscles maintains the stability of the joint. The glenoid fossa slopes in a posterior direction, and this also assists in maintaining the stability of the condyle. The tension generated by some of the masticatory muscles which stabilize the joint may explain why these muscles may become fatigued and painful. Pain in the masticatory muscles may be referred to the joint. The joint itself is seldom the source of pain unless it has experienced some trauma. In spite of this pain in the masticatory muscles and limited movement of the jaw, this condition is usually referred to as temporomandibular joint dysfunction or disorder. There has been considerable attention paid to this so-called dysfunction of the joint. Invasive treatments have been popular in the past including surgery to the joint. There is now reliable evidence that reversible noninvasive management of dysfunction is successful. The essential component of psychosocial factors in pain has to be recognized.

Keywords: TMJ mechanics, load bearing, joint reaction, joint stability, clicking, power muscles, control muscles, TMJ structure, disk displacement, temporomandibular dysfunction, Research Diagnostic Criteria

9.1 The Mechanics of the Temporomandibular Joint

9.1.1 A Load-Bearing Joint

The load lifted by a class 3 lever is applied at the end of the lever, separated from the fulcrum by the lifting force. The forearm, lifting a weight in the hand is an example. The further away the load is from the lifting force, the greater the reaction at the

fulcrum in order to keep the lever stable (▶ Fig. 9.1). If we transfer this analogy to the jaws, the articular eminence acts as the fulcrum. The load is the point on the arch of teeth, where the bite is applied. There is no muscle force which acts directly through the load, as all the teeth are anterior to all the muscles. The

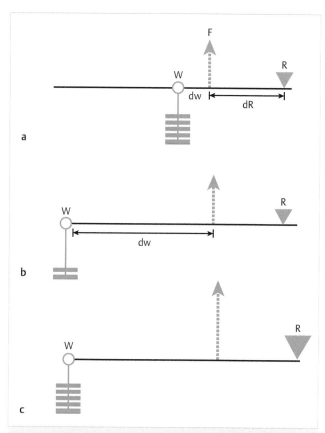

Fig. 9.1 Diagrammatic representation of a class 3 lever and the forces required to keep it stable. (a) Diagram of a class 3 lever. When the lever is stable, the force (F) is balanced if the load (W) × the distance (dw) is equal to the reaction force R × dR. **(b)** If the load is moved further from the fulcrum, it has greater leverage and would pull the lever down. To keep the lever stable, the load must be decreased so that W × dw remains the same. **(c)** An alternative to balancing the system as the load moves away from the fulcrum is to increase the force (F). As F increases, it must be balanced by an equal increase of dR × R. As dR is constant, it is the reaction at R which is increased when the load is moved further from the fulcrum.

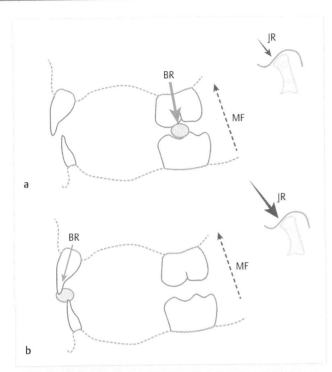

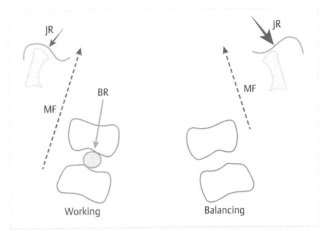

a

b

Fig. 9.2 Diagrammatic representation of the mechanics of the human jaw which works as a class 3 lever. (a) The fulcrum is at the joint (JR). When the jaw is stable, the muscle force (MF) is balanced by the bite reaction (BR) and the reaction force at the joint (JR). **(b)** If the bite action moves to the incisors, and the muscle force remains the same, the bite reaction (BR) decreases, but the reaction force at the joint (JR) is increased. The temporomandibular joint is thus a stress-bearing joint, and it receives its greatest forces when the bite is forward of the molars. A lack of posterior teeth may therefore stress the joint more than would be normal.

Fig. 9.3 Diagrammatic representation of the mechanics of the human jaw in a coronal plane. The jaw can be viewed as a triangular plate with a fulcrum (joint) on two corners. The muscle force (MF) on the **working** side is stabilized partly by the joint reaction (JR) and the bite reaction (BR) through the bolus. However, on the balancing side, even though the muscle force (MF) is slightly less, there is nothing but the joint reaction (JR) to stabilize the muscle force on this side, if there is no tooth contact. This suggests that for man the balancing condyle is under a greater load than the working condyle, unless there are balancing side contacts during function.

muscle force is therefore partly resisted at the TMJ and partly at the teeth. In equilibrium, the reaction at the joint plus the resistance to the load is equal to the force applied by the muscle (▶ Fig. 9.2). As the load moves forward toward the anterior teeth, the bite force on the bolus decreases, but there is a greater load on the TMJ. The TMJ, like the fulcrum of a lever, is always under load whenever any bite force is applied.

This analogy of the TMJ to a class 3 lever assumes that there is a single fulcrum, but of course, there are two condyles. We now have to view the jaws as a curved plate rather than a beam. The plate has a triangular shape, with a fulcrum at two corners, and the teeth along two edges. The muscles of mastication pull upward on both sides of the plate, slightly more powerfully on the chewing side (▶ Fig. 9.3). There is therefore a reaction at both joints during the generation of a bite force on one (working) side. On the balancing side, if no teeth meet, the reaction of the bite force is resisted only by the joint on that side. On the working side, the reaction is shared by the teeth and the joint. The simplified diagrams in ▶ Fig. 9.2 and ▶ Fig. 9.3 are accurate in that they identify the source of the three major vectors of jaw mechanics, namely the muscle force and direction, the reaction at the joint, and the load due to the resistance of the food bolus. They are oversimplified representation because all the component muscles are represented by a single force.[1]

9.1.2 Variable Forces at the Teeth

The load is not always a fixed distance from the joint and neither is the force generated by the masticatory muscle. Furthermore, the load may be applied to more than one tooth in the arch. By virtue of the arch of teeth being on a plane, which is offset from the joint, several teeth may contact at once. The requirements for efficient use of the teeth as tools may demand that forces are not always at right angles to the lever arm. For example, shearing forces at the teeth require forces applied at an angle to the lever. The most important consideration during chewing is to develop the appropriate magnitudes and direction of force at the teeth.

9.1.3 Joint Stability

The joint surfaces have an extremely low coefficient of friction; in other words, they are slippery surfaces. The joint surfaces therefore allow easy movement under load, but the slipperiness needs to be controlled. If you are skating on ice, you are most stable when your center of gravity is over, that is perpendicular, to your feet. The mandibular condyle is stable when the reaction at the joint is perpendicular to the surface of the eminence. In a simple masticatory system, with predictable muscle forces and a limited variation in load position and direction (e.g., a rat's incisor), the jaw could be stabilized if the contour of the joint surfaces was at right angles to the joint reaction. In humans, the jaw closing forces are generated by a number of muscles, each with a different origin, insertion, and direction of tension and each with more than one anatomically distinct part. Each anatomical section of a muscle has hundreds of separate functional units. It is clear that depending on which combination of these muscle units is active, a different force at the teeth and a different reaction at the joint will be produced.

The forces generated at the teeth will be influenced by tooth wear. The greater the cusp wear, the flatter the grinding surfaces and the more lateral the masticatory forces. It is not surprising, therefore, that the articular eminence has been found to remodel, becoming less steep as tooth wear occurs.[2] It is possible that this remodeling is a result of changes in the directions of forces applied to the teeth, which adapt to changes in cusp angles brought about by tooth wear.

Given the complexity of the force, load, and hence joint reaction in man, it is clear that the resultant of the three major force components is highly variable. If the reactions at the joint are not perpendicular to the eminence, then movement, either up or down the eminence will occur.

Such sliding movement may be contrary to that required at the teeth and would have to be controlled. In view of the complexity of the balance between the force components of the jaws, Osborn and Baragar developed a computer model of the forces involved in biting and have been able to predict those muscles which would be most efficient in producing a bite force at the molar and at the incisors.[3] The model also predicts what muscle action would be necessary to stabilize the jaw while the force was being produced at the teeth (▶ Fig. 9.4).

The two muscles, which may have the greatest ability to stabilize the reaction at the joint, are the lateral pterygoid and the horizontal fibers of the temporalis muscle. Contraction of the lateral pterygoid would resist the condyle sliding backward up the slope of the articular eminence; conversely, contraction of the horizontal fibers of temporalis would resist the condyle sliding forward. The muscles which are well positioned to provide powerful closure are the deep and superficial masseter groups, the medial pterygoid, and the vertical fibers of the temporalis muscle.

The muscles of the human jaw can be therefore be divided into two major groups. Firstly, those whose prime function is to generate forces in the desired part of the arch in the necessary direction and magnitude to allow the teeth to function. These could be called the *power muscles*. Secondly, there are those muscles which control the movement of the condyle up and down the eminence and thus stabilize the joint. These are the *control muscles*.[2] The jaw muscles are anatomically divided according to their ability to be visibly distinguished from each other. But we have noted that within muscles there are many functional units which can contract independently. The resultant of the activity of groups of these elements from different muscles is complex and continually alters as forces at the teeth are altered either in direction or magnitude.

9.1.4 Joint Instability and Muscle Fatigue

It follows from our analysis so far that as the destabilizing forces at the joint become more powerful, greater activity will be required by the stabilizing muscles to maintain condylar stability. This relationship between destabilizing forces and the activity of stabilizing muscles may be of interest in understanding the source of muscle pains associated with the TMJ. Temporomandibular dysfunction (TMD) is a syndrome of signs and symptoms. The chief signs are limited jaw movement, particularly opening, and tenderness to muscle palpation. The main symptoms are a diffuse, unilateral pain around the region of the joint and ear, which increases when biting hard, and which may radiate across the face. The source of the pain in most cases may be traced to trigger points in the muscles of mastication from which pain is referred to the joint area. The lateral pterygoid muscle, although difficult to palpate, is the muscle most commonly reported to be tender. There is no satisfactory explanation for why this particular muscle should be so commonly affected, but it may be related to its role in stabilizing the joint. Patients are able to chew more comfortably on the same side as the pain than on the opposite side. From what is now known about joint loading, it appears that the joint on the same side as the working side has a lower reaction force than that on the balancing side. It therefore requires less effort from the controlling muscles, one of which is the lateral pterygoid.

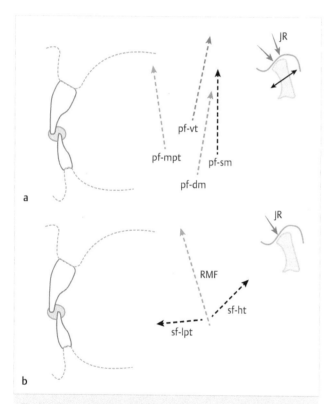

Fig. 9.4 Diagrammatic representation of the mechanics of the influence of control muscles on the stability of the temporomandibular joint. (a) The direction of some of the groups of jaw closing muscles which provide a power force (pf). They include vertical temporalis (pf-vt), superior masseter (pf-sm), deep masseter (pf-dm), and medial pterygoid (pf-mpt). The jaw joint slides readily and is only stabilized during a static bite force when the joint reaction (JR) is at right angles to the joint surface. **(b)** The control muscles are well placed to provide a stabilizing force (sf-) which influences the resultant muscle force (RMF) so that the joint reaction (JR) is at right angles to the joint surfaces. These stabilizing muscles are the lateral pterygoid (sf-lpt) and horizontal temporalis (sf-ht). (Adapted from Osborn and Baragar 1985.[3])

9.2 The Structure of the Temporomandibular Joint

The joint structure is unusual, in that a fibrous disk separates the two joint surfaces into two compartments[4] (▶ Fig. 9.5). The joint surfaces are also lined with dense fibrous tissue. This is in

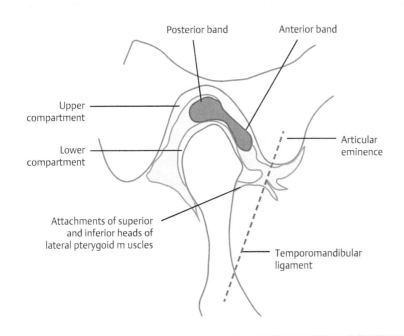

Posterior band   Anterior band

Upper
compartment

Lower
compartment

Articular
eminence

Attachments of superior
and inferior heads of
lateral pterygoid m uscles

Temporomandibular
ligament

Fig. 9.5 Diagrammatic representation of the temporomandibular joint. Note that the disk separates the joint into an upper and lower compartment. The superior and inferior fibers of the head of the lateral pterygoid muscle insert into the neck of the condyle and the anterior margin of the disk, respectively. (Adapted from Rees 1954.[4])

contrast to the cartilaginous disks and surfaces of other joints. While cartilage has a very high compressive strength, it has a relatively low tensile strength. As the human joint is loaded during sliding movements, shearing and tensile stresses are developed. The fibrous disk of the joint is therefore better suited to withstand these stresses than if it were composed of cartilage.

The purpose of the disk is to allow the condyle to roll and slide while under load and to provide a cushion to distribute the load more evenly. The disk is squashed between the two bony surfaces and being very slippery would escape like a squeezed pip from your fingers.[1] There is a raised ridge, the annulus, around the periphery of the disk which fits around the condyle like the band of a cap. Further anchorage is provided by attachment to the joint capsule. The posterior part of the disk extends into a highly vascular and elastic bilaminar zone. The bilaminar zone is richly supplied with sensory nerves, and unlike the disk itself is sensitive to compression.

The purpose of the articular eminence has been debated, but it would seem to increase the stability of the joint during the application of chewing forces in certain directions. The slope of the articular eminence may also act to guide the jaw during lateral movements; the separation of the posterior teeth during an incising movement is possibly assisted by the downward displacement of the jaw as it moves forward down the eminence.

9.3 Movement at the Temporomandibular Joint

9.3.1 Constraints of Jaw Movements

Imagine that you could manipulate the jaw of a sleeping subject. The upward movement of the jaw would be constrained by the presence and position of the teeth and the articular eminence of the joint. The horizontal movement, with the teeth close together, would be constrained by the degree of intercuspation and height of the cusps, but with the teeth apart, both lateral and forward (protrusive) movement would be possible. The jaw would be able to be protruded while the condyles slid down the articular eminence until they reached the limits imposed by the capsule and the lateral ligament. Likewise, the jaw could be retruded until the capsule and ligament limited it. This sliding movement of the condyle occurs in the upper joint compartment. Lateral movement is limited by the capsule and ligament of each joint. However, the jaw can rotate (swing) to each side, as the head of the opposite condyle moves forward down the articular eminence. The jaw joint does not allow the condyles to drop out of it. Both capsule and ligaments prevent this, but it does allow a certain amount of rotation. This allows the jaws to hinge open until the front of the capsule becomes taught and limits further rotation. This tension is relieved if the condyle slides forward down the eminence making some additional rotation possible (▶ Fig. 9.6).

Note that forward movement of the condyle during jaw opening is partly a mechanical event. The capsule becomes taught after a short period of rotation of the condyle. To allow further opening, the condyle head must slide toward the capsule. Hinge movement of the joint occurs in the lower joint compartment.

If you let go of the jaw and the patient was upright, it would not fall right open but hang near the closed position, possibly with the lips slightly apart. The tissue tone of the skin and muscle would be responsible for this neutral posture. If the subject awoke, the lips would meet and the jaw would close a little due to some muscle tone of the elevators, but a space of a few millimeters between the teeth would remain. This position of rest is called the *mandibular rest position*, and the space between the teeth is called the *interocclusal rest space*. If requested, the subject could voluntarily reproduce all the passive movements you produced while manipulating the jaw. It is important to realize that these constraints, or envelopes of motion, do not define or direct masticatory movements of the

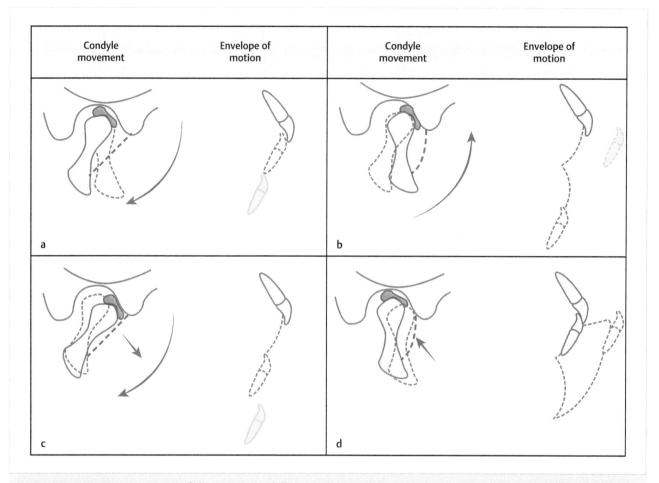

Fig. 9.6 Diagrammatic representation of the movements of the jaw within an envelope of constraints determined by the joint and teeth.
(a) Rotation of the condyle allows the jaw to open until the movement is constrained by the temporomandibular (TM) ligament (*red broken line*).
(b) Further rotation is possible provided the condyle translates anteriorly. With the condyle now constrained by the joint capsule and the TM ligament, the jaw is at maximum opening. **(c)** If the jaw rotates closed, without the condyle sliding posteriorly, the mandibular incisor teeth are anterior to the maxillary incisors. **(d)** As the condyle slides posteriorly, the mandibular incisor teeth pass under the maxillary teeth to return to a position of maximal intercuspation.

jaw, which are under neuromuscular control. They do define the limits of movements, such as yawning.

9.3.2 Disk Displacement

The disk may escape forward and lie anterior to the condyle head. This leaves the bilaminar zone as the intervening tissue between the condyle head and the articular eminence. The bilaminar zone is highly vascular, sensitive, and unsuited to transmitting loads through the joint. A consequence of the anterior displacement of the disk may, therefore, be pain during mastication. A more common consequence of anterior disk displacement is a clicking or popping sound during opening and closing movements. These sounds are caused by the head of the condyle bumping over the posterior band of the disk, as the condyle head translates forward during jaw opening. In the open jaw position, the condyle is temporarily in its correct position so the joint is "reduced." Hence, this is referred to as anterior disk displacement with reduction. When the jaw closes, the condyle bumps back over the posterior rim of the disk with

a second closing click. A progression of this disorder may be a failure of the condyle head, when sliding forward to regain, even temporarily its position beneath the disk, which becomes bunched up. This condition is described as anterior disk displacement without reduction, because the disk is never recaptured onto the head of the condyle, and there is limited capacity to open the jaw. There is no joint sound as attempts are made to open the jaw wide. If disk displacement occurs over a long period of time, the tissues of the bilaminar zone become fibrous and further adapted to function as a disk.

9.3.3 Condyle Position

Abnormalities in the position of the condyle have in the past been confidently proposed as a source of pain in the joint. The argument has been that the condyle should occupy a central position in the glenoid fossa. If it is displaced, particularly in a posterior superior position, there will be compression of the posterior part of the disk and pain. There is no evidence that this occurs or that there is an optimal position of the condyle in the fossa, so this theory has been abandoned by most authorities. There is also less emphasis placed on the diagnostic values of routine radiographs or magnetic resonance imaging (MRI) of the joint. Special techniques involving computer-assisted tomography (CAT) and the insertion of a radioactive die into the joint space (arthrography) are of some diagnostic value in situations where the disk is not normally related to the condyle head. In a recent study, MRI was used to investigate the disk position in normal volunteers. The authors found that 25% of the sample had abnormal disk positions. The definition of "normal" in this study was clearly too narrow, as all these individuals were without symptoms and required no treatment. It has been noted in *Chapter 8 Eruption, Occlusion, and Wear* that care must be exercised before constructing narrow definitions of normal. This practice is especially concerning if the use of sophisticated diagnostic techniques produces *false-positive* results, which may be used to motivate invasive treatment (*see section 9.4.7 Diagnostic Tests*).

Key Notes

The TMJ is driven through complex movements dictated by chewing activity under the control of masticatory muscles. It has evolved to support the loads applied during this activity and to remodel as the teeth wear. It is a robust structure which shows little evidence of dysfunction or degeneration.

Review Questions

1. How can it be demonstrated that the TMJ is load bearing?
2. Why would the joint be unstable if the reaction was not at right angles to the joint surface?
3. Why is the reaction in the joint so variable?
4. Why is the reaction at the joint higher when biting on an incisor that on a molar?
5. What do you think might be the main action of the lateral pterygoid muscle?
6. What do you understand by the term disk displacement without reduction?
7. What is meant by a false-positive result and why is it potentially harmful?

9.4 Temporomandibular Dysfunction

9.4.1 Diagnosis

The process of making a diagnosis involves the selection from a few possible options of the most likely classification for a disorder or identifying a known condition. Having identified the disorder, we then identify the most likely cause, if this is not well established. Both these processes, the classification and naming of the disorder, and identifying its cause, present problems when making a diagnosis of temporomandibular disorder (TMD).

Firstly, the selection of names includes myofascial pain dysfunction syndrome (MPDS), temporomandibular disorder (TMD), temporomandibular dysfunction (TMD), craniomandibular dysfunction (CMD), etc. which suggest that the disorder is not easily defined. Furthermore, within each of these names there are subtypes of the disorder, so it is clearly not a single condition. The term chosen for use in this text is temporomandibular dysfunction, as it does not imply any disorder of the joint itself.

Secondly, there is no consensus as to the probable causes. This leaves the practitioner uncertain about what is going on or how to control it. This review will introduce the Research Diagnostic Criteria (RDC) classification system for pain and dysfunction and review some of the current thinking on the cause for each of the related conditions.

The first description by Costen used the word syndrome to indicate its complexity. However, a syndrome does not take us beyond a mere collection of clinical symptoms and signs. If we want a holistic view of health and ill health, we have to accept that illness is more than a collection of clinical symptoms. There is a soul/mind in there, and it is inseparable from the body. So, illness is also about the host's state of mind. The data to support this ordinary wisdom are emerging in the relatively recent field of psychoneuroimmunology.

9.4.2 General Description of Temporomandibular Dysfunction

There are four main signs and symptoms which characterize TMD.

- The central theme and the most frequent presenting complaint is pain. This is usually unilateral, around the cheek, joint, temple, ear, and eye. It is dull, deep, may spread, and is persistent. Palpation over the TMJ or overlying muscle is painful. It is the second most common source of pain after toothache which presents to the dentist.
- It may be worse in the morning or at the end of the day, and when opening wide or biting hard. A history of this sort of pain immediately distinguishes it from the lancing, burning pain of the neuralgias (trigeminal and postherpetic).
- In addition to the pain in TMD, there may be limited mobility of the jaw.
- There may be grating or clicking of the TMJ.

9.4.3 Research Diagnostic Criteria

At the University of Washington in Seattle, a team of research workers in the Department of Oral Medicine developed a classification system for TMD.[5] Their leader, Samuel Dworkin, realized the need to recognize, and include, both physiological and psychosocial aspects to TMD pain and dysfunction in any diagnostic system. The team constructed two main axes to represent physical and psychosocial factors. They referred to the group of physical factors as Axis I and included classification factors based on signs, such as muscle and/or joint tenderness, limited movement, and joint sounds. They referred to a group of psychosocial factors as Axis II and included factors based on symptoms, such as pain and disability, depression, and other nonspecific complaints such as backache. This classification system was been styled TMD classification for the purpose of RDC. It is summarized in the following section.

9.4.4 Axis I—Physical Factors (Signs)

Group I: Muscle Disorders

These are of two types:
1. Tender muscles without limited opening.
2. Tender muscles with limited opening.

Group II: Disk Displacements

These are of three types:
1. Disk displacement (anterior) with reduction (click).
2. Disk displacement (anterior) without reduction (no click) and limited opening.
3. Disk displacement (anterior) without reduction (no click) and without limited opening.

Group III: Other Joint Disorders

These are of three types:
1. Arthralgia when there is pain over the joint on palpation.
2. Osteoarthritis when arthralgia is present with coarse crepitus in the joint.
3. Osteoarthrosis when there is coarse crepitus and no arthralgia.

9.4.5 Axis II—Psychosocial Factors (Symptoms)

- Pain intensity and disability graded on a visual analog scale.
- Psychological status as revealed by a depression score.
- The presence and prevalence of physical symptoms unrelated to the TMD, such as gastric acidity.

The Axis II factors are measured using a questionnaire which the patient completes. There are several inventories of anxiety and depression, some of them more suited to use by psychologists. The RDC recommend that the patient record chronic pain levels including disability. This is followed by a questionnaire which includes the Symptom Checklist—90, a series of reliable tests for measuring depression. The questionnaire takes about 20 minutes to complete, but as this can be done by the patient alone, it does not intrude on the dentist's schedule. It can be scored in a few minutes and the results shared with the patient. Some patients may find this degree of interest in their private lives rather intrusive. Shorter, single-page questionnaires can be useful if only to reflect to the patient the need to address stressful issues in their life. One simple inventory is called the Hospital Anxiety and Depression (HAD) index. It should be photocopied and folded so as to hide the scoring system. When the patient has completed the questionnaire, unfold the page and add up the scores for each question using the adjacent scoring system.

The development of the RDC has helped to reunite the two sides of the same coin. Illness is not either somatic or psychosocial, it is both, a continuum from one end to the other. We need to use a diagnostic system which helps us to focus our efforts in the most effective place, assuming that treatment should always be individualized. The RDC also offers the practitioner a reliable means of assessing psychological status. This helps us understand the patient better and gives us a guideline when we should be recommending that the patient also sees a trained counselor. The operative word is also. The RDC approach does not direct patients into one or other realm of therapy but keeps them on the same continuum. We still do not know why bite splints work, or why restoring posterior occlusal contact sometimes helps, but there is no doubt that physical therapy can be helpful.

9.4.6 Evidence-Based Etiology

Occlusion and TMD. A great deal of attention has been directed at occlusion as a causative factor in TMD. It has been argued that in order to avoid cuspal interference, the jaw assumes postures which are abnormal. It was thought that abnormal postures would cause pressure on sensitive parts of the joint, uncoordinated muscle activity, and muscle strain. There is a considerable body of evidence to support an association between occlusal disharmony and TMD, although little of this evidence has been derived from randomized and controlled studies.

- In a study by De Boever and Adriaens, no correlation was found between the numbers of occluding molars and levels of muscles dysfunction.[6]
- Experimentally placed occlusal interferences do not predictably cause signs and symptoms of TMD.[7]
- Patients with apparently severe malocclusion do not all develop dysfunction. Patients with TMD do not all have a malocclusion or even occlusal interferences.[8]
- Loss of vertical height does not appear to increase the risk of TMD.[9]

Muscle tenderness. Muscle tenderness is a frequent sign in TMD of muscular origin. Trigger points are especially tender to pressure. Muscle pain may be due to lactic acid buildup, which results from prolonged contraction of muscles. Masticatory muscles are particularly resistant to fatigue, provided that contractions are cyclic, tension followed by, relaxation. Sustained contraction, even though the force of contraction may be low, causes muscle ischemia and delayed-onset pain. Masticatory muscles may be under sustained contraction due to the following factors:
- Attempt to avoid gross occlusal interference, particularly lateral deviations from the centric relation position.
- Attempt to compensate for lack of posterior support.
- Mental stress causing raised muscle tone particularly in the facial and masticatory muscles.
- Nocturnal bruxism generally regarded as a sleep disorder and not related to occlusion.

9.4.7 Diagnostic Tests

Tests are available and have been promoted as more reliable than the rather simple observations we have so far made. However, are they of any use? The accuracy of diagnostic methods is indicated by determining how often they can correctly detect disease (*sensitivity*) and how often they can correctly detect the normal cases (*specificity*). In conditions which are not life threatening (like a displaced temporomandibular disk), it is not that important if the diagnostic test (e.g., MRI) misses a few abnormal disks. This would be expressed by a moderately high sensitivity. However, when a positive diagnosis might lead to invasive treatment, it is important that the test does not incorrectly identify normal disks as abnormal. This situation would be expressed by a poor specificity. Any such so-called false-positive results could lead to unnecessary surgery. It has been suggested that a *specificity* of at least 95% is acceptable (only 5% false positives) and that a *sensitivity* of around 80% (20% missed positives) is acceptable. Given these reasonable goals, there are no data to support the diagnostic accuracy of MRI or computerized tomography (CT) of the joint. The injection of radiopaque dies (joint arthrography) is more specific but invasive. Electromyography has also failed to emerge as a useful diagnostic test. The simplest techniques using surface electrodes are very susceptible to variations even between normal subjects. The most consistent diagnostic sign for TMD is a limited range of jaw movement, which can be measured with a ruler.

9.4.8 Illness Behavior

The team developing the RDC selected terms to define classifications which were directly related to observation, that is signs and symptoms. They avoided using terms which suggested an etiology. No suggestion is made about the origin of muscle pain or joint dysfunction, although those that exist, which are based on anecdotal evidence, are systematically disposed of. The RDC finds there is no evidence to support some of the favorite etiologies of the past, namely malocclusion, occlusal interference, or abnormal relationships between the condyle and the glenoid fossa (*see Appendix H.4 Anecdotal Evidence; a Poor Substitute for Science*).

Whatever the pathologies may be, which could account for the different aspects of TMD, a common theme joining them together is that individuals with chronic pain show some degree of illness behavior. It may be more productive to focus on the nature of this, for example, the degree of depression in comparison with stress in order to select the most appropriate treatment. Any physical treatment is at best taking a guess at what might work. No physical treatments have been found to be uniformly effective.

9.4.9 Management of Temporomandibular Dysfunction

The options for clinical management of TMD are beyond the scope of this text, though it is worth mentioning two broadly agreed maxims. They are that treatment should be reversible and noninvasive. While many dental problems are solved by some operative procedure, the treatment of TMD can be well managed without operative procedure other than the fabrication of an occlusal bite splint. The patient should take an active role in self management of this condition as lifestyle and stress are significant contributors. The dentist has an important role in educating the patient about the origins of TMD and in providing advice about its management.

Winfield gives us a refreshingly clear view of sickness and health. He asserts that we all suffer in varying degrees, on a continuum, from blissfully happy to chronically miserable.[10] The patients who come to chronic pain clinics do not have a discrete disease but are "simply the most ill in a continuum of distress, chronic pain, and painful tender points in the general population."

Key Notes

All classifications, including diagnostic categories, are of human construction. We should not be surprised, therefore, to encounter patients who do not fit readily in any particular category. We need to be cautious of diagnostic tests which have adopted narrow, restrictive criteria for defining normal, as these tests will give false-positive results and may drive unnecessary or invasive treatment.

References

[1] Osborn JW. The disc of the human temporomandibular joint: design, function and failure. J Oral Rehabil 1985;12(4):279–293
[2] Owen CP, Wilding RJC, Morris AG. Changes in mandibular condyle morphology related to tooth wear in a prehistoric human population. Arch Oral Biol 1991;36(11):799–804
[3] Osborn JW, Baragar FA. Predicted pattern of human muscle activity during clenching from a computer assisted model. J Biomech 1985;18:599–612
[4] Rees LA. The structure and function of the mandibular joint. Br Dent J 1954;96:125–133
[5] Dworkin SF, LeResche L. Research diagnostic criteria for temporomandibular disorders: review, criteria, examinations and specifications, critique. J Craniomandib Disord 1992;6(4):301–355
[6] De Boever JA, Adriaens PA. Occlusal relationship in patients with pain-dysfunction symptoms in the temporomandibular joints. J Oral Rehabil 1983;10(1):1–7
[7] Magnusson T, Enbom L. Signs and symptoms of mandibular dysfunction after introduction of experimental balancing-side interferences. Acta Odontol Scand 1984;42(3):129–135
[8] Shroff B. Malocclusion as a Cause for Temporomandibular Disorders and Orthodontics as a Treatment. Oral Maxillofac Surg Clin North Am 2018;30 (3):299–302
[9] Wilding RJC, Owen CP. The prevalence of temporomandibular joint dysfunction in edentulous non-denture wearing individuals. J Oral Rehabil 1987;14 (2):175–182
[10] Winfield JB. Pain in fibromyalgia. Rheum Dis Clin North Am 1999;25(1):55–79

Suggested Readings

Movement at the Temporomandibular Joint

Spruijt RJ, Hoogstraten J. The research on temporomandibular joint clicking: a methodological review. J Craniomandib Disord 1991;5(1):45–50

Temporomandibular Dysfunction

Clark GT. A critical evaluation of orthopedic interocclusal appliance therapy: design, theory, and overall effectiveness. J Am Dent Assoc 1984;108(3):359–364
Dolwick MF, Dimitroulis G. A re-evaluation of the importance of disc position in temporomandibular disorders. Aust Dent J 1996;41(3):184–187
Forssell H, Kalso E, Koskela P, Vehmanen R, Puukka P, Alanen P. Occlusal treatments in temporomandibular disorders: a qualitative systematic review of randomized controlled trials. Pain 1999;83(3):549–560
Luther F. TMD and occlusion part II. Damned if we don't? Functional occlusal problems: TMD epidemiology in a wider context. Br Dent J 2007;202(1):E3, discussion 38–39

10 Oral Sensations and Functions

Abstract

The dental patient is well equipped with oral sensory capacity. Touch, taste, and smell are all backed up and reinforced by sight and sound. To these five senses must be added several more, including pain. This rich, oral, sensory input has to be decoded and given meaning by the brain. The brain/mind may interpret the potentially fearful content of the incoming information as nonthreatening and ignore it. Or the sensory input may be magnified many times by stress, anxiety, and bad memories. Pain is not a direct sensory perception; it is an unpleasant emotional experience. Understanding pain would be impossible without joining up the sensations arising in the jaws and teeth with the patient's brain/mind. The "hot tooth" is the result of neurogenic inflammation, the transport of inflammatory chemical messengers inside the axons of the nerve fibers from the peripheral nervous system into the pulp tissue.

The functions of chewing, swallowing, and speaking are complex and require a rich source of sensory input from a variety of receptor types in the muscles of the jaw, the periodontal ligament, and the soft tissues.

Keywords: pain, experience, sensory, emotions, measuring, control, placebo, types, mechanisms, dentinal, neurogenic, gate control, taste, proprioception, reflexes, taste, swallowing, speech

10.1 The Nature of Pain

Several attempts have been made to define pain, none of which are entirely satisfactory. The definition adopted by the International Society of Pain Management is "an unpleasant sensory and emotional experience associated with actual or potential tissue damage, or described in terms of such damage." Note that this definition includes an emotional component of pain which is always present and in fact defines pain from other sensations. We should never be tempted to describe pain without both its sensory and emotional components.

10.1.1 Injury without Pain

The relationship between an injury and the pain it causes is usually obvious. Banging your hand against a door may cause a twinge of pain, but it is not comparable to the pain you feel when your fingers are caught in the door as it slams closed. Usually, the worse the injury, the worse the pain. However, there are many occasions when this is not so. There are recorded cases of congenital analgesia in which there is a total absence of pain, without any physical abnormality of the nervous system. These poor individuals injure themselves without knowing it and die rather young from chronic tissue damage. From this example, we can conclude that pain has survival value. Congenital analgesia is a rare condition, but not infrequently, individuals have short periods or episodes of analgesia immediately following severe injury. This unexplained absence of pain has been observed during conflicts when badly wounded soldiers, brought from the battle front, appeared to be free of pain from their wounds. Episodic analgesia has also been observed in industrial accidents free of the diversions of war. The analgesia commonly does not last longer than 24 hours. During this time, it is confined to the injured part, so the patient may complain of some mild injury elsewhere, like the prick of an injection. From this example, we can surmise that if our survival depended on it, pain might be temporarily suppressed.

10.1.2 Pain without Injury

One of the puzzles of pain is that it may be felt even when there is little injury. Tension headaches and low back pain cause misery in many individuals, yet there is usually little injury or damage occurring. The passage of a kidney stone down the ureter does insignificant damage, but the slight stretching of the smooth muscle wall causes the patient to double up with excruciating pain. It is also puzzling that pain may appear long after healing has occurred to damaged or severed nerves. Months after the stump of an amputated limb has healed, a constant searing pain may appear wherever the limb used to be. This phantom limb pain responds poorly to analgesics. Pain without injury seems pointless and perverse of nature to inflict it on us.

From these examples it is clear that pain mechanisms are complex.

10.1.3 Chronic Pain

Pain may be almost continuous or with only short remission for several years. It may be due to a chronic pathology (e.g., arthritis, vascular plaques around a ganglion) or a progressive cancer. However, the term chronic pain implies long-standing pain without any apparent organic cause which could account for its severity. The phantom limb pain mentioned above is an example. A similarly unpleasant cause of chronic pain is *causalgia* also known as complex regional pain syndrome. This pain is characterized by an intense burning pain in the area of a damaged peripheral nerve. It may result from trauma, such as a bullet wound, or fracture. Sometime after the injury, the skin becomes very tender to slight touching, which is followed after a slight delay by a most unpleasant burning or crushing pain over a wide area. The limb associated with the trauma may become swollen and stiff. Both phantom limb pain and causalgia are difficult to treat. Drugs and surgery, often performed at the request of the patient, are seldom successful.

We must avoid the temptation to assume that if we cannot find a cause for pain that it does not exist. Our ability to examine the nervous system is still very primitive. It is not like a network of telephone wires with direct links from receptors to a coordinating center. As more is understood about the complex changes in the nervous system following peripheral nerve damage, it becomes apparent that disruption in the central nervous system has also occurred.

Chronic pain sufferers tend to have signs of other conditions related to stress, such as depression, indigestion, constipation, and insomnia. Depression is a consistent feature of chronic pain. It may be argued that this is either secondary to the pain or that it is the primary condition and the most important to treat. The contribution made by physical and emotional factors to pain is illustrated by the Research Diagnostic Criteria classification of temporomandibular disorders (*see Chapter 9.4.3 Research Diagnostic Criteria*).

10.1.4 Measuring Pain

It is difficult to measure pain, because it is a private experience confined to the sufferer. We cannot examine the pain directly but have to rely on the patient's version of it. Sometimes, it will seem that there is no cause for the pain and we might want to conclude that the patient is imagining it. However, all pain is real to the sufferer. The causes may lie too deep for us to find. We can get an idea of the nature of someone else's pain by asking them to describe it. We will find it useful to pay close attention to the words they use. Some words may arise from a thoughtful, analytical process, so-called *cognitive* description. Other words which arise are an expression of emotions and from feelings, so-called *affective* descriptions. Examples of cognitive descriptive words are "sharp," "burning," "faint," "mild," and "intense" which suggest that the patient is describing the sensation of his or her pain. If affective words like "uncomfortable," "miserable," "unbearable," and "awful" are used, we know the patient's pain is affecting them emotionally.

A simpler, but less informative way of monitoring the levels of pain is by asking the patient to give it a rating on a scale from 1 (just perceptible) to 10 (unbearable). In experimental situations, the lowest intensity of a stimulus that produces pain is the pain *threshold*. The most intense stimulus that can be endured is the pain *tolerance*.

> **Key Notes**
>
> The brain/mind plays a selective role in determining the pain experience. We may suffer deeply in response to apparently quite trivial tissue damage, but we may also suppress pain if we think we can.

10.2 Psychological Factors and Pain

All pain has an emotional component. We have unhappy memories of being hurt and fear that pain may return. Pain is almost always unpleasant and we focus our efforts to avoid it. If we cannot avoid it, we want to make sure we get it under control as soon as possible. We usually welcome support from others who may help us to control our pain.

10.2.1 Culture

The attitudes to pain vary from one culture to another. Some individuals, such as the Native Americans, acquired a reputation for restraining their emotions, including pain. For them, it was not acceptable to show fear, suffering, or grief. These values became role models for the strong, silent cowboys, who the movies created into the heroes of the Wild West. In contrast, the individuals of the Mediterranean are less inhibited. It is not shameful for men to cry at the opera or for women to wail loudly in childbirth. Tests for pain threshold and tolerance for different cultural groups show marked differences, although the sensory threshold, that is, the ability to detect a stimulus such as a weak electric current or slight warmth is not different. This proves that the sensory apparatus of humans is essentially the same.

10.2.2 Past Experience

Attitudes to pain are shaped early in childhood by our parents' response to minor cuts and bruises. Learning about pain also occurs after having suffered from it, so that it may be avoided in future. Many adult dental patients who are afraid of dental procedures are able to trace their fear back to painful experiences as children. On the other hand, pain-free experiences in childhood pave the way for an easy relationship with dentists and dentistry in adult life. The experience gained by pain and learning to avoid it reveal one of its main purposes, that is to prevent recurring injury.

10.2.3 The Meaning of Pain

Pain is more bearable when its cause can be understood and the threat identified. Pain near the heart is frightening because of the possibility that a heart attack is coming. If the doctor can assure us that the source of the pain is indigestion, as it often is, the pain may become quite insignificant. Reassurance by the doctor or dentist that pain is not a sign of a sinister illness, like cancer, immediately reduces the level of pain in the sufferer.

In some circumstances, pain may carry such positive associations as to be ignored. In a few cultures, the pain of childbirth is welcomed and celebrated as it brings promises of birth and new life. Such is the conviction of their women in labor that they laugh with pleasure and excitement at their birth pain.

10.2.4 Control over Pain

Following severe burns, the dead skin must be removed to allow healing. This wound debridement is very painful but is bearable if the patient can assist in the work of pulling away the dead tissue. The importance of control can be verified under experimental conditions. Volunteers allow themselves to be given an electric shock to find out how much they can tolerate. If they are able to manipulate the controls which increases the voltage, they are able to tolerate higher levels of stimulus than if this control is manipulated by anyone else. Some dental patients find that having their teeth cleaned with an ultrasonic scaler is uncomfortable and at times even painful; it helps the patient to put up with some discomfort, if there is some agreed way of giving the dentist a sign that the pain is more than the patient wants to tolerate.

One of the strategies for helping patients to deal with chronic pain is to give them control over their drug doses and to help them to take control of their lives rather than allow the pain to become their master.

It is possible to reduce awareness of pain for a while by diverting attention from it. Dancers and athletes are able to concentrate so fully on their performance that they can put pain out of their mind. Even mental arithmetic or visual and auditory distractions may for a while be effective in reducing pain.

Pains which are readily understood, and which over time are reduced, are reasonably well tolerated. Examples are birth pain and injury or inflammation, which are relatively short lived and can be reduced with suitable treatment. When the pain is out of the patient's and the doctor's or dentist's control, it is said to be intractable and is highly distressing.

10.2.5 Suggestion and Placebo

The mere suggestion that pain will be taken away has a powerful effect on the sufferer. So, a tablet which contains nothing more than flavoring, a *placebo*, often succeeds in reducing pain if the patient is told it is a powerful analgesic. It is still more effective if the tablet looks impressive (capsules are better that tablets) and if two are given. It is most important, though, for the therapist also to believe that the patient is being given an active analgesic, and that it is a strong one. When clinical trials are designed to compare an analgesic with a placebo, they are so-called "double-blind," meaning neither the patient nor the doctor knows whether the tablet has the active ingredient or not. Under these conditions, 35% of patients given a placebo report that their pain goes away. The powerful effect of placebos extends to somatic illness. It does not imply that the patient's complaint must be imagined but illustrates the complexity of illness, and how it is influenced by the reaction of both our minds and immune systems to it.

Experiencing pain and illness is worrying, and so it comes as a great relief to be in the care of someone who wants to help. It is likely that any benefit patients receive from homeopathic remedies is due to the care, compassion, and companionship, which the therapist provides.

10.2.6 Hypnosis

The exact mental state during hypnosis is not clear, but it seems to be a sort of trance during which the subject is particularly susceptible to suggestion from the hypnotist, yet not under his or her control. Some individuals are unable to be hypnotized, but about 30% can be induced into a deep trance during which some painful surgery can be performed. These subjects are receptive to suggestion and also inclined to benefit most from placebos. Some individuals are able to induce trance-like states in themselves and then walk over hot coals or lie on beds of nails and even cut themselves without bleeding. An essential requirement of performing these challenges is training. So, these individuals do not possess some unusual physiological resistance to pain but must be trained to ignore it. Volunteers who are complete novices may be trained in a few days to walk over hot coals.

10.2.7 "Psychological" Pain

Unfortunately, many normal patients may have been told their pain is "psychological" because the doctor or dentist could not find a reason for it. All pain is strongly influenced by psychological factors; it is a highly emotion-filled experience, but what these therapists are really wanting to say is that the pain is imagined and not really there. As providers of health care, we have to be careful not to invest too much confidence in our own healing powers. We have some tools in our bag, but when it comes to management, particularly of chronic pain, the bag soon empties, and we may feel powerless and frustrated. Then, it is tempting to dismiss the problem by ruling that it does not really exist. All pain is real to the sufferer, whether or not the therapist can make any sense of it.

There are cases of patients who seem to need to have pain. They may be able to nurture it from within, or they may seek out painful operations, one after the other. The need for pain seems abnormal in any context, but particularly so when it becomes a feature of sexual pleasure. In the past, self-flagellation (whipping) was a well-recognized pathway to spiritual purity in Christian monks. Self-harming is sadly not uncommon among today's troubled teenagers. There may be some sense of self-punishment in all these individuals, who feel better about themselves when some inner score is settled. However, the troubled mind of such individuals may work; it is probable that they have given pain a meaning, which somehow fulfils their emotional needs.

10.2.8 Pain at Death

The emergence of hospices followed the pioneering work of Cecily Saunders at St. Christopher's Hospice in London. Now, we know there is much more that can be done to manage pain in the terminally ill, not the least of which is a willingness to use as much morphine as is necessary, without fear of tolerance or addiction. It is well proven that when addictive drugs are used to control pain, the dose does not have to be progressively increased to have the same effect (tolerance), nor are there withdrawal symptoms (addiction) should the medical condition make it possible to reduce the drug. While pain in the terminally ill can cast a heavy shadow over the last few months, or even years, it seems that when very close to death, there is eventually some respite. Animals normally sensitive to pain become quite peaceful and free of agony when massive injury and almost certain death are close at hand. There are also many cases recorded of humans who have been declared dead yet survived to tell their experience. These so-called near-death experiences are remarkably similar; the survivors recall being quite free of pain and surrounded by wonderful music and warm friendly individuals. It is as if, in the last act, the shadow of pain melts away, and death is a welcoming end.

> **Key Notes**
>
> All pain is real to the sufferer. It always has both an emotional and a physical component. A placebo is not for imagined pain but offers hope, even belief, that the pain can be brought under control.

10.3 Some Types of Clinical Pain

While the brain or mind is the organ where pain is perceived, the tissue in which the pain originates makes a substantial difference to the experience. While some tissues have an unusual response to tissue damage, there are clinical types of pain which are common to all tissues.

Hyperalgesia: Tissues which have been subject to damage and painful for some time may become even more sensitive to stimulus than they were originally. An example of hyperalgesia is that experienced by light-skinned individuals, who have been sunburnt. The same day, they may feel pain getting into a hot bathtub. The next day they may feel pain in getting into even a slightly warm bathtub. The pain brought on by levels of a stimulus which are normally low enough not to cause pain is called *allodynia*. Both hyperalgesia and allodynia are brought about by an accumulation of pain and inflammation-stimulating chemicals in the damaged tissue and in the spinal cord. This is called

peripheral and central sensitization and will be described in further detail below.

The pulp–dentin: The pulp–dentin is densely supplied with free nerve endings which are specialized (not specific) to conveying pain. The role of this sensitivity to pain is unclear. There are patients who feel very little pain during cavity preparation to remove dental caries, but most are only too happy to have as much anesthetic as is needed to ensure that cavity preparation is pain free.

The pulp–dentin is particularly sensitive to increase in pressure as it is a confined tissue space. Inflammation of the pulp rapidly causes a raise in tissue pressure, which leads to allodynia and hyperalgesia. In an allodynic condition, the pulp–dentin is sensitive to even slight changes in temperature, either hot or cold.

When enamel protection is lost or removed, the exposed dentin is sensitive to changes in osmotic pressure which may be brought about by sweet or sour foods. Pulp–dentin is also sensitive to electrical stimulation. The mechanisms which are thought to cause pulp–dentin pain are discussed in the next section.

Visceral pain: The gut and urogenital organs of the body are surprisingly insensitive to cutting or even burning but exquisitely sensitive to pressure or tension. As we have noted, the mild distension of the ureter, as a kidney stone is passed, causes severe pain. So does distension of the uterus during the contractions of menstruation or childbirth. Dilation of the cervix during childbirth may cause quite severe pain, but when the dilation is sudden, as may occur during rape, the pain is excruciating. If any of these organs is even slightly inflamed, the pain threshold to tension or pressure is very low.

Muscle pain: All types of muscle tissue are sensitive to ischemia. This is a reduced blood supply which may occur after sustained periods of muscle contraction which progressively interrupts the circulation. Ischemia causes a build up of metabolites, particularly lactic acid which may cause severe cramps and acute pain. A deeper and more diffuse muscle pain may occur after gradual and low-grade tissue damage to muscles. This damage may occur due to prolonged tension of the muscle, such as occurs with bad posture. For example, the neck muscles of dentists may ache after a day's work, if the neck is not held in an upright posture at all times during operative procedures. There are usually tender areas of the back muscles, which are detectable as small lumps or ridges within the muscle mass. They have been called trigger points, as pressure on them triggers an episode of pain. Muscle pain is diffuse and may be felt some distance from the sight of a trigger point. Painful muscles of the jaw often refer pain to the area around the ear and the temporomandibular joint (TMJ) (*see Chapter 10.4.8 Trigger Points in Muscles*).

Peripheral nerve pain: Neuralgia is caused by viral infection or degeneration of peripheral nerves. *Causalgia* is more commonly caused by damage to peripheral nerves. During infection by the herpes zoster virus, inflammation of peripheral nerves occurs with blisters (shingles) on the skin over the affected nerve. During the active infection, a burning pain is felt, which usually subsides when the infection is resolved. In some patients, the pain persists (postherpetic neuralgia) and may become worse. This pain is similar to *causalgia*, in that the skin is hypersensitive to light stimulation, such as mild heat. For the first few seconds nothing is felt. Then a rush of burning pain follows which has a particularly unpleasant nature.

Trigeminal neuralgia is confined to the sensory distribution of the trigeminal nerve. Gentle stimulation of a usually well-defined trigger point on the face provokes a massive stabbing pain. Local anesthesia of the trigeminal nerve branches produces temporary relief. Other procedures which block the nerve for longer periods work temporarily, but the pain recurs. A frequent finding at autopsy or operation is a demyelination of the roots of the trigeminal nerve. This may be due to compression from the surrounding blood vessels. In many cases, relief is obtained by surgical decompression of the nerve roots. The pain may also be reduced by antiepileptic drugs (e.g., Tegretol), which decrease the firing of central brain cells.

An important factor which increases the response of all tissue to pain is inflammation. This is because many of the cytokines which promote inflammation such as prostaglandins, serotonin, substance P, and histamine all increase peripheral sensitization (*see Chapter 10.4.6 Neurogenic Inflammation of the Pulp Tissue*).

Brain and bone tissues. Neither the brain nor bone tissues perceive pain. It is the membranes around these tissues which are sensitive to pain. The clinical implications for dental surgeons are that an implant osteotomy may be prepared in alveolar bone, provided that a local infiltration of anesthesia is used to reduce sensations from the periosteum.

10.4 Pain Mechanisms

The interactions between sensory neurons in the spinal cord which influence the pain pathway, together with the influences on these neurons of a large family of neurochemicals, are complex. It is therefore not possible to present a comprehensive or succinct summary here. The reader interested to pursue a fuller understanding of pain mechanisms is referred to a group of reviews which present the latest levels of understanding.[1,2] What follows is an abbreviated overview which is designed to provide the practitioner with a working understanding which will support clinical practice.

10.4.1 Pain Pathways

Nerve cells (*neurons*) in the peripheral and central nervous systems have a single thin *axon* which may be several centimeters long and transports electrical and chemical messages over long distances. Neurons also have hundreds of shorter projections called *dendrites*, which communicate with neighboring nerve cells. Bipolar neurons have two long axons, one receiving nerve impulses from the periphery and the other carrying impulses toward the central nervous system. The cell bodies of bipolar neurons are situated in peripheral nodes called *ganglia*. Nerve fibers serving the teeth and jaws have their cell bodies in the *trigeminal* ganglion.

There are three main chains of neurons carrying messages from the periphery to the brain. The neurons whose fibers carry impulses from receptors in the peripheral tissue are called first-order neurons. Their journey toward the central nervous system continues only as far as the dorsal horn of the spinal column or in the case of the trigeminal nerve to the subnucleus caudalis in the brainstem. Here, the central part of the axons of

the first order neuron forms junctions with the second-order neurons of the trigeminal nucleus in the brainstem. These second-order neurons convey the impulses onward along their axons toward the third-order neurons in the thalamus from which axons project to the cortex (▶ Fig. 10.1). These are the three main levels in the pathways of the nervous system, but there are also interneurons, which carry impulses between the spinal neurons at each level and between each level in the main pathways.

The junctions between the nerve axons and the cell membrane of the next order neuron are called *synapses*.

Nociceptors are sensory nerve cells with receptors which detect tissue damage and are responsible for transmitting pain impulses to the brain. The cell bodies of nociceptors are the first-order, bipolar neurons located in the dorsal root ganglia of the spinal cord and the trigeminal ganglia of the trigeminal nerve.

There are two main types of nerve *axons* (fibers) associated with nociceptive neurons.
- The C fibers have a small diameter and are nonmyelinated. They conduct impulses slowly, from 1 to 3 m/s. They are very numerous.
- Aδ fibers are also small diameter (0.2–1.5 μm), but they are myelinated and conduct impulses at 3 to 30 m/s.

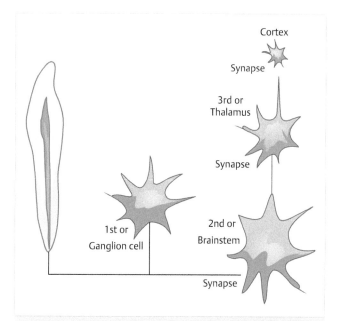

Fig. 10.1 A diagrammatic representation of the three orders of neurons in the nerve pathways of the trigeminal nerve. The nerves of the dental pulp have their cell bodies in the trigeminal ganglion. These first-order nerve cells (1st or) are bipolar, that is they have two axons, one leading toward the periphery, in this case, the dental pulp, the other leading toward the brainstem, where they synapse with the second-order (2nd or) nociceptive specific neurons (NS) of the trigeminal nucleus. Should the membrane of the NS depolarize, an impulse will travel along the cell's axon to the next level, a synapse in a third-order neuron (3rd or) of the thalamus. If this neuron depolarizes, an electrical impulse travels down its axon to synapses in the cortex. The route for a single nerve impulse from a receptor in the dental pulp must then pass through three orders of neuron. These synapses may be likened to gates, which may or may not transmit the impulse onward.

There are other fiber types (Aβ), mainly concerned with non-pain sensation such as mechanoreception and proprioception which are up to 50 times faster than fibers which convey pain impulses. They are of importance in the pathway of pain as they may modulate pain transmission.

The first sharp stinging pain after injury (such as touching a hot cooking pan) lasts a few seconds only and is carried fast enough along myelinated Aβ fibers to ensure a rapid response (withdrawal). This first pain is followed by a poorly localized deeper pain which is carried by the nonmyelinated, C fibers. The impulses carried by C fibers also alert the slower metabolic responses required for inflammation and healing. The pain response to sudden injury changes in the seconds, hours, and days after tissue damage.

Nerve axons are two-way transporters of both electrical and chemical messages. They carry electrical impulses toward and away from the nerve cell. Nerve cells are polarized, the outside of the cell membrane being relatively positively charged. The nerve impulses start as a reverse in the polarity, just at one site of the membrane. This reversal of polarity triggers a cascade of depolarization events along the nerve axon, and like a wave, this electrical pulse passes down the nerve axon (▶ Fig. 10.2).

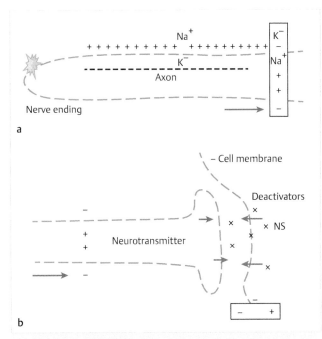

Fig. 10.2 A diagrammatic representation of a nerve impulse propagated by depolarization of the axon membrane. (a) The nerve cell membrane and its axon are highly polarized. Stimulation of a nerve ending sends a wave of electrical depolarization caused by the rapid exchange of sodium (Na) and potassium (K) ions through channels in the cell membrane. The wave of depolarization moves toward a nociceptive specific (NS) neuron in the spinal cord or brainstem. (b) At the NS neuron, the electrical impulse causes the release of neurotransmitter substances into the synapse gap. If the concentration of these chemicals reaches a critical level, and if the NS neuron is already in an excited state, its membrane may depolarize and send an impulse toward the brain. The NS neuron also secretes deactivators into the synaptic gap which break down the neurotransmitters and deactivate them. It is here that opiates and serotonin reduce the influence of the neurotransmitter substances. Here, even at the first synaptic junction, there are neurochemicals which are associated with emotions, fatigue, or anxiety, which influence the excitability of the NS neuron.

The electrical potential of this depolarization is constant in the peripheral nerve axons, but the frequency of the impulses varies, and it is this variation which conveys the nature of the information being carried.

If the axon is more than 1 µm in diameter, it is covered by a sheath of *myelin*, an insulating material. This material is formed by a *glial* (nerve-supporting) cell, called a Schwann cell. These cells wrap their cell membranes, which contain myelin around the nerve axon. There are gaps in the myelin between each cell, called nodes of Ranvier, which allow the nerve impulse to jump across from one node in the myelin sheath to the next, thereby increasing its speed of conduction several times.

10.4.2 Nerve Synapses

A nerve impulse that originates from the periphery travels as far as the spinal cord where it has to be carried across a space between the nerve axon and the cell membrane of the spinal cord cell. This space is called a *synapse*. The synaptic space is crossed, not by an electrical discharge, but by chemical transmitters released from the end terminal of the axon. These *neurotransmitters* accumulate in the narrow synaptic space, and when the concentration is high enough, they cause the adjacent cell membrane of the spinal cord cell to depolarize and send an electrical impulse along its own axon.

Impulses from pain receptors traveling along C fibers or Aδ fibers synapse with *nociceptive specific* (NS) neurons in the spinal cord. These neurons are dedicated to pain impulses. There is a second type of neuron in the spinal cord which receives pain and non-pain impulse of varying ranges of impulse intensities. This is a called a wide dynamic range (WDR) neuron.

These WDR neurons also receive impulses from viscera. This association is thought to account for the pain, for example, from angina (visceral) which may become associated with somatic tissues (the shoulder) and produce the sensation of shoulder pain, which actually originates from the heart. This is called *referred* pain.

Nerve axons not only transmit electrical impulses but also carry chemical messengers. These messengers are *neuropeptides*, protein-like molecules used by neurons to communicate with each other. Neuropeptides are carried in both directions within the axon along a transport route of microtubules. This transport may take days, whereas the nerve impulse takes a few seconds. Some of the neuropeptides are transported from the ganglion cell to the synapses with the spinal cord NS neuron. Neuropeptides are also transported toward the peripheral nerve endings and released into the tissue where they mediate inflammation and lower the threshold of the receptor to excite further depolarization. The inflammation mediated by this release of neuropeptides into the tissue is known as *neurogenic* inflammation. The influence of released neuropeptides on the threshold of the receptor is one of the causes of *peripheral sensitization*.

Pain fibers not only transport peptides to the peripheral end of the nerve axon but also to the central end where they increase the excitability of the spinal nociceptive neuron. This process is called central sensitization (*see Appendix G.1 Peripheral Sensitization and G.2 Central Sensitization*). The clinical manifestation of peripheral and central sensitization is *hyperalgesia*. Hyperalgesia is an increased sensitivity to pain caused by heat, chemicals, or mechanical trauma.

The pathway of pain impulses toward the brain is complex. There are many levels through the brainstem and midbrain where impulses are diverted and subject to modification before continuing eventually to the cortex. The simple observation which can be made is that there is no center in the brain or brainstem where pain is specifically experienced (*see Appendix G.3 Central Connections of Pain Impulses*).

10.4.3 Innervation of the Pulp–Dentin

The pulp is extremely highly innervated. Beneath the layer of odontoblasts there is a rich plexus of nerves described by Rashkow. Nerves which are continuous with this plexus penetrate into the dentinal tubule for a short distance (about 100 μm). If cross-sections of dentin are viewed using a transmission electron microscope (TEM), the unmyelinated nerves can be seen lying next to the odontoblast's process (▶ Fig. 10.3). At those places, where the nerve and process are close, there is evidence of a *gap junction* which would allow electrical communication between the two membranes but no synapse between the nerve and odontoblast. The nerve axons contain mitochondria and microfilaments and both these can be observed to disappear after experimental inferior alveolar nerve section. Not every tubule has a nerve, only about 40% do in the densest areas around the pulp horn. The incidence of nerves in tubules falls to 5% around the sides of the pulp chamber and drops to less than 1% in root dentin.

10.4.4 Dentin Sensitivity

A number of facts make it impossible to offer a simple explanation for sensitivity of dentin:
- The distribution of nerve endings in dentin is sparse and virtually absent in root dentin and deciduous dentin, but both are sensitive.
- Nerve fibers penetrate a very short distance into dentin from the dental pulp, yet dentin is sensitive right up to the amelo-dentinal junction.
- Pain is not blocked by the application of topical anesthetic to the exposed dentin.

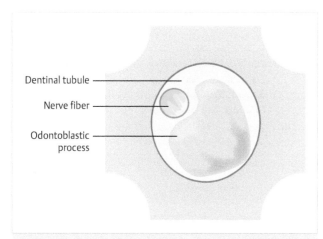

Fig. 10.3 Diagrammatic representation of a cross-section through a dentinal tubule containing the odontoblastic process and nerve fiber.

- Substances such as histamine, which cause pain when applied to nerve endings in the skin, would not be applied to exposed dentin.
- Exposed dentin is sensitive to changes in osmotic pressure, for example, the sudden application of something sweet.

Dentinal tubules contain fluid in the periodontoblastic space. This fluid is probably derived from pulp capillaries but may arrive via the odontoblast. According to the *hydrodynamic theory*, a stimulus applied to the dentin surface induces fluid flow in the dentinal tubules (▶ Fig. 10.4). This flow causes distortion of the peripheral pulp tissue and consequent activation of nerve endings at the pulp–dentin border. The theory is supported by a number of in vivo observations. If the passage of fluid is blocked, then dentin sensitivity is reduced. This happens if after cutting dentin with a bur, the layer of smeared debris is left on the dentin surface. Reduced sensitivity also occurs if the flow of fluid is reduced by the deposition of peritubular (intratubular) dentin. If, on the other hand, the passage of fluid is increased, so is dentin sensitivity. This occurs if the surface of the dentin is etched with acid, which opens up the tubule.

The flow of fluid in the dentin tubule can be measured in vitro and can be experimentally increased by applying a strong osmotic solution to an exposed dentin surface. This experimental observation may explain the pain which occurs when cement-denuded root surfaces are in contact with sweet food which has a high osmotic pressure. Although the initial stimulus to the dentin may be sensed by mechanical displacement of fluid in the tubule, it must eventually be transcribed into a nerve impulse. How and exactly where this occurs is not certain, although the rich nerve plexus of Raschkow just beneath the layer of odontoblasts must be involved. What is evident is that dentin sensitivity is dependent on the condition of the pulp. Hence, some patients are able to tolerate tooth preparation without an anesthetic, and on the other extreme, a tooth whose pulp is already inflamed may be so hypersensitive that pain is felt in spite of several injections of local anesthetic. There is no proof of the hydrodynamic theory, but it fits the observations better than any other at present.

A knowledge of the mechanisms and pathways of dentinal pain allows dentists to take rational clinical steps to reduce dentinal sensitivity. The main thrust is twofold. Firstly, to reduce fluid movement and secondly to reduce inflammation of the pulp. The dentist can reduce root dentin sensitivity by applying adhesives which will block the exposed dentinal tubules. At present, there is no medication that has been found to be reliably successful for home use, although toothpastes containing potassium oxalate and stannous fluoride are available. The response of the pulp can be reduced by applying sedative dressings to the floor of deep cavities. Eugenol causes reversible sedation of the pulp.

10.4.5 Pulp–Dentin Pain

Dentin which has been recently exposed is usually sensitive to a variety of stimuli, heat, cold, osmotic pressure, drying, and mechanical stimulation. These stimuli all cause pain, no other sensation. Dentin which has been exposed for some time, such as might occur after gradual tooth wear, is not sensitive.

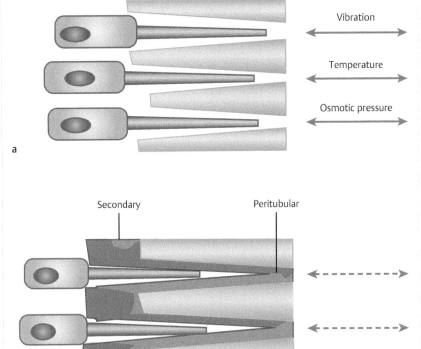

a

b

Secondary   Peritubular

Vibration

Temperature

Osmotic pressure

Fig. 10.4 Diagrammatic representation of flow in the dentinal tubule. (a) In the young tooth, dentinal fluid flows back and forth in the tubule in response to mechanical and thermal stimuli causing stimulation of pain receptors in the dentin and pulp. **(b)** In the older tooth, the tubules become narrower and are eventually blocked with peritubular dentin and secondary dentin, which progressively reduce the flow of the dentinal fluid and reduce the sensitivity of dentin to mechanical stimuli.

However, root dentin often is sensitive (one in seven complaints). The root dentin is covered with only a thin (100 μm) layer of cement which may be removed during periodontal surgery or by incorrect tooth brushing. The exposed root dentin is sensitive to brushing, cold and sweet foods.

Bacteria in carious lesions produce acids, which diffuse through sound dentin to reach the pulp tissue. The acid irritation causes pain and inflammation of the pulp and increased sensitivity to stimuli which would not normally cause pain, such as hot or cold beverages. If bacteria in dentin continue to advance toward the pulp, inflammation progresses and the tooth begins to ache continuously. Other nearby teeth may also ache. This is the typical response of C fibers in promoting further inflammation, sensitivity, and healing. In softer tissues, these responses produce the cardinal signs of inflammation, redness, swelling, heat, and pain. However, in the pulp chamber, no swelling is possible. The pulp tissue pressure increases, as the inflammatory exudate accumulates in the confined space of the pulp chamber. The increased pressure causes further pain. At this point, the pulpal damage may be considered irreversible; the pulp tissue must be removed by root canal treatment.

The dentist and patient are concerned with reducing dentinal pain during cavity preparation. This is usually successfully achieved by blocking the nerve impulse on its way to the trigeminal nucleus using a local anesthetic. Not everyone finds an injection of local anesthetic essential, even though they have a normal pain response elsewhere. On the other hand, sometimes it is difficult for the dentist to achieve anesthesia, even after

several injections. It does not help to apply the local anesthetic directly to the dentin, but it may be applied under some circumstances directly to an exposed pulp.

An aching tooth may not be that easy for the dentist to locate, because the pain may be referred from another tooth or even from one of the muscles of mastication.

10.4.6 Neurogenic Inflammation of the Pulp Tissue

It has been noted above, that neurogenic inflammation may be promoted by the release of chemical at the nerve endings. This component of inflammation is caused by the releases from the terminal ending of the nerve axon, substance P and calcitonin gene-related peptide (CGRP). These peptides cause extravasation of plasma proteins and vasodilation of the blood vessels. These processes would together normally result in tissue swelling, but the compliance of the pulp tissue is very low and does not allow an increase in tissue volume. The result is that pulpal pressure builds up. This contributes to the tooth becoming sensitive to temperature changes which are normally tolerated. This is described as *pulpal hyperalgesia*.

This cycle of peripheral and central sensitization has been called "wind up" as the process is a positive feedback. The more advanced the neurogenic inflammation, the greater the sensitization, which increases the neurogenic inflammation. Wind up is responsible for the clinical presentation of the "hot tooth." This is a tooth causing constant severe pain but which may appear to be clinically normal. This phenomenon is important to recognize, otherwise it may lead to the extraction of a sound tooth.

10.4.7 Facial Pain of Muscular Origin

Acute muscle cramp may be brought on by a buildup of lactic acid, due to failure to remove metabolites during prolonged muscle activity. Prolonged activity may also result in muscle pain and stiffness 48 hours after the activity. This so-called, delayed-onset muscle stiffness (DOMS) is quite similar to facial pain of muscular origin. The muscles of mastication are surprisingly resistant to fatigue due to sustained function, as long as it is cyclic. They are more susceptible to fatigue due to clenching. Clenching involves sustained contraction, without the beneficial effect of adequate circulation, which is provided by cyclic patterns of contraction and relaxation. The delayed effect on the masticatory muscle may be responsible for pain and stiffness sometimes experienced by individuals who clench and grind their teeth. Sustained light tension of muscles, which occurs during sustained postures, such as bending over a patient, may be responsible for chronic neck and back pain (*see Chapter 9.4 Temporomandibular Dysfunction*).

10.4.8 Trigger Points in Muscles

There are often well-localized areas where a muscle is particularly sensitive to pressure, which have been called nodules. These tender areas have subsequently been called *trigger points* to indicate that while they are tender, they also appear to set off pain somewhere else (► Fig. 10.5). Travell and Simons confirmed that this *referred pain* from muscles does not follow a simple neurological pattern.[3] It is important for the clinician to be familiar with these mapped patterns of referral. They alert the clinician, to the possibility, that pain which appears to be localized to an anatomical area does not necessarily originate there. A common example is the pain which appears to be localized around the TMJ, but which originates in the muscles of mastication and neck muscles. If this referred muscle pain is not recognized, it may result in misguided and ineffective treatment to the joint.

Suppressing the neural activity at these trigger spots with local anesthetic may serve as a diagnostic confirmation of referred pain. Stimulation of the trigger point using acupuncture needles appears to be effective in reducing the sensitivity of the trigger point. A further option is to pass a light oscillating current down the needle. Other alternatives include massage and intermittent periods of sustained pressure on the trigger spot. Trigger points may be located in skeletal muscles and tendons, capsules and ligaments of joints, periosteum, and the scar tissue of skin. They are most likely found at the free borders, belly, origin and insertion of muscles, and at the motor point.

Trigger points tend to be in similar places for many individuals; for example, a common trigger point location is the midpoint on the anterior border of the trapezius muscle. Some trigger points may be latent, that is painful if touched, but not otherwise generating spontaneous pain. Latent points may become active as a result of direct injury, sudden stress, unusual exercise, cold, nervous tension, and febrile illness. Latent points may also become

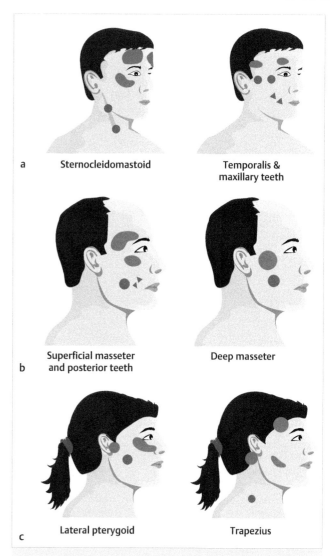

Fig. 10.5 A diagrammatic representation of the origins of trigger zones (*purple*) and their referred areas (*red*). (a) Trigger points in the sternocleidomastoid muscle refer pain to areas above and below the eye. Trigger points in the vertical temporalis muscle and the maxillary teeth refer pain to the area of the temple and above the eye. (b) Trigger points in the superficial masseter muscle and the posterior teeth refer pain to areas above and below the eye. Trigger points in the deep masseter muscle refer pain to the side of the face. (c) Trigger points in the lateral pterygoid muscle refer pain to the temporomandibular joint and below the eye. Trigger points in the trapezius muscle refer pain to an area behind the ear, the cheek, and above the eye. (Adapted from Travell and Simons, 1983.[3])

activated by neighboring trigger points. Travell and Simons call these secondaries "satellites" because a whole series of them may occur due to a domino effect.[3] Such a series can be plotted, and when this is possible, it often corresponds to the pathway of a traditional acupuncture tract. The structural changes in trigger points vary, but common findings are an increase in platelets and mast cells. These cells produce serotonin and histamine, respectively, both of which are powerful pain-producing substances. There is also an increase in tissue proteoglycans including hyaluronic acid which is associated with swelling due to fluid retention.

10.4.9 Referred Pain

The patterns of referred pain related to muscle trigger points of the jaw and neck are not unique. The referred pain in the jaw and left arm, associated with cardiac pain, is also well described. So is the referred pain which is located in a limb which has been amputated, so-called phantom limb pain. A common finding is that referred pain is a one-way diversion. While a trigger point in the sternocleidomastoid muscle may be referred to a maxillary molar, the reverse referral does not occur. Referred pain is also characterized by a delay in the referral. It takes several minutes to take place.

There is no universally agreed explanation for referred pain although we have noted that WDR neurons may play a part. Further support for an explanation which involves spinal cord cells is that referred pain is observed in tissue whose sensory nerve spinal connections are not far from each other.

10.4.10 Nerve Injury

Some of the most intractable pains are caused by nerve damage. When a peripheral nerve is damaged, there is an immediate volley of impulses to the central nervous system, and then all falls quiet. A severed nerve axon soon begins to grow and bud, in search of protective nerve cells (Schwann cells). If it can find support, and the previous myelin sheaths are not too far away, it may grow out along the old nerve fiber. If it cannot find supportive cells, it may bunch up and form a *neuroma*. At this stage, it is very excitable and may spontaneously discharge impulses to the peripheral and central nervous systems. It is possible that extraction of a vital tooth could cause a neuroma to form where the nerve fibers are separated from the root apex, but there are little recorded data of this occurring.

10.4.11 The Gate Theory

It used to be thought that pain was the result of nerve impulses generated in specific pain receptors which were carried to the brain along specific pathways to a central pain area of the brain. We now know that the situation is more complex than this, and that pain does not result from a linear chain of events, rather emerges as the outcome of many factors which are all part of a network.

What sort of mechanism could account for the variety of responses to tissue damage? The theory of gate control put forward by Melzack and Wall attempted to account for the observed responses to pain.[4] Both pain and non-pain impulses converge at different but interconnected NS neurons, which control the ascent of a new pattern of nerve impulses to second-order neurons. The interaction of all these converging impulses at the NS neurons was called a "gate," because it appeared to be a site at which impulses were either blocked or allowed through, an ascending pain pathway (▸ Fig. 10.6). Opening and closing of the "gate" depends on the relative levels of activity of all the converging impulses. The impulses which may influence the transmission of a pain impulse come from a number of axons.

- Arriving from the periphery are the C and Aδ fibers carrying pain impulses.

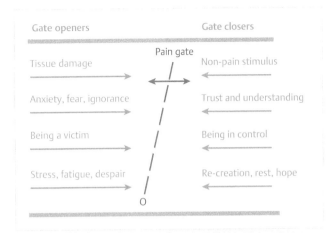

Fig. 10.6 A diagrammatic representation of the factors which influence the transmission of pain impulses. The pain gate may open or close depending on a variety of factors.

- Also arriving from the periphery are large-diameter Aβ fibers, carrying impulses caused by gentle brushing or rubbing of the skin, which reduce the excitability of the NS neurons.
- A steady inhibition of the excitability of the NS neurons descends from the reticular formation in the medulla.
- Nerve fibers from the cortex and thalamus descend through the medulla and synapse on the NS neurons of the trigeminal nucleus and spinal cord. These fibers convey influences such as fear, memory, anxiety, and depression. They may either inhibit or excite the NS neurons.
- A continual discharge from interneurons in the gate circuit inhibits the firing of the NS neuron which may, or may not, transmit the collective influence at the gate neurons forward to the next level neuron.

The value of the gate theory is its contribution to the direction of continued research into the further understanding of pain mechanisms. For the clinician, it provides a framework into which all the factors which influences the experience of pain may be brought together.

- It provides an explanation for the observations that simultaneous non-pain stimuli, in particular, the effect of light touch and vibration, influence pain perception. This simple knowledge is put to good use when administering an intraoral anesthetic. If the lip is vigorously vibrated as the needle is inserted into the oral mucosa, the unpleasant pricking of the needle is hardly felt.
- It provides an explanation for the observation that emotional factors, such as anxiety and fear, contribute directly to pain perception and reaffirms the value of developing trust in reducing pain experience in patients.

10.4.12 Pain and Stress

Stress can be defined as a perceived inability to cope with an unpleasant or painful life situation. The definition is broad as we must include stress due to physical deprivation or abuse and stress arising from within, such as anger, anxiety, or grief. Like pain, there is no direct relationship between the stressful situation (tissue damage) and the stress (pain). It is the mind which decides whether a situation is stressful or not. Memories of past experiences are called up, cultural and social norms apply, and these factors build up a perception of our ability to cope with a situation. Stress is a very personal experience. What may be stressful for one individual is not for another.

The physiological response to stress includes an increase in activity of the sympathetic nervous system and the release of increased levels of epinephrine and norepinephrine into the bloodstream. It also includes raised activity in the hypothalamus due to emotions of anxiety and fear. Nerve fibers from the hypothalamus project to the pituitary gland, which releases increased levels of adrenocorticotropic hormone (ACTH). The resulting raised levels of cortisol affects metabolic, psychological, and immunological functions. Mood is altered, behavior disrupted, and serotonin synthesis reduced. Reduced serotonin causes sleepless nights, an unsatiated appetite for food, and a drop in the pain threshold. Drugs which prevent the breakdown of serotonin (and thus keep its levels high) have been widely used to fight depression (e.g., Prozac). Another consequence of prolonged stress is depression of the immune system. It illustrates one of the many biochemical pathways which link our emotional state to our susceptibility to some if not all illnesses.

> **Key Notes**
>
> The gate control theory brings into focus the variety of influences on the pain experience. All these influences, even those of thought and emotion, modulate via the same family of neurochemicals at the synapses of the nociceptive pathways.

10.5 Oral Pain Control

There are two different but equally important parts to pain control. They address the two dimensions we expect to be present, the body and the mind (cognitive and affective responses) of the patient. They apply equally to acute and chronic pain, although some forms of pain control are obviously more appropriate for acute than for chronic pain.

10.5.1 Controlling Sensations

In order to reduce the sensory origins of pain, treatment should be directed toward reducing the pain stimulus. The following techniques may contribute to pain management:
- *Pharmacological methods:* Analgesic and anti-inflammatory drugs; local and general anesthetics to perform operations.
- *Physical measures:* Operative procedures to control or remove infection and promote healing, particularly of acute pain. The skillful use of operative techniques is crucial to the management of acute pain. Of prime importance is the effective use of local anesthetic.

10.5.2 Controlling Emotions

These objectives are directed at modifying the psychological factors described at the beginning of this chapter. We can make a significant contribution to reducing the emotional (affective) aspects of acute pain by careful patient management.
- Reassurance from the operator that anesthesia will be effective and confidence that the pain can be resolved are of great comfort to the patient. As much as possible should be done to reduce the patient's anxiety before any steps are taken.
- Put the patient in control if at all possible. A simple agreement that a raised hand will signal to the dentist to stop is a great reassurance to the patient.
- Keep the patient informed. The unknown is a powerful source of fear. Patients who do not understand what will be done become anxious and intolerant to pain. The importance of using a language familiar to the patient cannot be overemphasized.

10.5.3 Chronic Pain Management

The behavioral aspects of chronic pain must be controlled by the patient with the advice of the dentist, who should offer the patient a strategy to help them cope with the pain.
- *Increase level of activity:* Frequent pain may easily dominate one's life, so that all else comes to a halt. The pain is then in control and the sufferer in its grip. By a conscious effort to keep going, to take exercise and to make time for hobbies, the pain can be put aside for a time. The value of choosing not to let the pain dominate should be explained to the patient. Pleasure is an antidote to pain.
- *Decrease stress level:* Pain is stressful in its own right, but it is made worse by other sources of life stress. Death of a loved one, divorce, job loss, family abuse, and financial worries are just a few common life events which can be overwhelming. The first step toward coping better with stress is to acknowledge it, and, next, to identify its source. Talking about grief and suffering helps the patient to think more clearly about it and allows some changes in attitude to emerge. Thinking differently leads to feeling differently, which leads to adaptive behavior, coping strategies, and eventually stress reduction. Taking time to listen to a patient talk through some of these processes may be the greatest contribution the practitioner can make.
- *Pain diary:* Monitoring the levels of drugs needed and the daily variation in pain levels gives patients a sense of control and encouragement when there are remissions.

10.5.4 Pain Control Mechanisms

Prostaglandins are one of a number of naturally occurring peptides (e.g., histamine, kinins) which are found in inflammatory exudates. The analgesic effect of aspirin, like drugs, is to suppress the synthesis of prostaglandins. In view of the important contribution to pulpal pain made by neurogenic inflammation the use of nonsteroidal anti-inflammatory drugs (NSAIDs) is particularly effective. Topical cream containing steroids is used to apply directly to pulpal tissue in an effort to reduce inflammation.

Local anesthetics act by interfering with ionic mechanisms involved in nerve impulse conduction. They block the flow of sodium ions through membrane channels of the nerve axon which is part of the process of depolarization and repolarization of the axon.

Morphine acts at two distinct sites:
- One of *these* is in the midbrain, where cells of the periaqueductal gray produce enkephalins and endorphins. These

natural opioids stimulate nerve impulses which descend in the nerve bundles of the spinal cord and reduce the excitability of NS neurons. Morphine adds to this mechanism, an artificially high level of descending inhibition of NS neurons.

- Morphine also acts at a spinal cord level where it directly inhibits the release of peptides at the terminal of the incoming pain fiber. In technical terms, it causes *presynaptic inhibition*. This action of morphine has made possible a technique for injecting quite low concentrations of the drug into the epidural space around the spinal cord producing profound analgesia from the waist down without blocking other motor nerve functions. *Epidural anesthesia* is a safe and successful way of controlling childbirth pain, without the mental side effects, such as drowsiness which morphine tablets or intramuscular injections produce.

There has been, in the past, a reluctance to use morphine freely for the control of acute pain and to allow patients to have as much as they need because of the fear of addiction. There is in fact no grounds for such fears. Morphine, given to control acute pain, is rarely addictive and it is not necessary to keep increasing the dose because of tolerance to the drug. Clinical guidelines for prescribing opioids for chronic pain include the importance of assessing the patient for the risk of substance abuse, misuse, or addiction. A personal or family history of substance abuse is the strongest predictor of aberrant drug-taking behavior.

Key Notes

The role of C fibers explains the progression of symptoms from a tooth mildly sensitive to hot and cold to one which causes continual pain. The low compliance of pulpal tissue and the increased tissue pressure brought about by neurogenic inflammation support the use of non-steroidal anti-inflammatories in pain control.

Review Questions

1. Think of an example, perhaps from your own history, of an experience which was painful and has left you with a fear of a similar experience.
2. How did your parent's reaction to your injury as a child shape your response to injury as an adult?
3. If a placebo is effective in a pain control study, can it be concluded that the patient's pain may be imagined?
4. What aspects of C-fiber functions are unique to them?
5. Who proposed the gate theory and why did they call it a gate?
6. Describe the distribution of nerve fibers in the pulp–dentin.
7. Why does the neck of the tooth sometimes become sensitive to sweet and cold food?
8. What observations make it difficult to offer a simple explanation for dentin sensitivity?
9. What is neurogenic inflammation and how could it affect the dental pulp?
10. What steps could you take to help a patient control the emotions which contribute to the pain experience?

10.6 Taste

10.6.1 General Features of Taste

The sensation of taste is special, in that it is restricted to oral tissues. In common with pain there is an emotional aspect of taste. Humans have both an innate and acquired taste preferences; for example, a liking for sweet foods appears to be inborn, but it can be increased by habits and persuasive advertising.

10.6.2 Modalities and Distribution

There are at least four taste modalities: sweet, salt, sour, and bitter. There may be others; some experiments show that individuals can "taste" water. The tongue is the major site for taste sensation, though the palate, pharynx, and larynx provide additional sites for taste sensation. It has been traditional to recognize a distribution pattern for the four tastes. Sweet and salt appear to be better perceived at the tip of the tongue, sour at the sides, and bitter at the back of the tongue and the palate, pharynx, and larynx. However, it now seems that each of these regions is sensitive to all taste qualities; it is just the thresholds which differ.

Food flavor is of course dependent on both taste and smell. Hence, food loses its flavor when we have a head cold because aromas are blocked from reaching the olfactory receptors in the nasal mucosa. The tastes, however, remain unaffected.

10.6.3 Taste Buds

Taste buds are found especially in the fungiform, foliate, and circumvallate papillae of the tongue. Their numbers are reduced in the elderly. Only some of the cells making up the taste bud may be receptor cells; the rest are supporting cells. The life span of the taste cell is only a few days; it apparently reverts to a supporting cell while another supporting cell becomes a taste cell. By some means, perhaps by molecular "lock and key" processes, or by synchronous oscillation frequencies, the cell membrane of the taste cell recognizes the molecule of, for example, salt, and transduces the chemical message into a neural message. The relationship between the taste cell and the nerve endings next to it is similar to that of the odontoblast and the nerves of the pulp. The nerves appear to have more than just a sensory function; they also have a neurotropic function. That is, the nerve supply is essential for the proper development and regeneration of taste buds.

Measurements from isolated taste nerves show that while the response of the taste cell to say salt is greatest, the same cell can respond to other taste modes.

The chorda tympani branch of the facial nerve supplies the taste buds of the anterior two-thirds of the tongue, the glossopharyngeal nerve innervates those of the posterior one-third and the pharynx, and the vagus nerve supplies those in the larynx. The trigeminal, facial, and glossopharyngeal nerves are probably all involved in supplying the palatal taste buds. Gustatory afferent fibers relay in the solitary tract nucleus in the lower brainstem. From there they pass to the thalamus and finally to the sensory cortex.

Several factors modify taste sensations. Oral factors include the food temperature, smoking and alcohol consumption, amount of saliva, age, and dentures. The ability to taste phenylthiocarbamide is confined to a certain percentage of the population and appears to be genetically determined.

Review Questions

1. What is the difference between taste and flavor?
2. Are taste buds specific to one taste mode only?
3. In what ways are taste sensations modified?

10.7 Oral Proprioception

10.7.1 Skin and Mucosa

There are two basic histological types of touch and pressure receptor: the corpuscular type and the free nerve ending. Receptors can also be divided into two functional types: those which are *rapidly adapting* and those which are *slowly adapting*. Rapidly adapting receptors fire for a short burst and then stop firing, even though the stimulus, for example pressure, is still being applied. They provide information about how the environment changes. When receptors take some time to adapt or continue to fire while stimulated, they provide a different sort of information, which is about the current state of the environment.

The corpuscular type of receptor consists of epithelial or connective tissue cells around the enlarged ending of the nerve. Corpuscular endings are of at least four types, each with a specific sensory function.

The Merkel cell neurite complexes and Ruffini endings are position sensors found in the skin, oral mucosa, the periodontium, and the TMJ. They are slowly adapting and hence provide information about the quality, intensity, and location of a mechanical stimulus (▶ Fig. 10.7).

The lanceolate corpuscles are wrapped around a hair shaft and are rapidly adapting as are the pacinian corpuscles, which resemble onions. They provide information about change in touch and pressure, which conveys information about movement, velocity, and direction.

Receptors for touch and pressure are particularly numerous in the skin around the mouth and the intraoral mucosa. The density of receptors is indicated by the minimum distance between two points of pressure which can still be separately distinguished. Two-point discrimination on the tongue is about 2 mm. This is similar to that of the finger but less than the mouth, face, hands, and back, in that order. The threshold for pressure on the oral mucosa is a force of about 10 to 20 g. This is at least 10 times less sensitive than an incisor tooth to pressure (0.5–1 g).

10.7.2 Periodontal Receptors

Receptors in the periodontal ligament provide information about the magnitude, direction, and duration of forces applied during chewing. Most of the receptors in the ligament are in the apical third. Their distribution allows direction of the force to be perceived. The force threshold is lowest for incisors and is lower for labially directed forces than axial forces.

The ability to detect a very thin metal strip placed between the teeth is called the size threshold. It is partly a function of periodontal receptors. At least, this ability is reduced if the periodontal ligament is anesthetized.

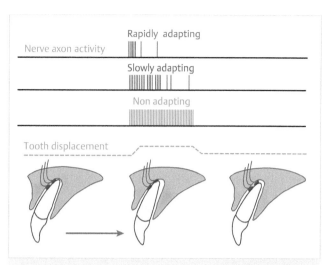

Fig. 10.7 **A diagrammatic representation of rapid, slowly adapting, and nonadapting receptors in response to displacement of a tooth.** An anterior tooth has been displaced toward the palatal by a labial force. The broken blue line indicates the period of displacement. Pressure receptors in the periodontal ligament have been stimulated. The nerve axon activity from these receptors has been plotted and shown above. The rapidly adapting receptor soon stops firing while the slowly adapting receptor fires for a few seconds. The nonadapting receptor fires until the force is removed, when all impulses cease. These three receptors provide different types of information about the force applied (after Anderson and Matthews, 1976).

The ability to discriminate between smaller and larger sizes of objects is called size discrimination and is not reduced if the periodontal ligament is experimentally anesthetized; nor is size discrimination reduced in denture wearers. The perception of size discrimination is a function of receptors in the muscles and joints.

10.7.3 Altered Feedback

There has been interest by dental scientists in the possible hazard to chewing function and muscular balance of the TMJ of disruptive information from the periodontal ligament receptors. This disruption is said to arise if there is any occlusal interference with the smooth working of the teeth against each other. Even one tooth, a little proud of the others, could cause this disruption. The receptors in the periodontal ligament of this tooth would presumably be excessively stimulated, thereby producing an abnormal feedback from that tooth. This abnormal feedback would have to be so disruptive as to disturb the normally well-coordinated pattern of jaw movements during chewing.

The role of the neural feedback from periodontal receptors has been investigated. Most of the conclusions are as yet tentative as there are many pitfalls in investigating jaw function. As we have seen, anesthetized teeth have an increased size threshold, but in experimental conditions, this limitation does not appear to influence existing chewing patterns. Additions to the tooth surfaces have been experimentally placed in order to determine whether the chewing pattern would be altered. The results are conflicting, an indication that feedback from the periodontal ligament has a variable effect on jaw movement. It has been suggested by Dubner et al that there must be a number of factors which determine the influence of altered feedback from the periodontal receptors.[5] These include the following:

Magnitude: The magnitude of the force will determine the intensity of the receptor response. *Direction.* The direction of the force will influence the amount of displacement of the tooth. Lateral forces cause greater tooth displacement than apically directed forces, hence would provoke a response from receptors more easily than an apical force.

Duration: The duration of the force applied will determine the duration of the feedback. A fleeting tooth contact is less likely to have a major influence on the total feedback message than a prolonged force.

Frequency: The frequency of the force applied will determine the frequency of the response. An interfering tooth contact which often occurs is more likely to be a significant feature of the feedback than one which seldom occurs. For example, an interference on the side of the mouth not normally chosen for chewing would have less impact than one which occurred in the most favored area for tooth contact.

Effective root size: The effective root size and shape influences the ease with which displacement under load occurs. Short, single, conical teeth move more easily than long, parallel-sided, multirooted teeth do. The term effective root size is used because even a large rooted tooth will be displaced under load quite easily, if only 50% of the root is in bone. Hence, chronic periodontal disease has an impact on receptor threshold.

Threshold: The threshold of receptors is also reduced by the presence of acute inflammatory change in the periodontium. A tooth which is painful when touched will contribute a dominant part of the receptor feedback. Jaw movement will be altered to avoid further contacts with that tooth.

The subject's state of awareness influences the priority given to oral sensations. Change in the oral status tends to focus attention. For example, an extraction, or a new occlusal restoration, and especially a full-arch restoration increase oral awareness.

Most attempts to study the critical factors which control jaw function do not observe the jaws working at their full potential activity. Our diet does not demand it. Hence, little or no change may be observed by altered feedback while the jaws are working at less than maximum output. The methods for accurate observations of any response to altered feedback are underdeveloped. Minor shifts in the balance of activity in certain muscle groups change in the nature of the loads at the joint, and the resultant alteration in the pattern of movement may all occur following altered oral feedback, but they cannot be accurately monitored with existing technology.

10.7.4 Temporomandibular Joint Receptors

There are numerous free nerve endings in the capsule and round the periphery of the disk, especially the bilaminar posterior area. More complex receptors are in the lateral part of the capsule. Experimental anesthesia of these receptors has been used to determine the role they play in monitoring the position and movements of the jaw. Anesthesia of the lateral and posterior part of the TMJ capsule produced a slight increase in the size threshold and altered the ability of the subject to return the jaw to a reference position after moving away from it. There also seems to be a relationship between the position of the joint and the activity of the muscles of the jaw, which may have some influence in jaw posture. The joint contribution to the sense of position and movement is probably less important than that from the muscles. However, the receptors of the joint may have a more important role in providing sensory information about forces being applied at the joint, particularly those which tend to destabilize or damage it. Such sensory information would be important in protecting the joint structures by initiating protective or stabilizing reflexes. Presumably, as forces on the tissues reached a damaging level, the receptors would convey impulses which would be perceived as pain.

Key Notes

The physiological impact of altered feedback from the periodontal ligament, caused by occlusal interference, on a complex function such as chewing, will be determined by a combination of the six factors listed by Dubner.

Review Questions

1. Compare the information derived from slowly and rapidly adapting receptors.
2. What is the difference between size threshold and size discrimination?
3. What are the six factors listed by Dubner, which determine the level of feedback from periodontal receptors which may arise from occlusal interferences?
4. How important is the TMJ as a source of sensory information?

10.8 Oral Reflexes

10.8.1 Jaw Reflexes

The sensations which originate from the oral mucosa, periodontium, muscles, and joints comprise the afferent components of a wide variety of oral reflexes, most of which are protective. They may be quite simple, in that they involve only one synapse, no interneurons, and just one motor nucleus. Jaw opening and tongue protruding reflexes are simple. More complex reflexes like coughing and gagging involve more than one synapse, interneurons, and several motor neuron pools. Even more complex activities like swallowing and chewing have both involuntary and voluntary components. They are less predictable and can be modified by experience. Finally, feeding and all that it entails is a highly complex behavior involving a wide spectrum of activity. There is a thus a hierarchy of oral and facial reflexes, from the simple, monosynaptic to the most complex, which forms part of highly involved behavior. Common to all, from the simple to the complex, is a need for appropriate sensory feedback.

Jaw closing reflex: This simplest of jaw reflexes involves only one synapse. It occurs in response to a sharp tap on the chin or a tooth; the response is a short burst of activity of the jaw closing muscle. It should be remembered that this is not a naturally occurring reflex, but it is useful to illustrate important sensory pathways and motor responses. The response of the jaw closing reflex is dependent on the jaw being open; it is influenced by neck posture and depends on the central excitatory state. It provides an example of the interaction between all facial and jaw reflexes with other sensory and central influences.

Jaw opening reflex: The jaw opening reflex is a rapid contraction of the digastric muscle in response to a painful oral stimulus. It may occur during chewing, when a fish bone digs into the mucosa, or a piece of hard grit is unexpectedly found in softer food. The jaw opening reflex may also operate in response to nonpainful stimuli of the lips, tongue, and teeth as might happen when an infant was presented with food (▶ Fig. 10.8).

Jaw unloading reflex: When biting hard on a piece of brittle food, such as an unshelled nut, it may suddenly crack and no longer be of any resistance to the teeth. The jaws would crash closed, causing damage to the teeth, tongue, and cheeks unless at the moment of cracking through the nut, all further jaw closure was arrested. The jaw unloading reflex is dependent on sensory feedback from the periodontal ligament and other sources of feedback such as the muscle spindle. This reflex illustrates the importance of rapidly adapting periodontal receptors in the periodontium. It also illustrates the essential role of sensory feedback in permitting the use of maximum muscle force. If these receptors are experimentally blocked by anesthesia, the muscles of the jaw cannot exert more than about half their maximum biting force. This implies that positive feedback from receptors is such an essential component of muscle activity that without it a safe limit is imposed on the use of maximum muscle power.

One of the consequences of tooth loss is the reduction in maximum bite force. Denture wearers are unable to exert the same bite force that they were capable of when they had their own teeth, because the neural pathways of feedback from receptors in the periodontal ligament have been lost.

Inhibition of jaw closing muscles can be produced by stimulation of the mental nerve or other trigeminal sensory nerves. The inhibition is short, of the order of 20 to 50 ms. This inhibition is only detectable on an electromyograph trace, where it was once described as a silent period. It is now referred to as an exteroceptive suppression. The importance of this suppression is currently debated, but it was thought that it might be of diagnostic value in identifying patients with temporomandibular dysfunction (TMD).

Facial reflexes: The facial muscles may respond to cutaneous stimulation of the face. Interneurons would carry the impulses from the sensory nucleus of the trigeminal nerve (spinal tract part) to the motor nuclei of the facial nerve (solitary tract). An example of a facial reflex is the corneal blink reflex. If the cornea is lightly touched, the eyelid rapidly closes. The disappearance of this reflex is a useful indication of the depth of anesthesia. It is possible that facial reflexes may be important in maintaining the extraoral muscle tone, and so play a part in providing an adequate lip seal.

Tongue reflexes: Stimuli in the anterior oral region tend to have reflex effects favoring tongue retraction. This presumably helps protect the tongue during eating. In contrast, stimulation of deeper intraoral sites results in tongue protrusion. This would aid in the maintenance of a patent airway. A lowered threshold to this protrusive reflex may result in an excessive forward tongue thrust which may cause expansion of the mandibular and maxillary dental arches called an anterior open bite.

Coughing and gagging: The more complex reflex responses involve more than one group of sensory nuclei and more than one group of motoneurons. The protective responses of coughing, gagging, retching, and sneezing involve the trigeminal, facial, hypoglossal, vagus, and glossopharyngeal nerves. For this reason, they are referred to as *reflex synergies.* They are all concerned with preventing unwanted entrance of food or fluid into the trachea or esophagus. Stimulation of the pharyngeal and laryngeal mucosa by touch or fluid causes a reflex closure of the glottis and abrupt cessation of breathing (apnea). The response may be followed by a buildup of air pressure in the lungs followed by opening of the glottis. Coughing may be more

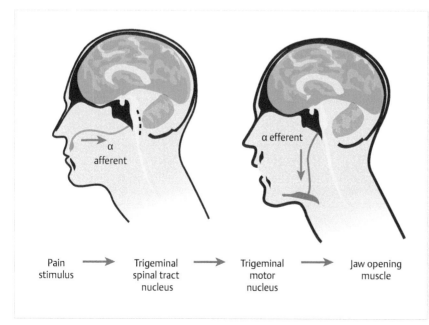

α
afferent

α efferent

Pain stimulus → Trigeminal spinal tract nucleus → Trigeminal motor nucleus → Jaw opening muscle

Fig. 10.8 A diagrammatic representation of the pathway of the jaw opening reflex. A painful stimulus to the palatal mucosa triggers pain impulses in the trigeminal nerve which travel along an afferent fiber, which then travels toward the sensory nucleus in the trigeminal spinal tract. An interneuron conveys the impulse to the motor nucleus of the trigeminal nerve. The motor neuron depolarizes and sends an efferent impulse which travels away from the nucleus to the jaw opening muscles which contract and open the jaw.

voluntary when a deep inspiration of air precedes the cough. The threshold to the cough reflex may be reduced during social stress when coughing occurs due to embarrassment.

Stimulation of the mucosa of the back of the tongue, faucial pillars, and soft palate may cause gagging. In many ways, gagging represents a reversal of swallowing; gagging may in fact be followed by vomiting. It is not an uncommon response of the dental patient, particularly to having impressions made. As with other oral reflexes, the threshold to gagging may be reduced by anxiety and fear. A calm and reassuring manner may be the most effective way to reduce gagging, but there are many other recommended solutions.

Key Notes

The threshold of the gagging reflex will depend on the level of sensory input from the receptors in the mucosa of the oral cavity and pharynx, but, like pain, the reflex is also under central cortical influence. The individual's past experience, level of anxiety, and confidence in the operator have decisive influence on the short-term challenges of having impressions made.

Review Questions

1. What is meant by a hierarchy of oral/facial reflexes?
2. Why does periodontal anesthesia reduce the maximum bite force?
3. What effect do higher centers have on reflexes?
4. Why do we refer to reflex synergies?

10.9 Mastication

10.9.1 Evolutionary Aspects

Mastication or chewing is one of the distinctive characteristics of mammals. It is a vital function for most of them, without which they starve. It may have been a vital function for primitive man, but his modern diet hardly requires chewing at all. The modern adult chewing apparatus is thus unpracticed, of weak muscles, and unworn teeth. Perhaps, for this reason it gives more trouble than it should.

The masticatory apparatus has a long pedigree, over 50 million years, and so we might begin by assuming there have been evolutionary opportunities to refine its structure and function. This conclusion is supported by the trouble-free service the dentition gives other mammals. Veterinary surgeons are seldom required to perform dental procedures. The breakdown of the human dentition is therefore more to do with diet than design.

Dental scientists have been studying human chewing by examining this rather pale relic we see in modern man. This may have been useful in the sense that it is man whose chewing apparatus gives him so much trouble. However, it has also been misleading, as we have tended to assume that we have always had available "normal" individuals to provide a benchmark for comparison. This is where the error may lie, as the only "normal" individuals would be found in the few remaining peoples of the world, who still live a primitive lifestyle. As we study human chewing in this section, we will have to bear in mind that we are not observing human mastication at its most optimum.

10.9.2 Suckling

Chewing is a complex process, and for this reason, it is not one of the capabilities of the newborn. This may be because infants have no teeth, but even when the teeth arrive, the toddler still needs rather mushy foods, and in unsophisticated societies he or she is at the mother's breast until 2 or 3 years old, by which time it has a full complement of deciduous teeth. During the early years the feeding method is suckling. It involves rhythmical movements of the jaw and tongue, with each cycle lasting 1 to 2 seconds. Swallowing seems to merge with it rather than being a separate event. It seems likely that many of the central reflex connections described for simple reflexes and reflex synergies are involved. An additional component would be a central pattern generator to produce the rhythmical series of muscle contractions.

10.9.3 Masticatory Efficiency and Digestion

Masticatory performance or efficiency may be assessed by giving a subject a weighed quantity of a firm food, such as nuts, to masticate, and after a fixed period, recovering the food. The food particles are then passed through a graded series of mesh sizes or measured using image analysis. The proportion, by weight, of fine particles to course particles is a measure of masticatory efficiency. It does not appear that masticatory efficiency is influenced by the area of occlusal contact, provided there are no missing teeth. Those whose masticatory efficiency is less effective than average seem to chew longer before swallowing, but they still do not compensate enough and swallow larger-sized particles. Large particles of uncooked vegetables and nuts are poorly digested, but even large particles of unchewed meat are completely digested. Some masticatory ability is therefore necessary for some foods, although thorough chewing seems to offer no advantage to digestion, as it does in dedicated herbivores. Man does require grains and some other starches to be cooked to allow them to be digested.

10.9.4 Masticatory Forces

The forces developed on a molar tooth during normal mastication are between 5 and 10 kg. Biting hard would generate from 20 to 200 kg. It has been noted that a tough diet will increase the normal and maximum biting forces. Loss of periodontal support and sensation decreases the ability to bite hard.

The jaw is a class 3 lever, and it is therefore to be expected that the nearer the load is placed to the bite force, the greater is the force applied. The biting force is thus greatest at the molars and least on the incisors. Biting force is also greatest at an optimal amount of jaw separation, about 3 mm. Tooth support for the forces generated by chewing comes from the periodontium. If the force is applied apically (toward the apex of the root), the entire periodontal ligament and bone socket contribute to the support. If the force is applied at an angle to the root, then the area of ligament providing support is reduced, and it is consequently under greater compression or tension. If this maldistribution of load is frequent and of long duration, damage to the periodontium may occur, and the tooth may become abnormally mobile. The direction in which chewing forces are applied is partly dependent on the direction of jaw closure but also depends on the angle of the tooth surfaces. If these occlusal services are flat, or consist of a stable cusp in a fossa, the force will be applied down the root (apical). However, if the tooth surfaces meet at an incline, only part of the force is apical, the rest tends to drive the tooth sideways. The way the teeth meet during function is called occlusion and is a subject of a separate chapter (see *Chapter 8 Eruption, Occlusion, and Wear*). When contouring the occlusal surfaces of a restoration, we try to ensure that forces on the tooth during mastication will be mostly apically directed.

10.9.5 Functional Jaw Movements

There are several devices for tracking the movement of the jaws during mastication. The sirognathograph is a device invented by Professor Arthur Lewin of the University of the Witwatersrand.[6] The movements of a small magnet cemented to the lower incisors are tracked by aerials sensitive to changes in magnetic field. The device samples the position of the magnet every 10 ms and records the coordinates for later computer analysis. The results of studies using this and other jaw tracking devices show that jaw movements are extremely varied. They reveal intraindividual variation depending on the type of food, the state of the bolus, and the chewing side used. There is even greater variation between subjects. Each masticatory cycle lasts 0.5 to 1.2 seconds. It consists of an opening phase, a closing phase, and a contact phase. The closing phase is usually the fastest. If viewed in the frontal plane, a typical cycle has been said to resemble a teardrop, the width depending on the texture of the food. Masticating raw carrots requires a chopping stroke, but tough meat would require more lateral grinding of the teeth against each other.

There is a wide range of jaw movements which occur during normal mastication, and this presents a problem when attempting to establish or define what might be described as normal movements. Computer analysis of jaw movements is essential in order to process the large volumes of data and to filter out movements which are unusual or infrequent. A core which represents the essential characteristic of movements may be generated and measured (▶ Fig. 10.9). It is possible to discriminate between a subject's left- and right-sided chewing, provided several characteristics are measured. A fast moving, lateral approach to, and away from, the intercuspal position with little hesitation has been found to be associated with improved masticatory efficiency (▶ Fig. 10.10).[7]

10.9.6 Muscle Activity

It seems reasonable to assume that a single muscle always exerts a force of contraction in the same direction. However, each muscle has well-defined anatomical sections, such as the superficial and deep parts of the masseter muscle. Each anatomical section has hundreds of functioning motor units which function separately. Coordination of all these components is necessary to effect skilled movement and to generate powerful biting forces at the teeth. In general, there are some muscle suited to particular actions. The masseter muscles are well placed to provide a powerful bite force, while the temporalis and lateral pterygoid are better aligned to position the jaw and line up the teeth onto the bolus.

Within a single muscle such as the temporalis, there are sectors more suited to some movements than others. For example, contraction of the vertical fibers of temporalis are effective jaw closing muscles, while contraction of the horizontal fibers tends to retrude the jaw. The direction of pull, of a muscle like the temporalis, can therefore vary considerably. Further variation is possible if the temporalis on one side contracts before the other. The muscles on the side on which food is being chewed are called the ipsilateral muscles, and the muscles on the nonchewing side are called the contralateral.

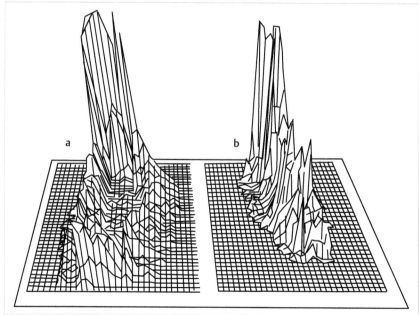

Fig. 10.9 A plot made of the tracks made by a magnet, cemented to a lower incisor, while 20 jaw cycles of mastication were recorded. The height of each plot represents the number of milliseconds the magnet spent in each sector of a grid. The speed of the jaw may be estimated by the height of the plots in an area. Around maximum intercuspation, the plots are high, indicating there were many milliseconds spent in these sectors as the jaw movement slowed down. In the middle of the opening or closing sectors the plots are low indicating rapid movement. The jaw slows down as it reverses its direction of movement from opening to closing. (a) This subject has a fast, smooth flowing, broad cycle associated with good chewing performance. (b) This subject has a slow, hesitant, limited movement associated with poor chewing performance.

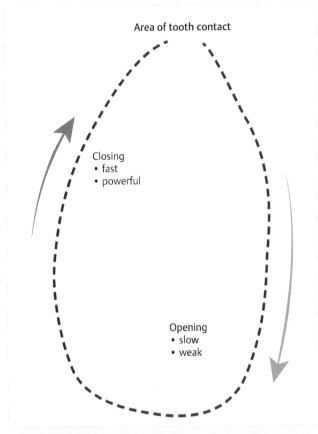

Fig. 10.10 A diagrammatic representation of a single jaw cycle in a frontal plane during mastication which is characteristic of optimal masticatory performance. This cycle is deep and wide indicating a smooth transition from balancing to working side. There is a rapid acceleration during the opening phases and a long, slow slide into a region around maximum intercuspation.

The timing of contractions of ipsilateral and contralateral muscles of the jaw allows smooth and fast opening followed by powerful grinding movement through the area of maximum tooth contact.[8] The muscles which close the jaw, the adductors, stop closing after the teeth have penetrated the bolus. They then allow the opening muscles (abductors) to open the jaw without resistance (▶ Fig. 10.11). When muscles fail to relax, coordination is disturbed, the muscles may even act against each other. For example, closing muscles may fail to relax at the right time to allow opening muscles to be active. This lack of coordination causes muscle stiffness and fatigue.

Key Notes

Mastication requires the accurate application of forces which bring the teeth together in crushing and grinding movements. As with other precise movements, it is not achieved by only one or two major muscle contractions, but by the interaction and rapid adaptation, during each movement, of hundreds of muscle units. Infants and the edentulous take time to master these skills.

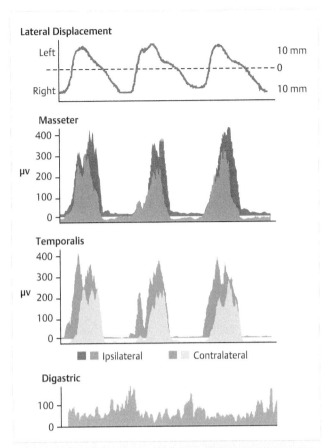

Fig. 10.11 Plots of the electrical activity of masticatory muscles and the jaw movement during three cycles of mastication. At the top of the figure, the lateral movement of the jaw is plotted. The electrical activity of the masseter and temporalis muscles is plotted for both the ipsilateral (chewing side) and contralateral (nonchewing side). The digastric activity plot is reproduced at the bottom of the figure. The movement toward intercuspation from the right side is initiated by the ipsilateral temporalis muscle. As the lateral jaw movement plot indicates an approach to the midline, both ipsilateral and contralateral masseter muscles become dominant. The contralateral temporalis muscle becomes dominant in the final stages of the lingual phase of mastication before jaw opening begins.

Review Questions

1. Could elderly individuals become malnourished as a result of inadequate chewing?
2. Palpate your own joint and feel the movement of the condyles as you open wide, and swing the jaw from side to side. What do you notice?
3. How do just a few major muscles of mastication achieve the fine movement and control which occurs during chewing?
4. Clench your teeth together very hard for 30 seconds. What do you begin to feel?

10.10 Swallowing

Swallowing, like suckling, is an innate capability immediately necessary for the survival of the newborn. Swallowing is essential, not only for food ingestion, but also for the equally critical purpose of protecting the airway, by clearing away fluids such as saliva and nasal secretions, and preventing them entering the larynx. Fluid contact on the laryngeal mucosa is an effective stimulation as is mechanical stimulation of the tonsillar pillars and the posterior pharyngeal wall. Swallowing is also under voluntary control although it appears that some supportive sensations from the mucosa are needed.

Dryness of the oral cavity or local anesthesia may make voluntary swallowing difficult. The decrease in the rate of salivary flow during the night may explain the drop in the incidence of swallowing from 500 events during waking hours to 50 events during sleep.

Once initiated, swallowing proceeds to completion. The sequence is usually divided into an oral phase followed by a pharyngeal phase ending with an esophageal phase.

10.10.1 The Oral Phase of Swallowing

During the oral phase, the tongue forms a lubricated bolus and pushes it upward and backward toward the pharynx. This movement is achieved with the help of the intrinsic and extrinsic muscles of the tongue which are effectively braced against the palate by the contraction of the jaw closing muscles. The purpose of this activity is to reduce the oral volume and squeeze the food backward.

A simple exercise will illustrate the activity of the jaw closing muscles during swallowing. Place the tip of your little finger between your teeth and try to swallow. The pressure exerted on your finger by the jaw closing muscles may be painful.

The circumoral muscles contract, helping to reduce the oral volume. To ensure the bolus or fluid does not enter the nose, the soft palate is lifted against the posterior pharyngeal wall, and the velopharyngeal sphincter is closed. The mechanical stimulation of the food bolus on the mucosa of the soft palate, pharynx, and faucial pillars initiates a series of reflex contractions, and the second phase begins.

10.10.2 The Pharyngeal Phase

The response of the pharyngeal muscles is to begin a series of contractions starting at the velopharyngeal sphincter, which pass down in a ripple toward the esophagus. The elevation of the larynx helps the epiglottis to tip over to protect the airway. Any fluid escaping past is trapped by the vocal cords which close as well. During this short period, breathing is stopped (apnea). The bolus enters the esophagus as the sphincter relaxes.

10.10.3 The Esophageal Phase

The bolus is carried by peristalsis to the relaxed gastroesophageal sphincter and into the stomach. The process is assisted by gravity. This sphincter is normally closed to prevent regurgitation from the stomach.

10.10.4 Muscle Activity of Swallowing

The perfectly timed sequence of muscle contractions is, like chewing, the result of a central pattern generator. This central control for swallowing is little influenced by external factors,

except perhaps bolus consistency. It controls the sequence of movements in a swallow by causing a series of bilateral contractions and relaxations in 30 different muscles. Most of these muscles are always involved, their participation is essential, and they are mostly insensitive to sensory feedback. These are the *obligate* muscles, under direct central control. Other muscles respond to sensations arising in the mouth and are under voluntary control, the *facultative* muscles.

The infant swallow, and that of the edentulous, non–denture-wearing individual, makes use of the facial muscles and tongue protrusion to aid swallowing, whereas the adult swallow makes more use of the jaw closing muscles. A persistent infantile swallow during development of the dentition may cause protrusion of the anterior part of both dental arches.

10.10.5 Forces during Swallowing

The teeth may come together while swallowing, depending on the consistency of the food bolus. When they do meet, the forces on the teeth are about 6 to 8 kg. There are also labial and lingual forces produced by the tongue and lips. It used to be thought that these forces balanced each other and so guided the arch into a neutral position. It has been shown by Proffit that the lingual forces produced by the tongue are much greater than those of the lips and that no such balance occurs during swallowing.[9] The forces generated during normal swallowing may not be of sufficient duration and frequency to displace the teeth out of the arch. However, if the tongue thrust during swallowing is excessive, both maxillary and mandibular incisors may be displaced forward. During resting posture, equilibrium between lingual and labial forces may occur and are important in influencing the labio-lingual position of the dental arch. Note, that these postural forces, although light, are continual. Thus, the duration of forces acting on teeth has a more decisive effect on tooth position than the magnitude of the force. The subject of equilibrium of forces on teeth is also discussed in *Chapter 8 Eruption, Occlusion, and Wear.*

Key Notes

Reduction in oral volume is an essential event in the initial phase of swallowing. This requires elevation of the tongue and with it the floor of the mouth and the mandible. The peripheral border of a mandibular denture may impinge on the elevation of the floor of the mouth, and if the occlusal vertical height is excessive, it may prevent adequate elevation of the mandible, thus making swallowing difficult.

Review Questions

1. Swallow several times. Why does it get more difficult each time? What do you notice about the activity of the circumoral muscles?
2. Place your little finger between your incisors and try to swallow. Why is it difficult?
3. Can you swallow while standing on you head?
4. Do swallowing patterns influence the position of the teeth?

10.11 Speech

The development of normal speech in the child requires the adequate maturation of the following anatomical, physiological, and psychological factors.

Hearing: Deaf children need intensive speech therapy. They have to be taught to copy their teachers' example as they cannot correct and control their own sounds.

Muscle control: Children who lack muscle coordination may slur words and are unable to sing.

Oral nasal seal: The speech of children with an unrepaired cleft palate has a nasal sound as these children are unable to build up air pressure inside the mouth.

Emotional stability: Autistic children may be withdrawn and do not wish to communicate. A severe shock may leave you "speechless."

10.11.1 Phonation and Articulation

Phonation is the production of sounds by vibration of the air passing through the vocal cords. As the cords are tightened, the vibrations have a higher frequency and the sound gets higher. The vocal cords are tightened by activity of the laryngeal muscles. Variation in the pitch of the voice conveys not only color but its own range of messages.

Articulation is the modification of the sound as it passes from the larynx through the velopharyngeal valve and the oral cavity (▶ Fig. 10.12).

- Modification through the larynx occurs when sounds are not voiced at all. When air passes though the relaxed cords, the speech emerges as a whisper. Some speech sounds are recognizable because they begin voiceless and then are voiced. For example, "P," "T," "S," "Sh," "F," "Th (ing)" begin voiceless, whereas "B," "D," "Z," "Zh," "V," "Th (is)" begin voiced.
- The velopharyngeal valve separates the nasal and oral cavities and is formed by the apposition of the soft palate against the posterior pharyngeal wall. It is usually open during vowels and some consonants like "M," "N," "NG" but closed during the remaining consonants.
- Several types of complete or partial obstruction to the sound may occur in the oral cavity. The sounds are classified by speech therapists according to the nature of the obstruction.
  - Plosive sounds are temporally, totally held back; for example, "P, "B, "T, "D.
  - Resonant sounds are diverted around the tongue and lips; for example, "R, "L.
  - Nasal sounds are diverted through the nose; for example, "M, "NG.
  - Fricative sounds are in two parts; they start with a partial obstruction which is then cleared as in "Show, "Sew, "Few.

10.11.2 Defects in Speech

Speech is severely distorted by loss of mobility of the tongue. This may be the result of surgery for tongue cancer or due to motor nerve damage which occurs during a stroke. It is also quite obvious in someone who has had too much alcohol or drugs. A common speech defect in the young children learning to speak is a lisp. It is caused by an inability to retract the tongue behind the front teeth when making an "S" sound. The sound produced is "Th" such as "thixty thix."

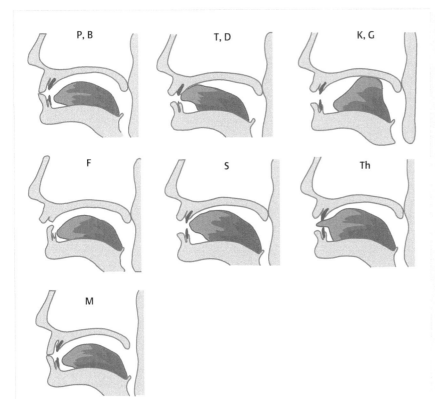

Fig. 10.12 A series of diagrammatic representations of the position of the tongue and soft palate during the articulation of consonants. Note that the velopharyngeal valve is closed for most speech sounds except vowels and the nasal consonants "M, N, NG." In individuals with an unrepaired cleft palate, this valve is unable to close.

The loss of velopharyngeal competence causes alteration of plosive sounds which become nasal and breathless speech. This is usually the result of a cleft palate which has only been partially repaired. Speech therapy with the aid of intraoral devices which help close the sphincter may be of help.

Loss of the vocal cords may occur due to cancer surgery leaving the patient incapable of producing voice sounds. However, these patients often develop such burping skill that adequate sounds are made by the esophagus. Alternatively, a small sound resonator is handheld against the throat and its sound modified in the normal way. Most speech sounds are unaffected by tooth loss except the fricative sound "F."

Review Questions

1. Why is the speech of an individual with an unrepaired cleft palate nasal and breathless?
2. How would you classify the sounds "K" and "N"?
3. What defect causes a lisp?
4. What effect on speech would the loss of the central incisors have?

References

[1] Basbaum AI, Bautista DM, Scherrer G, Julius D. Cellular and molecular mechanisms of pain. Cell 2009;139(2):267–284
[2] Moayedi M, Davis KD. Theories of pain: from specificity to gate control. J Neurophysiol 2013;109(1):5–12
[3] Travell J, Simons DG. Myofascial pain and dysfunction. The Trigger Point Manual. Baltimore, MD: Williams and Wilkins; 1983
[4] Melzack R, Wall P. The challenge of pain. 2nd ed. London: Penguin Books; 1988
[5] Dubner R, Sessle B, Storey A. The neural basis of oral and facial function. London: Plenum Press; 1978
[6] Wilding RJC, Lewin A. A computer analysis of normal human masticatory movements recorded with a sirognathograph. Arch Oral Biol 1991;36(1):65–75
[7] Wilding RJC, Adams LP, Lewin A. Absence of association between a preferred chewing side and its area of functional occlusal contact in the human dentition. Arch Oral Biol 1992;37(5):423–428
[8] Wilding RJC, Shaikh M. The relationship between muscle activity, jaw movements and chewing performance in normal subjects. J Orofac Pain 1997;11:24–35
[9] Proffit WR. Equilibrium theory revisited: factors influencing position of the teeth. Angle Orthod 1978;48(3):175–186

Suggested Readings

Oral Pain Control

Baldry PE. Acupuncture, trigger points and musculoskeletal pain. London: Longman; 1993
Grushka M, Sessle BJ. Applicability of the McGill Pain Questionnaire to the differentiation of 'toothache' pain. Pain 1984;19(1):49–57
Lund JP, Lavigne GL, Dubner R, Sessle BJ. Orofacial Pain; From Basic Science to Clinical Management. Illinois, IL: Quintessence Books; 2001
Trowbridge HO. Review of dental pain—histology and physiology. J Endod 1986;12 (10):445–452

Oral Proprioception

Berkovitz B, Moxham B, Linden R, Sloan A. Oral Biology: Oral Anatomy, Histology, Physiology and Biochemistry. 3rd ed. London: Churchill Livingstone; 2010
Nauntofte B, Svensson P, Miles T. Clinical Oral Physiology. Quintessence Publishing; 2004

Oral Reflexes

Anderson D, Mathews B. Dentinal and periodontal sensory mechanisms. Front Oral Physiol 1976;238–250

de Laat A. Reflexes in jaw muscles and their role during jaw function and dysfunction: a review of the literature part III. J Cranio 1987;5(4): 333

Türker KS, Jenkins M. Reflex responses induced by tooth unloading. J Neurophysiol 2000;84(2):1088–1092

11 Aging

Abstract

When treating any patient, but in particular, one who is elderly, it is necessary to consider the needs of the whole person. Management of the elderly requires more than just carrying out repair work to dental tissues which have broken down as a result of aging. Elderly people have special needs, which are partly due to the biological effects of aging, but equally due to a series of social and behavioral changes in their life. This chapter cannot do justice to these aspects of aging but is important to be aware of them. The dentist/therapist must be sensitive to the influence these age changes might have on the resilience of the patient. Treatment must therefore take account of each patient's needs and be personalized and appropriate.

For example, expensive procedures, which involve long chairside hours, are not suitable for a pensioner who tires easily and finds it difficult to use public transport. The approach to the elderly patients must take account of their need to retain their personal dignity and respect. They do not want to be hurried or talked at; of all age groups they are least likely to tolerate being persuaded against their will.

Keywords: general features, cell metabolism, teeth, abrasion, attrition, tooth support, saliva, nutrition, forensic

11.1 General Features of Aging

Some aspects of biological age changes in the dental hard tissues are unique to the oral environment, but mostly, aging of the structures of the oral cavity occurs just as they do elsewhere in the body. Some of these age changes can be accounted for by a reduction in the rate of cell metabolism. Thus, a reduced mitotic rate causes thin epithelia and slow repair; a reduced cell synthesis causes less bone, saliva, collagen to be produced; a reduction in cell contraction ability causes muscle weakness. These events affect the whole system (e.g., poor circulation, reduced hormone secretions) and they also affect the local oral tissues (e.g., causing thin atrophic mucosa, alveolar bone loss, poor healing). So, changes in the oral cavity occur in association with general

biological events of aging; they are not necessarily related to the chronological age of the patient. However, changes in the teeth are a useful (and almost indestructible) guide to the age of an individual and are important for forensic purposes (▶ Fig. 11.1).

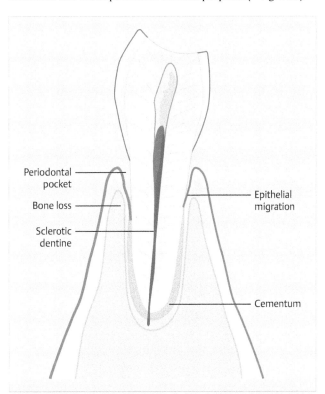

Fig. 11.1 A diagrammatic representation of age changes in the teeth. Wear of the enamel causes dentin to be exposed. The pulp chamber has been largely replaced with secondary dentin, and there is narrowing or complete obliteration of the root canal. Loss of epithelial attachment has resulted in a periodontal pocket with epithelial migration down the root face. Loss of alveolar bone height has occurred. The dentinal tubules in the root dentin have become filled with peritubular dentin giving the root dentin a translucent appearance know as sclerotic dentin. Cementum has been deposited around the apex of the root.

11.2 Age Changes in the Teeth

Aging is associated with a progressive loss of the teeth. The life expectancy of the dentition varies all over the world, and is not, as one might expect, always related to the level of social welfare. The percentages of edentulous individuals are falling in many developed nations. In the United States, it decreased from 54% who were edentulous in the age group of over 65 years of age in 1960 to 14% edentulous in the same age group in 2010.[1] In poorer nations, whose populace has limited access to dental treatment, the percentage of edentulous individuals is higher than in the United States.

Loss of teeth in the elderly used to be thought to be mainly due to periodontal disease, though this assumption has been recently challenged. Where dental services are rudimentary, or unaffordable, dental caries, which goes unrepaired, takes a greater toll. Partial loss of the dentition may increase the risk of further tooth loss, as it imposes a greater strain on the periodontium of the remaining teeth.

11.2.1 Abrasion and Attrition

Generalized tooth abrasion is a feature of a course diet and has not been seen in Europe since steel was used instead of stone to mill flour. Stone-milled flour contains stone dust which is highly abrasive and gives the bread an unpleasant gritty quality. Attrition is not always related to aging but may be seen on the few remaining teeth of a reduced dentition. The vertical facial height may become reduced if wear is rapid, but it is more common for the facial height to increase with age, as eruption continues without equivalent wear.

11.2.2 Stains and Discoloration

Enamel becomes more translucent with age and allows the underlying yellow-colored dentin to be more visible. The enamel also tends to develop cracks which may cause incisal edges to chip off the teeth. The cracks also harbor stains, particularly from tea and tobacco. If enamel has been worn away, as happens on the tips of the lower incisors, the exposed dentin usually becomes darkly stained. These oval-shaped stains are also prominent in the lower incisors of a horse and are known as "marks." The number of incisors with "marks" is used as an indication of the horse's age.

11.2.3 Secondary and Sclerotic Dentin

The deposition of secondary dentin increases the thickness of dentin over the pulp causing the teeth to be less sensitive. The size of the pulp chamber and the diameter of the root canal are reduced, and this may cause difficulty during endodontic treatment. While secondary dentin is a feature of old age, it is also seen in younger patients as a response to caries and attrition. Peritubular deposits of calcified tissue cause the dentin to become less porous and more brittle, which may lead to fracture. This *sclerotic* dentin begins at the apical part of the root and spreads coronally with age. The increasingly brittle nature of root dentin of the elderly patient may lead to root fracture during extraction of the tooth, should this be necessary.

11.2.4 Age Changes in the Dental Pulp

The pulp becomes less cellular and more fibrous. This may be related to the decrease in vascular supply, reduced metabolism, and slower turnover of collagen. The reduced pulp metabolism reduces its capacity for recovery from inflammation and repair of pulp exposures. Intracellular vacuoles are found within the odontoblasts, and large extracellular vacuoles can be seen throughout the pulp tissue of elderly individuals.

11.3 Age Changes in Tooth Support

11.3.1 The Periodontal Ligament

In elderly individuals, who have not suffered from periodontal disease, the teeth may show some wear and be firmly attached to alveolar bone with a narrow periodontal space. In many individuals, there would be some degree of gingival recession with root exposure and mobility, giving rise to the expression "long in the tooth." The junctional epithelium migrates progressively apically with age.

11.3.2 Cementum

The deposition of cementum is closely related to aging and is a useful guide to the forensic aging of teeth. The deposition is mostly around the apical third of the tooth and around the apex of the tooth. The cementum is cellular and shows lines of incrementation. An increase in apical cementum may cause problems if a tooth requires extraction, as the increased bulk of cementum locks the root into the bony socket (▶ Fig. 11.2).

11.3.3 Alveolar Bone

As a general rule, decreased functional loads on bone cause its resorption (*see Chapter 7.7.7 Response of Alveolar Bone to Dentures*). Patients, who have lost all their teeth, tend to lose the bone of the residual alveolar ridge and this may present problems in wearing dentures. Aging bone is also characterized by an increase in bone resorption called osteoporosis. It is particularly common in women during menopause. This combination of tooth loss and osteoporosis accentuates the resorption of the residual alveolar ridge. The resorption may not be regular or uniform; sharp remaining spicules are a frequent cause of denture pain.

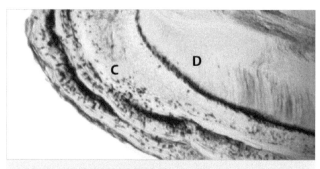

Fig. 11.2 A decalcified histological section through the root apex of a tooth from an elderly individual. An accumulation of cementum (C) is confined to the apex of the root dentin (D).

11.3.4 Oral Mucosa

The epithelium of mucous membranes becomes poorly differentiated in old age. The distinction between oral mucosa types becomes less noticeable. The submucosa becomes more fibrous and less elastic than it is in younger individuals. The amount of elastin is said to increase, but this may be a type of converted collagen which is not very elastic. The tongue becomes smooth and fissured.

The tongue and oral mucosa are dry and poorly lubricated due to the reduced secretion of both minor and major salivary glands. The relative dryness of the mouth of the elderly patient may reduce the comfort and retention of dentures.

11.3.5 Changes in the Temporomandibular Joint

Flattening of the articular surface as a result of remodeling of the condyle is related to wear of the teeth. The disk becomes thinner and may perforate, often without any clinical signs or symptoms. Islands of cartilage and the development of clefts in the fibrous joint surface and disk are features of aging. Proprioceptive activity and hence neuromuscular control is diminished in the elderly. Mandibular movements may be involuntary and less well coordinated.

11.4 Age Changes in Saliva

The reduction in cell mitosis leads to a reduction in the cellular component of many tissues including the salivary glands. Cell synthesis is also reduced, leading to a reduction in salivary flow. Older individuals may need to take sips of water while eating, as there is not enough saliva to lubricate their food.

The elderly people are at risk for developing dental caries, which occurs around exposed root surfaces more than it does on enamel. The enamel, after many years of remineralization, is robustly acid resistant, but the newly exposed root surfaces are vulnerable.

Denture wearers are particularly affected by a reduction in saliva, as retention of dentures depends on a film of saliva between the denture and the mucosa.

11.5 Nutritional Changes in Aging

Tooth loss, muscle weakness, and poor coordination make it difficult for older individuals to masticate adequately. This reduced ability influences the selection of their diet. The reduction in the number of taste buds and the decrease in taste perception also affects food choices as well as reducing the stimulation of saliva. Tactile sensation is diminished, which reduces efficiency in food management and control.

All these challenges are compounded in elderly denture wearers. Reduction in saliva production reduces the protection of the oral mucosa which may develop a burning sensation or become easily ulcerated by wearing dentures.

These factors contribute to others, which collectively, may be responsible for poor nutrition of the elderly. Some elderly individuals may depend on a state pension which may not be generous enough to allow the more expensive foods to be purchased,

such as meat and cheese. If the elderly individuals live alone, and get tired easily, they may not want to go out shopping for fresh fruits and vegetables. They are inclined not to bother with cooking, and so make do with food which is easy to prepare but has limited nutritional quality such as toast and coffee. It may be useful to suggest to elderly patients, whose diet may be inadequate, that they purchase a protein supplement which is pleasant to eat, easy to prepare, and ensures an adequate nutrition.

11.6 Forensic Features of Eruption and Wear

The sequence of eruption of the deciduous teeth, through the eruption of the last molar, may give an indication of the age of a child, accurate to within a year. Age changes in dentin are used to make age estimates of older individuals. The amount of peritubular dentin, the thickness of cementum, the amount of secondary dentin, and reduction of the size of the pulp cavity are all reflections of aging. The soft tissue changes are the apical migration of the epithelial attachment and the decrease in the cellular components of the pulp.

11.7 Emotional Changes in Aging

The changes in the oral environment brought about by cellular events are more predictable than emotional changes, but there are some which will be familiar to those with elderly relatives.
- *The world becomes more threatening:* The fear of being lost, robbed, falling over, poverty, illness, and being lonely all increase the anxiety of the elderly.
- *Change is unwelcome:* The familiar friends, home and belongings, including dentures are precious. They bring comfort and security. Learning new skills and making new friends is more difficult.
- *Reliability* becomes more important. People must do what they promise to do, keep appointments and be on time.
- There is less energy for long journeys or long appointments.
- There is a lower tolerance to discomfort; being cold, hungry, in pain and tired are all unwelcome. Being unable to enjoy food without pain is miserable. Rudeness is poorly tolerated. Respect and good manners are much appreciated.

These features of aging should direct certain modifications in clinical practice. These include planning as few appointments as possible, which are early in the day and short. Procedures which may suit some elderly patients include repairing or relining an old denture and using a resilient lining to reduce pain.

Key Notes

A little extra chair-side time is required for the elderly to explain and consider treatment options. The busy practitioner may be tempted to move along, but an unhurried approach will be rewarded by the patient's appreciation. Many elderly folks are more grateful, than they were when youngsters, of the good things that come their way, like being treated with honesty, good manners, and respect.

Review Questions

1. How can changes in cell metabolism explain the events of aging?
2. What is the difference between chronological and biological age?
3. How can the teeth be used for forensic purposes?
4. What are the two reasons elderly people may lose alveolar bone?
5. Why should the submucosa and pulp become more fibrous in the elderly?
6. What are the consequences of a reduction in salivary flow for elderly people?
7. What factors, apart from difficulty in chewing, would influence the diet of elderly?

Reference

[1] Slade GD, Akinkugbe AA, Sanders AE. Projections of U.S. Edentulism prevalence following 5 decades of decline. J Dent Res 2014; 93(10):959–965

Suggested Readings

Bates J, Adams D, Staford G. Dental treatment of the elderly. Practitioners Handbook. Oxford, United Kingdom: Butterworth-Heinemann Ltd.; 1984:35

Hutton B, Feine J, Morais J. Is there an association between edentulism and nutritional state? J Can Dent Assoc. 2002; 68(3):182–187

Lamster IB, Northridge ME. Improving Oral Health for the Elderly: An Interdisciplinary Approach. New York: Springer; 2010

Mojon P, Thomason JM, Walls AW. The impact of falling rates of edentulism. Int J Prosthodont. 2004; 17(4):434–440

Seeman E. The structural and biomechanical basis of the gain and loss of bone strength in women and men. Endocrinol Metab Clin North Am. 2003; 32(1):25–38

Young MF. Bone matrix proteins: their function, regulation, and relationship to osteoporosis. Osteoporos Int. 2003; 14 Suppl 3:S35–S42

Appendices

Appendix A. The Origins of Teeth

A.1 Mastication and Mammals

A.1.1 The Evolution of Mammalian Teeth

The earliest origins of teeth were modified scales around the mouth of fish. Later versions in fish, mammals, and man have become more complex than scales, but their skin origins are still evident. During their development, human teeth still depend on the contribution of skin cells for their hard enamel covering. The function of teeth in sharks and early bony fish was to assist in feeding by holding the prey until it could be swallowed. Sharp teeth might have helped disable the prey and prevent it escaping but very little chewing went on. Even the large carnivore reptiles, like crocodiles, do not gnaw or grind, but tend to gulp the prey down after a few quick snaps of the jaw.

Fish teeth are more or less the same size and shape as each other, so are referred to as homodont. There are continually being shed and replaced, like their ancestral scales, and so they are referred to as *polyphyodont* (many generations).

The jaws of ancestral and modern reptiles are not particularly strong, as they are made up of several small bones fused together. The lower jaw serves two functions, firstly to bite food, and secondly as a route for sound vibrations to the inner ear. In reptiles, it is not particularly effective in either of these roles; chewing capability is minimal and hearing is poor. Snakes have poor hearing, but they can sense vibrations, such as the footsteps of an animal, provided their jaw is on the ground.

About 200 million years ago, in the Triassic period, before the great age of the dinosaurs, the synapsid reptiles were the major land vertebrates. These mammal-like reptiles began to show evidence that they actually used their teeth to chew. The synapsid jaws gradually became strengthened by increasing the size of the main bone, the dentary. The excluded small bones became incorporated into the middle ear as the incus and malleus, previously the quadrate and articular bones of the jaw. These small bones became dedicated to amplifying sound, leaving the dentary free to become a more specialized and effective part of the chewing apparatus. The increased size and area of the mandible allowed for greater muscle attachment and greater chewing power. The window in the skull which characterized synapsids, accommodated the coronoid bone of the jaw. This process provides attachment for the temporal muscle.

The teeth became fewer in number and more specialized (heterodont in size and shape), and instead of being endlessly replaced, they came in two sets: primary and adult (*diphyodont*).

A.1.2 The Mammalian Work Ethic

The relationship between the masticatory equipment of early mammals and their physiological changes was complimentary. Although fossil remains cannot reveal most of these changes, it is supposed that they were gradually occurring. Not all reptiles were cold, slow-moving, or inactive creatures dependent on the warmth of the sun. Those who were capable of longer working hours and night shifts were found to possess some advantage. This increased activity was made possible by an improved supply and storage of energy and temperature control. The four-chambered heart increased circulatory efficiency, by separating the pulmonary circulation from the rest of the body, and provided a higher oxygen content of tissues. Fur and subcutaneous fat stores retained heat and extended the working day. The senses of smell, hearing, and eyesight were more acute, which were an advantage in both hunting and defending. Rapid conduction of nerve impulses and an increased capacity of the central nervous system provided the coordination and balance needed for a life in the trees. The more ventral position of the limbs gave more agility and speed. The growth and development of young within the female demanded additional energy and nutrients but had the advantage of providing time for specialized organs to develop in safety.

A.1.3 A Voracious Appetite

An essential prerequisite for such a sustained supply of energy and a warm body was a generous supply of high-grade fuel. This was especially critical for the early small mammals whose heat loss was rapid. It is not surprising that small mammals have voracious appetites, and they may spend the entire day feeding, especially the vegetarians whose food source is not rich; an elephant needs 200 kg of fodder a day to stay alive. Not only vegetarians eat heartily. Moles consume their own weight in worms and insects every 24 hours. However, it is flexibility in the diet, which has been the characteristic of one of the most successful and ubiquitous mammals. The brown rat will eat anything from wax candles to lizards, from insects to garbage. The vegetarian mammals, by far the majority, require more specialized chewing apparatus than carnivores, and even then, needed a further mechanism for breaking down vegetable fibers. The ruminants enjoy a mutually beneficial relationship with bacteria in their stomachs. Their gut bacteria break down cellulose in exchange for a sheltered home and plenty of food. An effective chewing apparatus was therefore a selective advantage to the emerging mammals. The components necessary to achieve the desired food preparation vary, but there are some features common to the masticatory apparatus of all mammals.

A.1.4 A Robust Skeleton and Powerful Muscles

The application of powerful forces to bring the jaws together is common and characteristic of mammals. These are generated by a substantial muscle mass made up of several groups. There are broad areas of attachment of these muscles onto the mandible and the skull. In order to withstand the forces generated by the muscles, the skull is strengthened by an increase in mass of the facial bones and the buttress effect of the zygomatic arch. The maximum biting force of man is about 200 kg, and it is probable that a mammal such as the hyena would far exceed this. The jaws are moved by a variety of muscle groups so as to vary the direction of the applied force to suit the chewing requirements of the animal's diet, for example, cutting, grinding, shredding, or crushing.

Mammals possess an advanced nervous system, which enables them to generate rapid and powerful jaw movements with coordination and precision. A well-developed network of sensory receptors around the teeth and jaws provides the feedback for both reflexes and centrally (voluntary) controlled movement.

Mammals are able to breath during chewing, as the oral cavity is separated from the nose by the hard and soft palate. There is an active and flexible tongue with space within the lower jaw to accommodate it. The athletic tongues of the giraffe and anteater, in particular, need spacious accommodation. The cheeks and lips of some mammals are well supplied with muscles which contain or store the food. Hamsters fill up and hurry home to store, or chew, in peace.

A.1.5 Mammalian Teeth

The teeth of mammals have to be mechanically strong enough to withstand the forces generated by the increased muscle mass. They are all composed of a very hard but brittle outer layer of enamel and a highly compressible and more resilient inner core of dentin. The combination produces a hard wearing and tough tool. The teeth are usually of different shapes and sizes within the same jaw, sometimes being so specialized as to be hardly recognizable. The tusks of elephants and the long-twisted tusk of the male narwhal are examples of the specialization to be found in heterodont dentitions.

Instead of being constantly replaced throughout life, there are just two sets: one to be accommodated in the growing jaws of the immature animal and one for the adult. The opposing teeth meet together, in order to break down the food. This makes their position in each jaw critical enough to require some means of fine adjustment after eruption.

A.1.6 The Mammalian Tooth Socket

The teeth are firmly, though not rigidly, held in a socket lined by a highly cellular and fibrous tissue, the periodontal ligament. This method of attachment is unique to mammals and is called a gomphosis. The periodontal ligament provides the eruptive force for teeth (continuous in some mammals such as the rats' incisors) and allows the tooth to reposition as it wears, by remodeling of the bony walls of the socket.

A.1.7 The Mammalian Jaw Joint

The mammalian joint works like a class III lever (like the elbow). The joint acts as the fulcrum, where part of the biting force is resisted. The joints of carnivores confine movement of the jaw to a hinge type of opening and closing. Herbivores require more gliding lateral movements at the joint. The human temporomandibular joint has to resist loads and slide at the same time. It has evolved as an unusual disk of fibrous tissue, rather than the cartilage of other joint disks.

A.2 The Mechanics of Tooth Use

A tooth functions just like any other tool. It is a device designed to enable the application of force to a working surface. The term work will be used in the context of carpentry when it describes the material against which the tool is to be used. Chewing may involve a variety of processes such as piercing, crushing, cutting, shredding, and grinding, all of which require the application of force. The magnitude of the force will depend on the consistency of the food but the direction/s of the force will depend on the nature of the work to be done.

A.2.1 Piercing Food

Piercing requires the application of a force via a sharp pointed tool, in a straight line. Crushing can be achieved with a similar type of force applied via a blunt tool. These two processes are characteristic of animals which feed on insects. The earliest mammals were probably mainly insectivores; the shrew is an example of a modern-day insectivore. The premolar teeth are sharp and pointed, while the molars have pointed cusps and crushing surfaces. The jaw moves straight up and down with no sideways movement. Insect eating requires the least complicated masticatory apparatus and a simple tool type.

A.2.2 Cutting Food

Food can be cut by forcing a sharp blade through it while it is being held on a hard surface. The knife soon gets blunt and has to be sharpened frequently. Food can also be cut using a scissors-like action. The blades of this tool have to be forced sideways against each other as well as brought edgeways together. Consider why it is difficult, if you are right-handed, to cut the fingernails of your right hand with nail scissors. The application of the forces required for cutting with a blade–blade is thus more complicated. The performance of a scissors type of tool is not always satisfactory because of the following reasons:

- The work may slip along the edges if not trapped. (It is difficult to cut heavy nylon with tin snips).
- The cut work may prevent the blades coming close together. The tool is then clogged and must be cleaned before it can be used again. The blades in a well-made pair of scissors are hollowed out behind the cutting edge to prevent clogging.

- After some use, the edges of the blade become rounded instead of square and slip past each other without cutting. The tool then requires sharpening.

The carnivores of today have powerful jaw muscles. The mandibular arch of teeth is inside the maxillary arch. Were it not for a slight sideways approach as the jaw closes, the sets of upper and lower teeth would miss each other completely. In many reptiles they probably did. The cusps of the carnassial teeth trap tough tendons (▶ Fig. A.1).

A.2.3 Shredding Food

Shredding is a combination of tearing, cutting, and crushing. Forces must be applied to the tool in a variety of directions, but in particular, a side-to-side movement is necessary, while a force vertical to the work must be applied. Shredding is most efficient if there is a series of sharp edges to the tool. The problems with a shredding tool are as follows:

- It is very sensitive to clogging and must therefore be provided with escape ways for the shredded particles. Some types of work will always clog a shredding tool.
- The edges of the tool will eventually become rounded. They are almost impossible to sharpen individually, and the tool must therefore be discarded.

The teeth of mammals which shred food, such as those which browse on shoots and leaves, have evolved ranks of cusps along their molar teeth. When the enamel covering of each cusp has worn away, the inner core of dentin and cementum is exposed. The ranks of worn cusps provided an efficient tool for shredding fibrous food (▶ Fig. A.2).

A.2.4 Grinding Food

Grinding is a refined form of crushing. A grinding tool must generally reduce the work to a pulp, and this requires very closely fitting surfaces of the tool. The directions of the applied forces must allow almost circular movements. The problems are as follows:

- The work must be held in a depression so as not to escape before it has been properly reduced.
- The magnitude of the force required is unusually high, and considerable energy is needed to move the tool sideways while it is under a heavy vertical load.

The teeth of mammals which feed on a wide diversity of food types (omnivores) such as pigs, rats, grizzly bears, and primates, have evolved premolars and molars which have features of the sharp cusps of carnivores and the ranks of cusps of herbivores. When the human dentition has had a moderate degree of wear, the molar teeth have a circular depression of dentin surrounded by a periphery of enamel and provide a suitable tool for grinding food such as berries and seeds.

The processes described above would be suitable for the preparation of some foods and not others. Note that they are progressively more demanding to perform. Consider the capability of a preschool child to use a piercing tool, a pair of scissors, a kitchen grater, a woodwork plane, and a pestle and mortar.

The most advanced tooth design and jaw movement potential is necessary to shred grasses, stems, and wood or to grind seeds. For animals with this capacity, the teeth are such a vital requirement for obtaining food which can be digested that the teeth determine the life span of the animal. When they are completely worn away, for example, in elephants and sheep, the animal dies of starvation. Some of the most remarkable tooth tools are to be found in the order Rodentia. The speed with which beavers chisel through the trunks of large trees or the carefree way rats will gnaw away at cardboard boxes is unmatched by other mammals. The rodent's incisors are continually erupting at the rate of 0.5 mm per day, to compensate for wear.

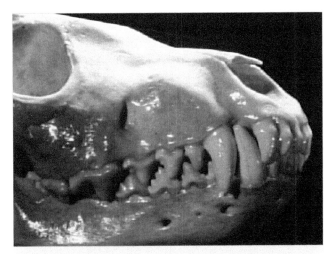

Fig. A.1 The adaptation of the mammalian teeth and jaws to cut through tough food. The skull of a dog shows the massive structure of the jaws and jagged profile of the cutting teeth which trap tough skin and tendons and bone. The canine teeth not only pierce and cut, but as they slide against each other, they guide the premolar and molar teeth onto trapped food allowing them to work as scissors.

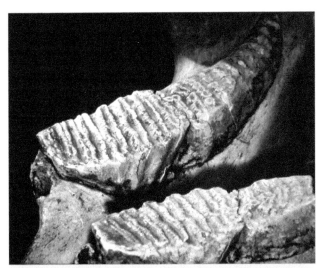

Fig. A.2 An elephant's mandibular molars reveal a series of cutting surfaces formed by folds in the crown during tooth development. The single molar is replaced when worn away by a replacement molar which erupts in a mesial direction into the same position the previous tooth occupied. The semierupted molars still have signs of the smooth enamel-covered ridges or cusps. When the final, sixth molar has erupted and worn away, the elephant is no longer able to feed and its life comes to an end.

Masticatory function developed to keep pace with the metabolic demands of the mammal. A generous supply of high-energy food which could be readily digested was essential. The scope of the diet was improved by more effective food preparation. This made available food sources previously untouched by any competitor, provided slight modifications were made to the chewing apparatus. Perhaps most important of all, an improved ability to chew permitted greater flexibility in the diet. This could have been of survival value if the supply of the favored food source diminished. However, there are always exceptions, anything goes attitude of the brown rat to food selection. The koala bear is dedicated and loyal to its special relationship with the leaves of certain species of eucalyptus tree. It will die of starvation rather than breaking the pledge and eating anything else.

Suggested Reading

Lumsden AG, Osborn JW. The evolution of chewing: a dentist's view of palaeontology. J Dent 1977; 5(4):269–287

Appendix B. Dental Hard Tissues

B.1 Physical Properties of Enamel and Dentin

Enamel is the hardest of all organic materials. It is about five times harder than dentin.

Young's modulus is a measure of the stiffness of a material. Enamel is 10 times stiffer or more brittle than dentin. The collagen fibers in dentin make it more flexible and less likely than enamel to fracture when compressed or under tension (▸ Table B.1).

B.2 Enamel Proteins

There are two main types of enamel proteins, amelogenins, which are hydrophobic, and a rather diverse group of proteins including enamelins, which are hydrophilic. Amelogenin is the protein first formed in the matrix of calcifying enamel and is essential for enamel mineralization. The amelogenins are secreted well before the enamel begins to mineralize and are to be found with fibronectin associated with the first mantel dentin to form. So, amelogenins are thought to be involved in the final differentiation of odontoblasts.

The very large size of enamel crystals is attributed to the special matrix for crystal growth which enamel proteins provide. Once the secretion phase of enamel is completed, and the tissue has reached its final shape, the transition phase follows, during which most of the protein matrix is progressively resorbed by the ameloblast. During maturation the remaining proteins are resorbed and replaced by minerals. Protein resorption is achieved by enzymes, which accompany the secretion of amelogenin. These enzymes are contained in lysosome vesicles and are not released until the enamel matrix has started to mineralize. They break down the original amelogenin molecule into a number of smaller proteins, and peptides, which are resorbed by the ameloblast or diffuse out of the maturing enamel. They may also be physically squeezed out in the channels between the crystals which are growing toward each other. The protein amelogenin is largely removed from maturing enamel, but enamelin remains as the main protein in the fully developed tooth.

Table B.1 Physical properties of enamel and dentin

Property	Dentin	Enamel
Hardness (Knoop)	62	296
Young's modulus	12 GN/m²	131 GN/m²
Compressive strength	262 GN/m²	76 GN/m²
Tensile strength	65 GN/m²	35 GN/m²
Abbreviation: GN/m², giga Newtons/meter².		

Enamel proteins have a role in the initiation of both dentin and enamel mineralization during tooth development and also support the growth of very large and orientated enamel crystals. They are also found in the adult cell rests of Malassez in the periodontal ligament where they play an important role in periodontal repair (see Chapter 3.5.3 Cells of the Periodontal Ligament).

The genes for amelogenins are found on the sex chromosomes, X and Y, and are slightly different (sexually dimorphic); perhaps, these differences account for the larger teeth of males. Amelogenins are a group of proteins, which show close similarity with those of other mammals. This conservation of genetic material during evolution is an indication of the structural importance of this protein in determining enamel structure.

Amelogenins are quite unlike collagen or keratin. They are not fibrillar and have few of the amino acids characteristic of collagen. They do, however, resemble salivary proteins in which they contain large amounts of proline and histidine.

B.3 Composites and Resistance to Fracture

A composite material is one in which there are two of more components which are intimately connected. Each component contributes different properties which complement the properties of other components. For example, the two components of a fiberglass resin produce a material which has greater application than either glass fiber or resin would have on their own. The dental restorative resins combine the excellent adhesion to tooth surface of the resins, with a hard-wearing quality of the filler.

Composite materials abound in nature and reach even greater levels of sophistication than the man-made analogues. Bone, for example, not only combines the hard surface and high compressive strength of apatite crystals with the tough elastic fibers of collagen, but it is responsive to changes in the way it is loaded. The orientation of collagen fibers is complex and serves to provide resistance to tensile and twisting forces which the long bones of locomotion must resist.

The combination of the hard and brittle outer enamel layer and the resilient tough inner core of dentin provides an ideal combination for tooth strength. When two hard materials like enamel come into contact with each other, there is a problem of dissipating locally applied and concentrated forces through the brittle enamel without cracking it. The orientation of enamel prisms which radiate inward toward the core of the tooth would provide little resistance to a crack developing into the tooth, just as a log of wood is most easily spit inward to the core of the log. Collagen fibers in dentin are orientated in a circular direction around the dentin core. They lie at right angles to the direction of a crack in enamel which is opening toward the core of the tooth. The dentin also contributes to arresting cracks as they begin. This property is due to the more resilient nature of dentin which acts as a crack stopper.

A crack stopper is an interface, weaker than the bulk of the material, which is opened up by the action of the stress concentrated at the tip of the moving crack. The opening up of the interface dissipates the stress, and this slows down or stops the continuation of the crack (*see Appendix H.1 Cracks Composites, and Teeth*).

Appendix C. Oral Mucosa and the Periodontium

C.1 Tooth Displacement

If the displacements of a tooth are plotted during loading, it will be seen that it does not displace in a linear way as the force applied increases, but it becomes progressively more resistant. When the loading force is removed, there is an initial rapid return to the original position, which slows down to a slow creep. The characteristics of the ligament under tooth loads may be described as viscoelastic (▶ Fig. C.1). It is therefore likely that both tension in the ligament fibers and compression of the ground substance contribute to tooth support.

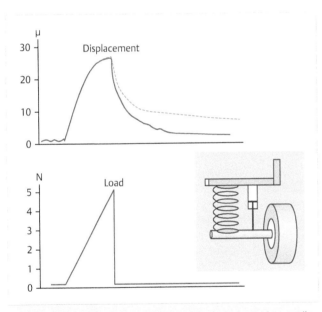

Fig. C.1 Response of the periodontium to loading. If a tooth is rapidly loaded with 5N, it offers progressively increasing, viscous resistance to displacement. If the load is rapidly removed, the tooth rebounds rapidly at first, but then takes some seconds to creep back to its original position. With age (*broken line*) the return is longer. Tooth and mucosa support are both elastic (spring) and viscous (damper), which are similar to the support of an automobile.

C.2 Tooth Mobility

After repeated loading toward its apex, a tooth becomes intruded and more rigidly held in the tooth socket. This progressive increase in resistance to displacement is due to failure of the tooth to rebound to its preloaded position before the load is applied again. It becomes therefore progressively less mobile. Teeth become less mobile during the day, presumably due to the regular light forces applied during swallowing. The mobility of the teeth returns to normal during the night.

The mobility of teeth has been shown to increase with vigorous chewing or with night grinding (bruxism). So, while light forces such as swallowing reduce mobility, heavy forces seem to increase mobility. Tooth mobility may be caused by local factors such as bone loss, loss of epithelial attachment, inflammation of the periodontal ligament, atrophy due to disuse, and physiological increase due to increased occlusal loads.

The presence of disruptive occlusal contact, or occlusal trauma, has been thought to be associated with increase in tooth mobility and loss of alveolar crest bone. There were claims that occlusal trauma could cause periodontal disease, though the evidence is that while mobility may be associated with alveolar bone loss and deep pocket depths, the mobility is a result not a cause of the disease. The role of occlusal trauma in periodontal disease and in temporomandibular joint disorders is unproven. There is no evidence that occlusal adjustment plays a significant role in the healing of periodontal disease.

Suggested Readings

Gher ME. Changing concepts. The effects of occlusion on periodontitis. Dent Clin North Am 1998; 42(2):285–299

Wills DJ, Picton DC. Changes in the force–intrusion relationship of the tooth with its resting position in macaque monkeys. Arch Oral Biol 1981; 26(10):827–829

Appendix D. The Ecology of the Oral Cavity

D.1 Saturated Solutions

A saturated solution can be made by placing crystals of a weakly soluble salt into water. Some of the crystals will become ionized and dissolve in the water, but after a while no more will dissolve. The solution is then saturated. If the solution is heated, more ions will dissolve into solution, but if it then cooled down, ions will precipitate back onto the crystals. If acid is added, it will also encourage more ions to form and dissolve into the solution, but if the solution is made alkali, salts will once more precipitate.

D.2 Salivary Gland Secretion

There are two types of cells which secrete saliva: mucous and serous. The secreting cells are grouped in clusters (acini) which are surrounded and supported by a basement membrane. The whole structure is enclosed in a fibrous tissue framework supported by septa, which join an outer capsule. The cells secrete fluid into a lumen which leads into a system of intercalated ducts.

Serous-secreting cells contain acidic granules which dominate the cytoplasm; the Golgi apparatus and endoplasmic reticulum are prominent. The cell membrane against the basement membrane is thrown into folds in order to increase the surface area for nutrition into the cell.

Mucous-secreting cells containing large pink staining droplets are closely packed and contain highly glycosylated proteins. The major salivary glands have distinctive proportions of these two major types of cell. The parotid gland is almost entirely serous. The submandibular gland is mixed, but mostly serous. The sublingual gland and the minor glands are also mixed, but mostly mucous. In the mixed glands, the serous cells are arranged like caps known as demilunes around the mucous acini.

From the intercalated ducts saliva enters a system of striated ducts. These ducts are so named due to the presence in the duct cell of plasma membrane folds adjacent to stacks of mitochondria which have a striated appearance. The saliva is modified as it flows through the striated ducts. The cells of these ducts remove sodium chloride ions and proteins and secrete potassium and bicarbonate ions (▶ Fig. D.1). The removal of sodium chloride causes saliva to be hypotonic in respect to plasma. For this reason, blood tastes relatively salty. Comparison of some of the constituents of saliva with serum will reveal the active and selective nature of salivary secretions.

The control of secretion is mediated by parasympathetic and sympathetic nerve activity. All secretory cells, whether serous or mucous, seem to receive a dual supply. It has been observed that if sympathetic activity predominates (such as in fear), the

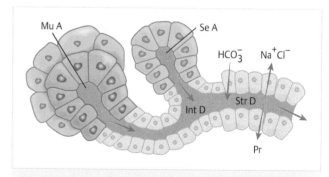

Fig. D.1 Diagrammatic representation of a mixed salivary gland. Each acinus contains both mucous (Mu A) and serous (Se A) acini. Secretions flow into the intercalated (Int D) and then through the striated ducts (Str D). Active transport of sodium chloride (Na$^+$Cl$^-$) and proteins (Pr) by the striated duct cells reduces their concentration in saliva. Bicarbonate ion (HCO$_3^-$) concentrations are increased by the cells lining the striated duct.

secretion is sparse and contains more mucous than normal (hence a dry, sticky mouth). In contrast, if the parasympathetic activity predominates, then the flow is copious and mostly serous (when feeling nauseous).

D.3 Gaia Theory

The Gaia hypothesis is the name given to a theory by James Lovelock that the earth is a self-regulating ecosystem. One of these systems within the complex whole is the oxygen cycle. It begins with the sun's energy, which plants' life uses in the conversion of carbon dioxide into larger carbon molecules with the releases of oxygen. Animal organisms feed off the carbon molecules and with the help of oxygen derive energy and release carbon dioxide. The system regulates itself, as the amount of oxygen released by plants influences the mass of organisms converting oxygen back into carbon dioxide. According to the Gaia theory, the oxygen level on our planet is maintained at a sensitive level to the general benefit of all living things. Any higher concentration would lead to spontaneous fires, and a lower concentration would stifle the life out of the planet. What keeps the levels of oxygen stable are complex interaction between many different forms of life, from forests of trees to oceans of algae. So, the life on earth drives its own precisely controlled environment.

This is just one of the main sources of controversy about the Gaia theory. The environment has been cast as the stage on which the struggle for survival of living organisms was played out. It was a given, apart from climatic changes. Life did not define the environment, it adapted to it. We have noted that a microbiome like dental plaque does, to a large extent, create its own environment. We see the relics of the structural and functional organization which results from the interactions between plaque organisms, in Fig. 4.7 of calcified plaque. This image encourages a new perspective on the relationship between life and its environment. The Gaia theory scales up this view we have of a microbiome and applies it to the whole earth.

Lovelock writes "The earth's atmosphere is not just life supporting, it is controlled by life. Life on earth is self-regulating." We depend on the biosphere of the earth, which is a complex system, for the stability required by all forms of life. We are an inseparable part of the biosphere, and what we do alters it in ways we cannot yet be certain off, though the signs of our pollution are worrying. If man interferes with this balance by destroying trees and by burning fossil fuels, the balance will be upset and the ecosystem will break down.

D.4 Gene Regulation in Biofilms

The change in *phenotype* from a plankton phase of a microorganism to a biofilm phase is brought about by the expression of about 80 genes which are associated with a large number of new proteins being formed. This change in gene expression is an indication that communal living calls for significant adaptations. Considering the relative mass of organisms which the biofilm sustains, this phase change to communal living is most successful. Further benefits of a life in the biofilm are that antibacterial agents are much less effective. It has been calculated

that it requires 1,500 times the concentration of antibacterial agent to have the same effect on the biofilm as it does on planktonic organisms. This is presumably due to the resistance to diffusion of the agent through the biofilm. This theory seems to be supported by an experiment in which it has been shown that an electric field developed through the biofilm helps to pull the agents through the film and therefore make it more effective. A method for sterilizing contact lenses has been developed in which an electric field is used to encourage the agent to penetrate the full depth of the biofilm.

The extent of order and structural design in biofilms has fairly recently been revealed. It is likely that further research will reveal some of the mystery surrounding the emergence of order in a complex system such as a biofilm. Such information might help to develop more effective strategies for controlling biofilms.

D.5 Strategies for Controlling Biofilms

Several methods have been proposed to control organisms in biofilm so as to eliminate or modify the biofilm. These include the following:
- Targeting the organisms in their planktonic phase.
- Targeting the organisms in the biofilm phase.
- Modifying the surfaces to discourage attachment.
- Modifying the environment to discourage growth.
- Disrupting preformed biofilms by physical or chemical means.

The use of an "artificial mouth" allows some of these variables to be controlled in laboratory experiments, so that the effectiveness of various strategies to control biofilms can be tested. The response of organisms to changes in the environment of an artificial mouth can be observed by measuring the growth rates of each species. If a neutral pH buffer is circulated around the growing plaque organisms, there is no change in growth, but if a low pH buffer is used, there is an increase in the total number of organisms in the system. It appears that a low pH is a major factor in encouraging organisms that cause dental caries because these organisms grow best in an acid environment. The environment of the plaque organisms is partially created and maintained by the organisms themselves. The drop in pH which occurs when acid-forming plaque bacteria metabolize sugars actively encourages their further growth. Acid formation therefore works as a positive feedback to stimulating an increase in the growth rate, and yet greater amounts of acid production.

A similar chain of events can be set in motion, under laboratory conditions, by circulating a higher pH buffer around organisms responsible for gingivitis. The concentrations, for example, of *Porphyromonas gingivalis* increase dramatically when the pH is increased from 6.0 to 8.0.

The artificial mouth has also been used to confirm the effect of even small amounts of fluoride on the plaque biofilm. Fluoride has a selective effect in preventing the rise in numbers of *Streptococci mutans*, which normally occurs when glucose is introduced into the environment. This dynamic response, characteristic of positive feedback systems, suggests that biofilms would be sensitive to small changes in the environment which could be responsible for shifts toward or away from diseased states. The benefit of plaque inhibitors in toothpastes and mouthwashes has been reviewed by Marsh.[1] These plaque inhibitors do not last long in the mouth at concentrations lethal to bacteria, but they do have an inhibitory effect at lower concentration for some time. While mechanical removal of plaque is essential, antimicrobial agents in oral care products can play an important supporting role.

D.6 Gram Staining Bacteria

One of the earliest, and still used, methods for staining bacteria was devised by Gram in 1884. Bacteria which stain violet are gram positive, abbreviated to Gm + ve. Those which stain red are Gm −ve. The different staining characteristics reflect differences in the composition of the bacteria cell wall and may be used to separate microorganisms into two useful categories. For example, the shift of plaque microbes' populations from gram + ve to gram −ve is an indication of increased pathogenicity in the development of periodontal disease. Gram stains are of limited significance in clinical diagnosis as there are some bacteria which cannot be classified using the stain. Most bacterial identification carried out in modern laboratories is achieved with genetic sequencing.

D.7 Microenvironments

The South African Cape Mountain Fynbos is an unusually old and mature ecosystem which supports more plant varieties, including reeds, Erica, and Protea, than any other ecosystem of comparable size in the world. There are hundreds of microenvironments on the mountains, and they partly account for the rich variations of plant life. These environments may differ in subtle ways, depending on sunlight, rain, mist, wind, soil type, and many other minor factors. Some species of orchid are found in only one particular valley which has just the right microenvironment to support its survival.

Some microbiologists suggest that there are microenvironments in the oral cavity, which may account for the distribution of periodontal disease when it is localized to just a few teeth.

D.8 The Vipeholm Study

This study in 1954 at the Vipeholm Mental Hospital in Sweden showed that taking sugar in between meals was an important cause of dental caries. Patients in separate wards had different diets. Some had sugar in between meals (they developed the most caries), others had the same amount of sugar, but with meals (they developed less caries), and yet another group had no sugar (they hardly had any new carious lesions). This study can be criticized, as the amount of caries in each group at the start of the observation period (1947–1951) was not controlled, but the final conclusions have since been confirmed. By current ethical standards, the study would not be permitted, as the researchers knowingly put some subjects, who were mentally disabled, at risk without their consent.

D.9 Fluoride Availability, Toxicity, and Fluorosis

D.9.1 Availability of Fluoride

Although fluoride is found in rocks, soils, and sea water, remarkably little is present in human diets. Most fluoride salts (e.g., NaF) are readily soluble in water and yield fluoride ions, but the calcium salts are virtually insoluble. In describing the amount of fluoride, the most important figure is the concentration of soluble fluoride ions; this is considerably less than the weight of the salt. Drinking water contains varying amounts, usually 0.1 part per million (ppm) (1 mg per liter) to 2.0 ppm. In parts of Kenya, the fluoride levels reach over 15.0 ppm. There is an unusually high level of fluoride in the tea plant. When prepared as a drink, it contains about 1.5 to 2.0 ppm. Milk contains very little; levels do not increase if the mother (or cow) drinks high levels of fluoride in water. Tablets (0.25 mg) may administered to children according to the level of the fluoride in the available drinking water.

Absorption of soluble fluorides is rapid through gut; it is inhibited in the presence of calcium ions (CaF_2 is insoluble). The plasma level is temporally raised but rapidly reduced by excretion in the kidneys and by skeletal storage. The concentration in plasma varies between 0.14 and 0.19 ppm but is stable between those limits even in areas of high fluoride levels. The concentration falls in the placenta and falls again in the fetus. Some fluoride is lost in sweat, feces, saliva, gingival crevicular fluid, tears, and milk. Children excrete less than adults.

The absorption of fluoride in the gut appears to be affected by climatic and geographical conditions. High altitude and a dry climate increase the absorption of fluoride. In a study of children in such an area, signs of chronic fluoride toxicity were found, even though the level of fluoride in the drinking water was optimal.

D.9.2 Toxicity of Fluoride

The optimum level of fluoride in water for dental health is between 0.7 and 1.0 ppm. It is estimated that 30 mg of fluoride ions per kg body weight would be toxic, that is approximately 3 g for a 100 kg adult. For a child of 10 kg, 300 mg would be dangerous. Fluoride is available in boxes of 150, 0.25 mg tablets (total 35 mg); in a mouthwash containing 2.2 mg/10 mL in a 500 mL bottle (total 110 mg); and in a large tube of toothpaste, there would be 220 mg. Thus, no single packaged source of fluoride would be toxic, even to an infant.

Chronic fluoride toxicity is most commonly due to raised fluoride levels in drinking water. It is also possible that incautious prescription of fluoride tablets to children and the unplanned dose of fluoride which they might get from swallowing toothpaste could mount up to excessive levels of fluoride intake in an area where the water content was already optimal. For this reason, the prescription of fluoride must take account of local levels of fluoride in water and other accidental sources.

D.9.3 Fluorosis

As fluoride is concentrated in hard tissues, it is the bones and teeth which show signs of chronic toxicity or fluorosis. The effect of fluoride on teeth is most profound during their development, and as teeth are formed only once during life, the effect of excessive fluoride on teeth is permanent. The mildest form of fluorosis is recognized by a mottled appearance due to scattered white flecks on the tooth surface. This may occur when the concentrations of fluoride in drinking water is above 2 ppm. It may also occur even if the water content is optimal, but there is a significant additional fluoride intake by accident or because of climatic factors. An index of fluorosis has been devised to categorize the severity of fluorosis into four levels. In moderate forms of fluorosis, the white flecks take on a brown stain. In severe forms, the tooth surface is pitted and misshapen due to interference with the process of enamel formation during tooth development. This is called enamel hypoplasia. Recall that during enamel maturation, enamel proteins, including amelogenin, undergo resorption in order to allow the enamel to fully mineralize. This resorption is achieved by enzymes which break down the enamel proteins. Fluoride interferes with these enzymes, and thus there are sites in the enamel where mineralization is incomplete leaving a chalky looking patch of enamel.

Review Questions

1. How is saliva modified in its passage through the striated ducts?
2. What general rule applies to the amount of fluoride which would be toxic?
3. What levels of fluoride cause fluorosis?
4. How could fluorosis occur when the fluoride content of the water was less than 2 ppm?

Reference

[1] Marsh PD. Contemporary perspective on plaque control. Br Dent J 2012; 212 (12):601–606

Suggested Reading

Prescott SL, Logan AC. The secret life of your microbiome. Vancouver: New Society Publishers; 2017

Appendix E. Cell Interactions in Embryology and Repair

E.1 Epigenetic Modulation

Not all genes carry information to synthesize structural or functional molecules. Many genes code for products which inhibit or facilitate the expression of structural genes. The expression of a structural gene therefore depends on interactions between inhibitors and facilitators. Furthermore, each gene has to be built up from a number of separate segments. The exact order of these spliced segments can be varied to produce slightly different proteins. To add to the uncertainty of the influence of a gene, it has been found that the expression of a gene's information does not usually lead in a *linear* way to some predictable quality of structure or behavior. In spite of much expectation and searching of the human genome, the best estimates are that there are more than 20 genes associated with height and that these 20 accounts for only about 3% of the variability found in humans.[1] There are relatively few genetically determined characteristics, either physiological or medical which can be attributed to a specific gene. Examples of diseases caused by a single gene mutation are sickle cell disease, cystic fibrosis, and Tay–Sachs disease.

The degree of expression or suppression of a gene is brought about by markers or tags known as epigenetic modulators which bind onto and suppress or enhance the gene's expression. Carey suggests that "cells read the genetic code in DNA more like a script to be interpreted than a mold that replicates the same result each time."[2] The role of these moderators may be even more decisive than the genes they control. For example, the gender of a baby crocodile is not genetically determined when the egg is formed after fertilization but by moderators which are affected by the surrounding temperature of the egg. Eggs in a very high or low temperature become male, while eggs in a medium temperature are all female. Moderators can be damaged by environmental hazards and fail to function effectively. That function may be to suppress cancer-forming genes. So, some cancers may be caused by moderators altered by factors such as age, diet, stress, or smoking. Some of the molecular tags which alter gene expressions are passed onto the next generation even if the genes are not. So, the effect of smoking might be passed on for generations. It may be that genetic determination of structure and function is not as linear a process as we have come to believe.

E.2 Morphogenesis

E.2.1 Adhesion and Contact Inhibition

It is possible to surgically remove a piece of tissue, separate all the cells using an enzyme, and then pick out cells of the same type from a growing mass. These separated cells when cultured together may move about until they contact another cell and then do one of the two things, either move together and adhere or move away from and inhibit further contact. Contact inhibition is seen in cells which are normally separated from each other, like fibroblasts and mesenchymal cells. On the other hand, if stratified squamous epithelial cells are separated from each other and cultured, they will stay together when they meet, and eventually pile up in a heap.

If two cell types are mixed together, like liver and kidney cells, they will eventually find each other again and reorganize into recognizable organ fragments. So, the general rule is that like cells adhere together more strongly than unlike cells. It is of interest that cells of a cancer are not strongly adhesive.

Cells may align themselves by attaching to recognizable tissues. Fibroblasts in tissue culture, placed between pieces of dentin and bone, recognize this environment and align themselves in sheets between the two hard tissues. The collagen fibers they secrete are also aligned between the dentin and bone, as they are in the natural situation where they anchor the tooth to the bony socket.

E.2.2 Apoptosis

During life there is death, not only by accident or exhaustion but by design. Sometimes, cells need to die in order to allow others to live or to complete the development of a structure. For example, when the fingers and toes are first formed, they are joined by a web of skin. The cells forming this web die, allowing separation of the fingers. Another example is the fusion of the horizontal processes of the maxilla to form the hard palate. The epithelial cells at the junction of these two processes must die in order to allow the connective tissue to fuse. If these cells do not die as planned, the two halves of the palate never meet, and the child is born with a cleft palate. This programed cell death is known as apoptosis and is under the control of at least 18 genes. One of these genes codes for an enzyme which splits up DNA, leaving ends which can be detected experimentally by labels. So apoptotic cell death can be experimentally distinguished from necrotic cell death.

An important example of apoptosis which occurs in the adult is the deletion of those clones of B- and T-cell lymphocytes which would otherwise attack the body's own cells. It is thus a process of protection against autoimmunity.

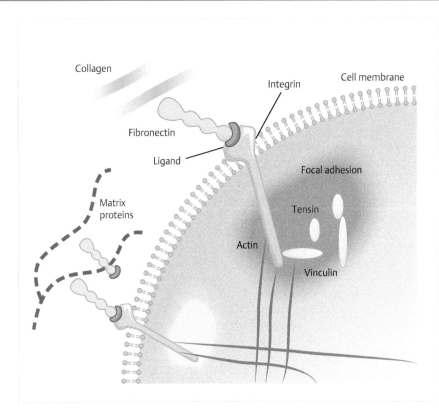

Fig. E.1 Diagrammatic representation of the structure of integrins. Integrins (*orange*) hold a cell in place by anchoring one end to a sack-like aggregate of molecules, the focal adhesions (*brown*). The cell's cytoskeleton of actin (*brown lines*) filaments is bound into the focal adhesion. The other end of the integrin is attached to molecules of the extracellular matrix such as fibronectin (*blue*) via ligands (*red*). Integrins not only hold the cell in place but also relay signals to the cell's nucleus.

E.2.3 Integrins

Most cells in multicellular organisms are anchored in place by a network of proteins. Collagen, lignins, and fibronectin are the proteins of the extracellular matrix, onto which tissue cells attach. There are special binding sites on the fibronectin molecule, called *ligands*, which bind specifically to special receptor molecules on the cell membrane called *integrins*.

Integrins are the cell surface receptor molecules which match up with parts of the matrix protein (ligands) to allow adhesion of the cell to the matrix (*see Chapter 6.2 Glycoproteins*). The attachment of cells to matrix proteins also influences the cells' behavior by the expression of genes.

The integrins are a family of proteins found performing the same functions on all animal cells. Their importance in maintaining the structural integrity of cells led to the name integrins. Some integrins help to attach cells to each other, but for the most part, that role is played by other proteins like cadherin, selectins, and immunoglobulin families.

Integrins go right through the cell membrane, so one end is outside the cell and the other inside. The outside part bonds onto the ligand receptor part of the matrix proteins. The cell membrane is physically quite fragile and would tear off easily at attachment sights. However, the integrin also binds onto the actin filaments of the cell's cytoskeleton, so the attachment is secure. The tails of the integrin and the ends of the actin filaments are held together in sack-like aggregates of molecules called focal adhesions (▶ Fig. E.1).

Apart from providing matrix adhesion, integrins have a second powerful function. They activate gene expression through a series of signals which start at the cell membrane and move in toward the nucleus causing transcription of specific genes. This role of integrins is also involved in the signaling of cytokines and hormonal messenger to the cell. Sometimes, the action of messengers, such as growth factors, depends on the cell being firmly attached to the matrix, so in this way, integrins also "integrate" the signals which cells receive from their environment.

Integrins not only carry messages to the cell but carry them from the cell. This inside-out signaling can cause the integrins to be more or less choosy about which molecules they bind to. For example, when platelets bind to thrombin, a signal is sent into the platelet cytoplasm, which then leads to an inside-out message which causes a different integrin to become adhesive to fibrinogen. The fibrinogen forms bridges between platelets to form a meshwork of cells and fibers, which prevents blood leaking out of damaged vessels.

References

[1] Goldstein DB. Common genetic variation and human traits. N Engl J Med 2009; 360(17):1696–1698

[2] Carey N. The epigenetics revolution: how modern biology is rewriting our understanding of genetics, disease and inheritance. Icon Books Ltd, London; 2012

Appendix F. The Physiology of Bone

F.1 Stress and Trabecular Orientation

In the 19th century, Wolff derived "laws" governing the direction trabeculae would align themselves in response to internal stresses in bone. He believed that they would orientate themselves at right angles to the lines of strain in a bone, so as to minimize further deformation (▶ Fig. F.1). Recent studies tend to confirm Wolff's laws with some modifications. Trabeculae do not always intersect at right angles, and minimizing strain does not appear to be the most important goal of bone remodeling, otherwise bone would become massive in order to minimize strain but at cost to the mechanical efficiency of the skeleton. In fact, bone appears to remodel, so as to sustain a certain optimal amount of strain. There has to be some safety factor built in, so that if the strain is temporarily very high, such as would occur during rapid locomotion, the bone will not fracture. If the safety factor is too high, the excess bone weight will deprive the animal of speed and agility.

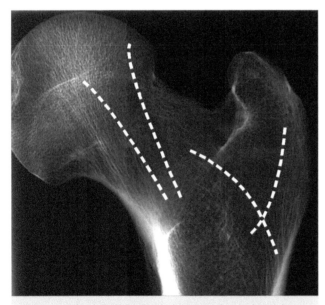

Fig. F.1 A radiograph of the head of a human femur shows the orientation of trabeculae in directions best suited to resist fracture. A prominent diagonal group of trabeculae resist compression of the inferior aspect of the femoral neck, a common site of fracture in the elderly who suffers from osteoporosis. The *broken lines* indicate some of the main trabecula groups. Some groups of trabeculae appear to intersect at right angles to each other, as Wolff observed.

McNiel Alexander in his book, "Bones," compares the weight of leg bones of regular and flightless birds. Birds that fly cannot afford to have heavy leg bones, so they must make them light but take the risk of fracture. Their flightless "cousins" such as the ostrich can afford to have proportionately much thicker and heavier leg bones.

The relationship between stress and design in nature was the life work of D'Arcy Thompson, who during the early part of the 20th century, drew attention to the similarity between manmade structures such as bridges and natural supporting structures like the femur.

Computer models such as finite element remodeling have confirmed Wolff and Thompson's basic assumptions that the loads applied to bone determine its shape and internal structure. A computer-generated design for a bone to transmit weight from the pelvis to the knee looks surprisingly like a femur. A criticism which has been made of this approach to understanding bone remodeling is that it is mechanistic and does not take into account the cellular processes involved in bone remodeling (*see Appendix H.2 On Growth and Form*).

F.2 Remodeling to Achieve Optimal Stress

From a structural point of view, the resistance of bone and stone, to tension, is particularly poor. In other words, they are both brittle. A problem in using brittle materials for support is illustrated by the limitations of stone and brick, as structural supports for buildings and bridges. A bridge may be made by placing a stone beam across two supporting piers. There are limitations in this design, because if the distance between the piers is too long, the beam collapses in the middle. This is because the stresses are concentrated in the center; there are mostly tensile stresses on the underside and compressive stresses on the top of the beam (▶ Fig. F.2). The tensile strength of stone is 20% less than the compressive strength, so fracture of such a beam would occur due to cracks developing underneath, before the upper surface collapsed. Roman and Arabian engineers solved this problem hundreds of years ago, by changing the shape of the beam to an arch, or a dome, thereby shifting the stress from the concentration in the center of the beam, and transforming the tensile stresses into compressive stresses. Their use of the arch and dome lead to new heights (literally) in architecture which reached a peak in the Gothic Cathedrals of Europe and the mosques of Arabia. The Gothic style is less affectionately referred to by some as "heap architecture," for it is just that a heap of stones, each one lying on the next, but by good design, reaching up to the sky.

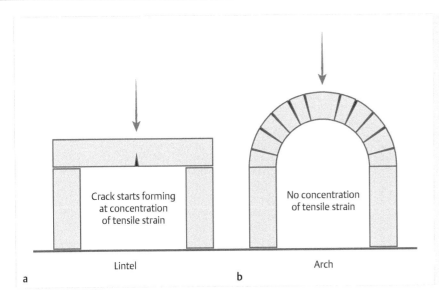

Fig. F.2 Diagrammatic representation of the conversion of tensile to compressive stresses by altering structural design. (a) Stresses on a **beam** are concentrated in the center. Tensile stresses on the side opposite to the load causes cracks and failure. Compressive stresses on the loaded side are better resisted. **(b)** The shape of the Roman **arch** allowed a beam to be made up of several parts with a keystone in the center, which transformed the tensile stresses into mainly compressive ones.

Crack starts forming at concentration of tensile strain

No concentration of tensile strain

Lintel

Arch

a

b

If bone remodels so as to reduce tensile strain concentrations, then deposition at sites of compression and reduction at sites of tension would have the effect of transforming a beam into an arch. This seems to hold true for the weight bearing long bones and vertebral bones. Compression stimulates bone formation. If it did not, our skeletons would not be able to withstand the forces of gravity. However, there are other situations where tension also appears to stimulate formation. Muscle pull causes tension on bone surfaces, and at these sites of attachment, bone formation occurs. The growing brain pulls apart the sutures between the skull bones and stimulates bone formation. Bone does not seem to resorb in response to tensile forces in these two examples.

The following may explain these observations. Bone cells are remodeling bone around them all the time. If they experience strains which are out of the normal range to which they have become "set," they either increase or decrease the net bone mass after remodeling. Therefore, bone remodeling takes place in order to optimize bone strain. A return to optimal strains can be achieved in two ways:

- An efficient and weight saving option is to alter the shape of the bone in order to transform tensile strains into compressive strains (e.g., change a beam to an arch). However, altering the shape of the bone may not reduce stress concentrations sufficiently. Unavoidable strains would be reduced by greater

distribution. Hence, the response of bone at muscle attachments is to increase the mass of bone around the insertion of the muscle tendon.

- If the bone became too robust with weight, there would be insufficient bone strain, and bone cells would respond by inducing bone resorption until they were in an optimal strain environment.

The response of alveolar bone to loads applied via the teeth is of vital interest to dentists. There is need to base clinical treatments on evidence-based science in order to work with and not against the dynamics of bone remodeling.

Suggested Readings

Frost HM. Skeletal structural adaptations to mechanical usage (SATMU): 1. Redefining Wolff's law: the bone modeling problem. Anat Rec 1990; 226(4):403–413

McNeil Alexander R. Bones, the Unity of Form and Function. Coopersburg, PA: Macmillan; 1994

Rubin CT, Lanyon LE. Regulation of bone formation by applied dynamic loads. Calcif Tissue Int 1985; 37:411–417

Thompson DW. On Growth and Form. Cambridge, United Kingdom: Cambridge University Press; 1942:958

Wilding RJC, Slabbert JC, Kathree H, Owen CP, Crombie K, Delport P. The use of fractal analysis to reveal remodelling in human alveolar bone following the placement of dental implants. Arch Oral Biol 1995; 40(1):61–72

Appendix G. Oral Sensations and Functions

G.1 Peripheral Sensitization

The deep, spreading pain and swelling, some minutes after deep tissue damage such as an ankle sprain, is due to the delayed response of C fibers, which mediate the inflammatory response to tissue damage. After further delay, the damaged tissue may become *hyperalgesic*, that is, highly sensitive to what would normally be a mildly painful stimulus. This hyperalgesia is caused by peripheral and central sensitization (▸ Fig. G.1). The first painful stimulus causes a release of neuropeptides from the ganglion cell, which travel inside the nerve axon. These peptides are carried by the microtubular transport system to the receptor terminal in the tissue. Here, neuropeptides, such as substance P and calcitonin gene-related peptide (CGRP), are released into the damaged tissue where they cause vasodilation and the extravasation of plasma proteins. The damaged

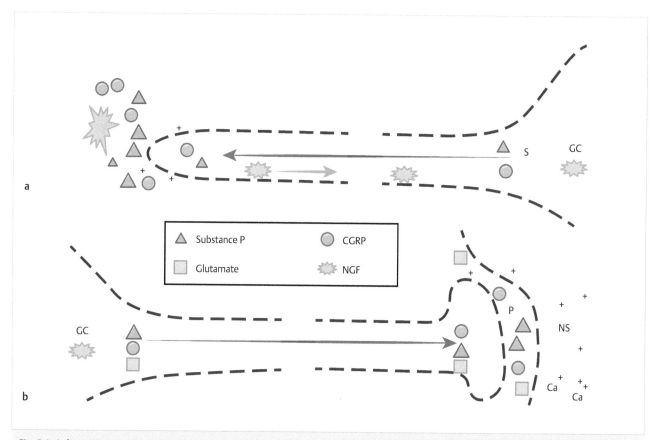

Fig. G.1 A diagrammatic representation of peripheral and central sensitization. This sensitization causes tenderness which develops hours after the injury. **(a)** Peripheral sensitization occurs due to transport from the ganglion cell (GC) and the release from the pain receptor endings of neuropeptides. These include substance P and calcitonin gene-related peptide (CGRP). These chemicals join many others released by the damaged tissue, all of which bind to receptors in the terminal cell membrane and open ion channels, which lower the membrane threshold to depolarization. Nerve growth factor (NGF) is taken up by the pain receptor and transported within the axon back to the ganglion cell. **(b)** Central sensitization is due to the transport inside the axon from the ganglion cell of substance P, NGF, CGRP, and glutamate which will all increase the excitability of the nociceptive cell and may even cause it to spontaneously discharge. Glutamate signals an increase in intracellular calcium ions (Ca$^+$) within the nociceptive specific (NS) neuron which reduces the threshold for depolarization and further amplifies the transmission of pain impulses. The increased excitability of the nociceptive neuron makes it more receptive to the interneuron connections with neighboring cells representing wider receptive areas.

tissue also releases inflammatory mediators from a variety of cells such as mast cells, macrophages, neutrophils, and platelets. The chemical mediatorsinclude histamine, bradykinin, prostaglandins from mast cells, and cytokines such as nerve growth factor (NGF), tumor necrosis factor (TNF), and interleukin-1β (IL-1β) and IL-6. These factors not only are powerful mediators of local inflammation, but also, they all act directly on the terminal of the nerve ending by binding onto their own specific receptors in the cell membrane. This binding process opens up the ion channels in the membrane which excite it to depolarize.

The pain receptor is thus excited by a mixture of chemicals, from both the damaged tissue and those released by the nerve ending itself. Peripheral sensitization increases due to positive feedback. The longer lasting the pain, the more neuropeptides are released which in turn cause sustained levels of pain. The inflammation mediated by neuropeptides has been described as neurogenic inflammation.

G.2 Central Sensitization

The peripheral sensitization, which increases the level of pain impulses from damaged tissue, is further amplified by an increase in the sensitivity of the spinal nociceptive specific (NS) neurons to continual pain impulses. This central sensitization is partly brought about by the transport from the ganglion cell to the NS neurons of the same neuropeptides exported to the periphery. In addition, NGF in the damaged tissue is transported in the nerve axon to the ganglion cell. Here, it stimulates the ganglion cell to increase the production of neuropeptides transported to the axon terminal at the synapse with the NS neurons. Among these peptides are substance P, somatostatin, CGRP, vasoactive peptide (VIP), and glutamate. These neuropeptides increase the excitability of the NS neuron, causing further pain and tenderness, and extend the area of tenderness far wider than the injured area, described as an expanded receptive field. When this group of peptides comes from injured muscle, the expansion of the receptive field is particularly extensive.

The presence of glutamate at the synapse has a further longer-term influence on the NS neuron. Glutamate signals an increase in intracellular calcium ions in the NS neuron, which reduces the threshold for depolarization and further amplifies the transmission of pain impulses.

Under normal conditions, inhibitory interneurons continuously decrease the excitability of NS neurons, an important inhibitory pathway which was described in the gate theory. Prolonged pain reduces the activity of these inhibitory interneurons which also reduces the inhibition of non-nociceptive A fibers. The consequence of peripheral and central sensitization is hyperalgesia which may lead to chronic pain.

G.3 Central Connections of Pain Impulses

Nerves supplying the oral cavity and face carry their information through the trigeminal ganglion where the cell bodies are located. They enter the brainstem and may ascend or descend in the trigeminal spinal tract before entering the trigeminal sensory nuclear complex. Fibers originating in the tooth pulp have a wide distribution in the nucleus and may synapse in the subnucleus oralis and the main sensory nucleus.

There are several areas in the brain which receive and process pain impulses. Spinal cord neurons project impulses to several areas of the cortex. Some of these pathways are routed through the thalamus and others through connections in the brainstem to the amygdala where they mediate aversive reactions to pain. The limbic part of the midbrain is known to be involved in feelings and emotions. The periaqueductal gray in the brainstem also receives connections from fibers carrying pain impulses, but here, the response is to generate a continuous stream of impulses back down the spinal column to the NS neurons which inhibit the generation of pain impulses to the brain. Several experiments have shown that profound analgesia can be produced by stimulating the periaqueductal gray matter in the reticular formation. The descending control from the brain to the NS neurons of the spinal cord and trigeminal nuclei provides another significant component of the gate theory.

It is becoming increasingly clear that the entire brain participates in pain perception, including memories, sounds, smells, thoughts, fears, and sights.

Depression is a predictable consequence of long-standing pain. It is a dark cloud which settles on the patient. Fear, anger, despair, hopelessness all add to depression. It is not surprising then that antidepressants are useful in controlling the despair of chronic pain. They do, however, also produce analgesia, apart from their antidepressant effect. Amitriptyline (a tricyclic antidepressant) is effective against migraine, chronic tension headaches, and facial pain due to temporomandibular disorders. Combinations of drugs are the most effective, for example, aspirin and codeine (a morphine-related drug) work well together. Morphine and amphetamine ("speed") are powerful agents against cancer pain.

Surgical approaches to pain control by cutting peripheral nerves, spinal tracts, or brainstem pathways have not been successful. The brain and spinal cord are complex structures, and they function in an interactive way. The processes of pain are too complex to be isolated to a particular area of activity. Therefore, a mechanical removal of parts of the complex has an unpredictable influence, often it makes pain worse.

Implants into the periaqueductal gray and the thalamus are quite promising though the early effects of pain reduction seem to wear of, and longer stimulation is required. However, a noninvasive and effective stimulation can be achieved through the skin using transcutaneous electrical nerve stimulation (TENS). The strength and frequency of the impulse can be controlled by the patient, and the device is small enough to allow for use at home or while at work. It is inexpensive and has no side effects. TENS has therefore used as an initial treatment for many chronic conditions, in particular, the facial pain which appears to be related to muscle trigger points (temporomandibular joint disorder [TMD]). It is particularly useful when other treatments have failed, for example, in postherpetic neuralgia and in amputation stump pain.

Appendix H. Endnotes

H.1 Cracks, Composites, and Teeth

One of my children seems to leave a trail of wreckage. Ordinary everyday items like door handles and toasters disintegrate in her hands. Her indignant defense is that it was already half broken anyway. It does seem as though nothing breaks with just one catastrophic rupture.

A block of homogenous material under a uniform tension has an even distribution of stresses through the material. If a small crack appears, perhaps due to a local flaw, the stress in the block tends to extend the crack even further apart. This happens because the stresses which were shared out evenly before the crack developed are now concentrated at the crack tip, making it more likely for bonds to break there than anywhere else. The crack may propagate very fast or progress in spurts as the pattern of stress in the block shifts, due perhaps to other cracks developing. Whatever way it goes, and however fast it happens, when a structure breaks, it happens as a series of developing cracks, not a simultaneous rupture of all its internal bonds. So, when the garage door finally comes off its hinges, we have all contributed a few cracks.

Stresses will only concentrate at the crack tip in a material which is very rigid and unyielding. Brittle materials like porcelain, glass, and cement, have very low tensile strengths because they crack so easily. In a material which contains sites of more ductile material, the crack opens by deforming the softer material instead of breaking the bonds of the more brittle parts. The inclusion of less brittle components in a material may therefore act as crack stoppers.

There are special advantages to be gained if the resilient component is a fiber. When fibers are dispersed in a matrix or binder, the properties of the composite material may be a useful blend of both fibers and binder. Even if a few fibers break in the path of a crack, they do not completely lose their contribution to resisting tensile forces, which they would do if not bound in a matrix. Composite materials are both strong and light, in comparison with single-phase materials. The newer carbon fiber and aramid fiber composites are stronger than steel, but only 20% of its weight. One of the requirements for a successful composite is good adhesion between the fibers and the matrix.

While glass fibers bond well to resins, they do not bond to builder's cement. The adhesion of some fibers can be improved by coating the fiber with an agent which will adhere to the matrix. The ceramic particles in dental restorative composites are coated with a silane coupling agent to improve their adhesion to the resin matrix.

Another requirement is that the fibers should be long. This is for two reasons. Firstly, if they are short, they may pull out of the matrix without breaking. Secondly, the orientation of long fibers can be controlled more easily than short fibers. When the composite is being made, the fibers can be placed in line with the expected tensions the structure will have to meet when it is in use. A woven fiber system, such as a fabric, resists tension best along the warp and the weft. Many composites are built like plywood, with several layers, each with its own specific contribution to overall strength.

The strategy of incorporating fibers into a brittle matrix can be traced back 500 million years. During the Devonian period, a new skeletal material appeared in the Osteichthyes which outclassed the other vertebrates who had skeletons of cartilage. These fresh water fish developed armor plates under the skin around the head, a successful form of protection for their brains, which to this day, we have retained. This crucial development required a new line of cells with a special capacity. They formed collagen fibers and a ground substance like cartilage, but in addition, they were able to concentrate calcium phosphate, until it would precipitate as crystals in between the collagen fibers. The resulting material was bone. It had the advantages of the compressive strength and hardness of the bone salts (apatites) and solved the problem of their brittleness by incorporating collagen fibers to act as crack stoppers.

The fibers of the first formed embryonic or woven bone are a tangle, giving no particular strength in any direction. The demands made by weight-bearing vertebrae and limbs would not be met without some refinements to such a disordered composite. A natural composite which is obviously more structured than embryonic bone is wood. The fibers of wood are orientated along lines of tension, which make it susceptible to splitting along the grain but very difficult to crack across the direction of the fibers. The fiber orientation works for trees, but when timber is used for building, it is often laminated to prevent it splitting. It is the orientation of each layer in plywood which contributes to its strength. Lamination toughens materials even if there are no actual fibers. Samurai swords were made by repeated softening, rolling, and folding of the steel blade, in the same way puff pastry is made. The result was a sword resilient enough to withstand the clash of armor in battle but so hard that it could be honed razor sharp. The legendry test of a good blade was that it should be able to slice through a silk handkerchief tossed into the air.

It is fiber orientation and laminar structure which takes the crucial step from embryonic, woven bone to the order and strength of compact bone. The metabolic unit of compact bone is the osteon, a rod with concentric laminations, like the layers of a leek. The collagen fibers run in a concentric direction around each lamination and in a longitudinal direction down the length of the osteon. Down the middle runs, a bundle of blood vessels provides the transport and energy required for the regular replacement of bone in the osteon. The osteons are packed together into compact laminated bone and aligned along the length of a thick tube, which makes up the shaft of long bones.

Synthetic composites follow the same rule of fiber orientation as bone does. The steel rods of reinforced concrete can be seen sticking out of the ground on building sites before the concrete is poured around them. A more sophisticated arrangements of fibers in a composite can be found in the drive shaft, which links the tail rotor of a helicopter with the motor. The shaft must be long and thin but not whip or wobble. A system of circular fibers prevents collapse in the middle of the shaft; a helical pattern of fibers resists twisting of the shaft, and longitudinal fibers prevent the shaft wobbling.

Teeth are composites of enamel and dentin, and each of these materials is itself a composite. Enamel consists almost entirely of hydroxyapatite crystals, but there is a regular alignment of the crystals within each enamel prism. Within each tooth, the enamel prisms radiate out at right angles to the dentin core. So, the crystal and the prisms of enamel comprise a sort of fibrous element rather like wood. And like wood, enamel is particularly vulnerable to splitting down its length. Every undergraduate dental student is taught to remove unsupported enamel from a cavity preparation, because if left, it will flake off later leaving a marginal defect. The earliest type of enamel, still found in sharks, has no prisms but is just a random arrangement of crystals which gives it great compressive strength. What selective advantage could mammals have derived from enamel prisms which were vulnerable to cracking off?

In order to chew food, mammalian teeth have to work like any other cutting or grinding tool. The cutting edge must be sharp, close to it must be an escape-way for food particles, so as to avoid clogging the cutting edges. Mammalian teeth are not made ready to use; they only become sharp after the rounded cusps have worn down exposing a hard edge of enamel and a depression of dentin next to it. Some small mammals actually grind their teeth in utero, so that when they are born, their teeth are ready to go to work. Enamel prisms lie at a right angle to the surface of a tooth. As wear occurs, the edges of enamel do not round off and get blunt, the way enameloid would do after small bits had flaked off; instead, a whole prism comes away the entire width of the enamel leaving a flat blade with a sharp square edge. The carnassial teeth of a carnivore will have just one sharp edge; the molars of an herbivore will have a whole battery of them. So, far from being a backward step, the enamel prism was a selective advantage to mammalian digestion (in whom food processing is a priority) because it maintained a sharp cutting edge to chew on, something enameloid could never have done.

Dentin is also a composite with the same bone salts as enamel, but in addition, there is a significant component of collagen fibers. While a crack proceeds rapidly down the length of an enamel prism, it is halted when it reaches dentin. The forces at the tip of the crack are dissipated by deforming the more resilient material. The enamel crack also meets up with a fiber system which is running at right angles to the crack. For the crack to continue, it would have to break through a web of collagen fibers. Thus, while dentin would crack at a tangent to the pulp, it is less likely to crack following the path of an enamel fracture. The combination of enamel and dentin results in a tough tool for cutting and grinding food. Consider that the forces generated by the human jaws may be as high as 200 kg, and that these forces must be quite insignificant in comparison to the bone-cracking power of carnivores like hyenas. The teeth are the tools which convey these forces, without showing any sign of breaking up under such stresses. Yet, the destruction of teeth does occur, not due to cracks and fractures, but in the silence of an attack by acids.

H.2 On Growth and Form

It makes a refreshing change to rediscover some old-fashioned, leisurely science. Just after the turn of the century, D'Arcy Thompson wrote "On Growth and Form" (it was revised and reprinted in 1942). His attention was drawn to the diversity of living forms which he observed and drew. His drawings not only reflect his love of nature, but also reveal an analysis of form which was quite mathematical. The diversity of his attention leaves one a little breathless, from shellfish to frogs, then snowflakes to bridges. It is just as well he was not dependent on the approval of a committee for his research funds, as he would surely have had all his proposals turned down. Firstly, because there were too many of them, and secondly, because his work is quite free of statistical analysis, an icon of modern science. His genius lay in making order out of the great diversity he recorded. All his observations seem to have been collected for the contribution they could make to his search for a unifying design in nature. He was looking for something which would tie all the repeated biological phrases together, a unity of purpose among all the diversity. And he found it in the mathematical expressions of the helix of shells and the shape of growing cells; he found it in the structure of snow flakes, the cracks in basalt, and the stripes of a zebra.

He argued that there were common laws at work. "*The search for differences or fundamental contrasts between the phenomena of organic and inorganic, of animate and inanimate things, has occupied many men's minds, while the search for commonality of principle or essential similarities has been pursued by few; the contrasts are apt to loom too large, great though they be."*

Thompson knew there were common principles among quite diverse forms of life, but he felt it necessary to be cautious about debating the philosophical or religious basis for this unity. The rigor of 20th century science would not tolerate a meaning or purpose to nature. Scientists at the turn of the century had only just shaken off the cozy ideas that Providence had indeed provided. In an essay called "Hutton's Purpose" Stephen Gould recalls the joy of a geologist, who in 1870 had written that coal was a wonderful gift Providence had made, so that we might keep warm. Yet more joy; Providence, with characteristic consideration, had arranged that this buried treasure, too deep for us to discover, occasionally rose to the surface and came peeking through, as if to say "Here I am"! So, Thompson was understandably wary of giving a purpose to the form and function of living things. However, he felt reasonably certain that the universality of the principles of physics and mathematics could be upheld. He wrote *"in general, no organic forms exist, save as are in conformity with physical and mathematical laws."* Here he was on safer ground.

He decided that the laws most commonly found to operate as unifying principles were those concerned with static and dynamic forces. *"The form of any particle of matter, whether it be living or dead, and the changes in form which are apparent in its movements and in its growth, may in all cases be described as due to the action of force."* Forces of tension, compression, and shear occurred in all living structures and influenced both growth, function, and form.

The bones of a museum skeleton would lie in a heap on the floor without the clamps and rods holding them together. In the living animal, tension holds the skeleton together as much as weight does. We have difficulty in remaining upright while we go to sleep, and so do most large mammals, because we have to keep our muscles active, in literally, pulling ourselves together. However, tension is not only developed by muscle pull. The ligaments of our joints are also vital structural elements, less obvious in man because our joints allow an unusual freedom of movement. The forelegs of a horse lock when bent slightly backward, preventing the leg from bending, thereby allowing the horse to sleep while standing up, without expending much energy in keeping postural muscles active. In this case, it is the ligaments of the joints of the foreleg which stop the skeleton from collapsing. Man-made structures are also held together by the same tension.

The towering medieval cathedrals were in fact heaps of stone without any significant tensile stresses. They were built on the Roman principle that arches are better able to support weight than lintels. While stone is brittle, steel provided a material which resisted tension. So instead of bridges resting on piles of stones, they could be suspended on steel cables, hung between concrete abutments; in the suspension bridge, the abutments are pulled inward. The Fourth bridge in Scotland is made from a series of identical units, each one consists of a concrete column with steel cantilevers on each side on which the railway runs. The cantilevers are held up by an arch made of radiating struts tied across the top.

D'Arcy Thompson believed that there was purpose in design in living structures which obeyed engineering principles. He cited as just one example the fore quarters of a buffalo, which are remarkably similar to the design principles of the Fourth Bridge. The sturdy front legs support the shoulder girdle from which the head and chest are suspended. The shoulders hang under an arch of high vertebral spines tied across by ligaments. Thompson believed that the use of bone and tendon in nature was related to the use of stone and steel by engineers.

There were common principles to be found at other levels. A useful structural element of bridges, plants, and animals is the tube. We are reminded of a reed, the quill of a feather, an antler, a long bone of a limb, a triple helix of collagen. Tubes are light and provide stiffness, although they do have a tendency to collapse and kink in the middle if they have to support any weight, especially if the tube is long. The weight a tubular column will support is in fact inversely proportional to the square of its height. The tall stem of a bamboo would collapse were it not divided into a series of short units by periodic thick bands, each unit being short enough not to collapse. The hollow shaft of the femur gets progressively thicker toward the middle to prevent collapse at this weak point of the tube.

Tubular structures can be strengthened by longitudinal fibers. Plant stems are responsive to the loads applied and can increase the amount of fiber if necessary. A peach stalk gets stronger (not thicker) as the peach grows heavier. Young sunflower stalks break if loaded with 160 g. If loaded, but not fractured, by say 150 g for 2 days, the load on the stalk can increase to 250 g without causing fracture. Thompson concludes that *"strain, the result of stress is a direct stimulus to growth itself. Growth may be coordinated with the structural adaptations required by mechanical requirements."* This principle is a fair prophecy of Moss's functional matrix theory, put forth in the late 60's which claims that bone grows in response to the functional demands of soft tissues. If lines of stress are studied by engineers, they can be used to predict the design required to relieve them. *"The skeletal form, as brought about by growth, is to a very large extent determined by mechanical considerations and tends to manifest itself as a diagram, or reflected image of stress."*

Structural adaptations to stresses may occur within a material, without change in its exterior size and shape. Shearing strain has the effect of displacing fibrous elements away from lines of stress. Examples are combing shanks of wool, drawing out wire, repeatedly folding a Samurai sword blade. The result of these shearing strains is that the fibers (or trabecula orientation) become aligned at right angles to the shear stress. So, Thompson concludes, *"there is a tendency for a material to be laid down just in lines of stress thereby avoiding the disruptions due to shear."* The trabeculae of the femoral head are indeed arranged along lines of stress; the pattern of one set crossing the other at right angles in accord with theoretical stress design.

The closing chapters of D'Arcy Thompson's work question the value of basing classification (taxonomy) on differences and similarities in structure. The structural shapes of living things have been used to place them into related categories; for example, carnassial-shaped teeth help us to classify carnivorous mammals. Such morphological characteristics are genetically determined and hence occur invariably among related mammals. However, *"heredity is not the sole determinant of morphology; it is one of the great factors in biology, but we cannot neglect physical and mechanical modes of causation."*

For example, some parts of whales look like seals, but that does not mean they are related by ancestry; they are related by their common need to adapt to stresses during function. Thompson argues that it is to be expected that unrelated animals would develop the same characteristics due to a common environmental need. Sophisticated eyes have developed separately in mollusks, such as squids, and quite separately in vertebrates. It is true that the morphology is not identical; in vertebrates, the light sensitive cells are deep to the nerve cells, whereas in gastropods the order is reversed. However, in both cases, an image is focused through a protein lens onto cells filled with rhodopsin, a light-sensitive pigment both phyla have borrowed from plant cells. So, the general structure and function is quite similar in two quite distantly related groups, the Chordata and the Mollusca. The chemistry and physics of vision are common and, in both cases, determine the structural elements.

The idea that there are a few generic shapes which nature keeps using and that these shapes are modified by their physical and chemical environment is a modern idea, eloquently set out by Goodwin. The studies of the basic patterns in limb and tooth morphology illustrate the enormous range of function which adaptations of these patterns can produce.

D'Arcy Thompson's outlook was shaped by religion, philosophy, science, and literature. It is quaint but humbling to come across footnotes written in Greek, Latin, German, French, and Italian, with the unselfconscious assumption by the author that the reader needed no translation. Are we less well prepared to understand the world around us because of our comparative illiteracy? Would D'Arcy Thompson have contributed more to our understanding if he had been able to use the fine tools we have today? What of all the Greek and Latin? Perhaps with all his wholeness, he would still have floundered had he been faced with today's dilemma in reconciling our ethical and religious values with space age biotechnology.

Such questions are too shrill. D'Arcy Thompson does not have to be measured up against anyone. While his insights were remarkably farsighted, they may eventually become quaint and old fashioned, or they may survive with greater prescience than he could have imagined. What lingers, regardless, is the celebration, the joy he found in the continual tension between the unity and diversity of life.

H.3 The Heritage of Fibrous Polymers

Before the days of synthetic fibers, man relied on both plants and animals for clothing materials. These natural materials have a great deal in common. Cotton and other plant fibers are all cellulose; wool, silk, furs, and feathers are all keratins; leather hide is mostly collagen. The common factor shared by cellulose, keratin, and collagen is that they all have similar molecular structures. They are all fibrous polymers. It seems as though silk worms, cows, and cotton plants, in spite of being very distantly related, have independently evolved the same recipe for making a tough fiber.

First, you take some carbon atoms and make a long thin chain using the very best covalent bonds. Next, they need to be stacked alongside each other and packed tight using more covalent bonds. Then, they must be tied in a bundle and the bundles be positioned all along the line of tension. Lastly, the free ends of each chain in the bundle need to be linked up to those in the bundle in front and behind. The recipe is the same whether it is for a spider's web or a bird's feather. Darwin and D'Arcy Thompson would surely have been delighted by this evidence of natural selection and common purpose at work. Several unrelated organisms, with the same problem to solve, and quite independently, arrived at the same answer. What works well is worth keeping, and it survives.

Some of these natural materials have synthetic equivalents, but it is still hard to find anything quite like Angora wool or silk or just plain shoe leather. A craftsman who builds string instruments insists that there is nothing comparable with animal glues for joining the panels of a violin or a harpsichord. So, he boils apart the collagen fibers from animal bones and puts up with the smell. There are others of us, perhaps just as old fashioned, who insist on cotton underwear.

Long before the complexity of the natural fibrous polymers was understood, chemists were taking the first steps toward copying their molecular structure. The first plastics were produced by joining together many small single units (mers) like ethylene into fewer large molecules (polymers) like polyethylene. The early synthetic polymers were brittle and affected by heat; they were called plastic, because they could be made plastic by heating, and while still hot, the material could be forced into a mold. Modern plastics are of sterner stuff and more properly called resins. The latest techniques used to make very strong, heat-resistant resins are based on principles of polymer mechanics which owe their heritage to living organisms.

Like the natural polymers, an essential requirement of a synthetic fiber is its ability to resist tension. If a material is being pulled out, it is less likely to break if it is made from a bundle of long fibers than if it is one solid block. A metal rod is more likely to snap under tension than a wire cable of the same dimension and made from the same metal. The components of the cable may in turn be smaller cables which in turn may be made from fine wire. This hierarchy from the smallest unit to the larger units of the structure is also found in animal tendons. The advantage of a hierarchy is that if one level breaks, the fault is contained there, while the next higher level merely takes a bit more strain. A small fault in a monoblock material tends to spread as a running crack through the entire structure. The fiber, or cable, is strongest, if all the units, even down to molecular size, are long chains, all orientated along the lines of tension. Consider the strength of a piece of wood under tension along the grain; but if pulled across the grain, it is very weak. These observation about fiber orientation and tensile strength of materials hold true at different scales of size, that is, they are also true at a molecular level.

The strongest bonds between molecules are those provided by the sharing of electrons which occurs in covalent bonds. The more electrons shared, the stronger they are, so elements like carbon, silica, nitrogen, oxygen, and aluminum make strong covalent bonds. Examples are the ceramics, aluminum oxide (the basis of rubies and sapphires), silicon carbide (abrasives), silicon dioxide (glass), and of course the hardest material of all, diamond. Baer (1986) explains that molecules linked together in a chain by covalent bonds are very difficult to break if pulled along their length, so the orientation of the chain when tension occurs is crucial. If several chains are stacked next to one another, the bundle (or fibril) will be a useful unit for building a fiber, provided that the chains of molecules cannot slide past each other. In order to prevent this, they need to be tied to each to each other by cross-linkages and at least reasonably long. It is worth looking closer at these three requirements for a strong molecular fibril, that is stacking, cross-linking, and length.

If uncooked spaghetti is spilled on the table, it is easily gathered and returned to the box; it would be impossible to bring such order to the pieces once you had cooked them. Stacking of long molecules cannot be achieved unless they are stiff, and cross-linkages are impossible to achieve unless the chains are packed close to each other. The first formed molecular chains of collagen and keratin are stiffened in places by the rigid nature of some of the amino acids which form the links of the chain. The important one is proline, an amino acid with an aromatic ring which becomes part of the backbone of the chain.

Commercially made polymers, like the aramids, also contain polyaromatic amide rings in the chain to make it rigid. However, molecular stiffness is only the beginning. While they are still in the production line, within the cell, the collagen chains are woven together into a rope. Recall that if you unwind the end of a rope, the three strands flop about and will not lie together again. You can reform the rope end by twisting each of the strands. Strange that you have to twist them in the opposite direction to the way they lie in the rope. Well, the primary unit of the collagen chain (protocollagen) has a twist to the right, and three of these chains join together to form a rope, like molecule (procollagen), with a twist to the left. No sooner is this done, than some cross-linking bonds are added to keep the coiled chain together. The longer each chain unit is, the greater the opportunity each has to bind against its neighbor and the greater the tensile strength of the entire material. However, there is a diminishing return from excessive length. When chains get too long, they are difficult to stack and orientate. The length to width ratio of the collagen molecule is about 100 to 1. In his review Baer (1986) tells us that polymer chemists have calculated the ideal ratio between length and width of a molecular chain and, not surprisingly, have come to the same conclusion; 100 to 1 is best! The collagen subunits are 300 nanometers long, but they are joined end to end with others making a continual chain throughout the entire length of a fibril. Keratin fibers are only one-third the length, and not surprisingly, keratin is less strong in tension than collagen.

If chains lying next to each other have cross-linkages, they are unable to slip past each other, and this increases their resistance to being physically torn from each other. Cross-linkages also occupy chemically reactive sites on the chain, and this increases their resistance to being chemically separated by enzymes. Collagen chains are cross-linked with the help of vitamin C. If there is a dietary deficiency of vitamin C, as in scurvy, the newly formed collagen is weak and easily breaks down. Collagen is normally being constantly turned over; the older fibers are resorbed and replaced with new ones. The new defective collagen in scurvy causes a breakdown of previously healed wounds, which open, even years after having completely healed. The complex system of gingival and periodontal fibers also breaks down causing a gingivitis and tooth mobility.

Keratin chains are also frequently cross-linked by disulfide bridges, which contribute to its extreme insolubility. Not surprisingly, it is to be found as an all-weather covering for mammals in the form of hair, hooves, and horns. Not the least of its vital roles is in skin, where it provides an effective barrier to the invasion of microorganisms.

The plant kingdom arrived at the same conclusions about cross-linking fibrous polymers. The insolubility and strength of the cellulose in plant fibers is due to the frequent cross-linking which occurs between strait, long chains of sugar molecules. Anything less thorough, and cellulose would be structurally weak, and all too easily accessible as a source of food for animals, considering all the glucose it contains. The cross-linkages of cellulose make it so tough and insoluble that only a few bacteria (sheltering in the stomachs of cows and termites) can break it down and get to the sugar. Starch has a very similar chemical makeup to cellulose, but because the molecule curls up into a ball, there is no opportunity for chain alignment and cross-linkage, so starch has no structural strength and is reasonably accessible as a food source. Finally, mention must be made of chitin, the remaining great fibrous polymer, which is the main structural material of the insect world. Once again, it consists of long fibrous polymers, closely packed and cross-linked.

Cross-linkage also provides stability for synthetic and natural rubbers. Vulcanization is a mechanism for cross-linking natural rubber fibrils with sulfur, a process which was patented by the Goodyear rubber and tire company in the 1850s. For many years, complete dentures were fabricated by vulcanite; the dental technicians paid a license fee to Goodyear for the right to use its patented material. Until acrylic denture base polymers were cross-linked, they were affected by heat and the surfaces were crazed by organic solvents. Many commercially made polymers which lack cross-linkages are easily softened by heat.

We have unpacked the chains of both living and synthetic polymers to find that they satisfy the mechanical requirements of strong fibers. The final step in reconstructing a cable or tendon is to orientate the fibers along the lines of tension. Polymers which have long rigid chains may be aligned by squeezing them through a narrow opening, rather like logs in a river, which would tend to line up as they flowed fast down a narrow waterfall. Spiders squeeze out a long thin silk filament to construct their webs. They have no inner store of ready-to-use web, but make it up from a bag of liquid containing long-chained polymers. The liquid is forced through a fine tube, which aligns the chains parallel to each other so that they can form cross-links and join head to tail. A fine filament emerges which has a tensile strength five times that of high tensile steel. Not content with this supreme feat of real-time material synthesis, the spider adds a touch more class, by eating up unused web, so as to recycle the raw materials.

Polymer chemists have been successful in mixing two different polymers during the molding process. The first material is extruded and then the second is placed over it, followed by a layer of the first and so on to form a laminated structure. Dentin is also extruded from the end of each tubular odontoblast, and the collagen orientation tells us that it is laminated. The laminations of both living and synthetic polymer composites are specifically orientated to provide the most effective resistance to stresses which might disrupt the material. The terminal peptides at the end of each tropocollagen molecule prevent any alignment from happening until the peptidase enzymes split them off outside the cell. Some factor in the extracellular environment (perhaps minute piezoelectric currents set up during stress) can control the alignment of the molecules into a fibril. This is clearly seen in tendons, where the lines of tension are most simple. However, collagen fibers are also a vital strengthening element in bone and dentin. Their orientation in bone accounts for the plate-like (lamella) structure of compact bone. Collagen fibers in dentin are most favorably orientated to prevent enamel cracks from continuing right through the tooth. Fibrous polymers in tendons, bone, and dentin are blended, stiffened, stacked, packed, and orientated according to the stresses they must resist. Their organization is reflected in the highest technology found in commercially produced polymers. And then some for the living polymers are responsive to changes in their environment; they are forever remodeling in response to altered demands. The "heritage award" for fibrous polymers could certainly be given to collagen, but there is an even more deserving candidate. The fibroblast is the real source of the magic.

H.4 Anecdotal Evidence; a Poor Substitute for Science

H.4.1 Convictions and Reality

Our reality is shaped more by what we want to believe and what fits our world view than the cold evidence of facts and numbers. Even the minds of scientists can be led astray by belief. There is still a large following for Rupert Sheldrake's conviction that our dog knows we are about to return home before we arrive. It is a seductive idea that appeals to all dog lovers. Their pooch so loves them, it longs for, and anticipates that important home coming. The excited tail wagging, barking, and chasing its tail are all unmistakable signs. As with other forms of anecdotal evidence, it resists any challenge, because it rests securely on and within a growing pile of similar stories. And it contributes to our need for a comforting certainty, which like all dogma rests quietly within. And as for the challenge that it might be wishful thinking, well, if so, many people have found this to be true how can it be imagined. The so-called "evidence," which Sheldrake cites, is based on thousands of anecdotes from all over the world. However, sadly, there is no well-conducted trial using controls and numerical analysis.

Ridding ourselves of deeply held convictions does take a long time, and it is often never achieved in a lifetime. We know how it may take generations to rid our society of prejudices such as misogyny, racism, and homophobia.

We might view the history of science, as a landscape, through which we have made our comparatively recent journey. There are raised hills on the landscape which are visible from afar and stand as landmarks, such as Newton's laws of motion or more recently quantum theory. There are also depressed basins in which science has languished for many years without being able to arise from it. One of these basins is the sad history of bloodletting. Sad because so many died unnecessarily. There is no doubt that science today has its basins where progress appears to be on hold. Mental illness is an example; there is no coherent understanding of its causes or even universal agreement on a scheme of diagnostic criteria. If we are to escape these basins of our present scientific quests, we must learn what we can from the circumstance which entrapped science in our recent history.

H.4.2 The Lessons of Bloodletting

One of these lessons which stands out is the long but eventually successful challenge to the practice of bloodletting as a means of treating the unwell. Bloodletting was a well-established and highly respected form of treatment which was recommended and used by Greek, Egyptian, Arabic, Indian, Roman, and European medical practitioners. It was founded on a conviction that illness was caused by too much blood or bad air. It seemed plausible that if you were ill, there was something inside which needed to be removed, let out, discharged, expelled. The conviction was reinforced by the practical intervention it offered, when there was a strong desire to do something to help the seriously ill, but few options were in hand. Practitioners defended its success, even in cases which today would horrify us. For example, a soldier, badly wounded and unconscious from blood loss, immediately had a vein opened, and blood removed. A few hours later even more was taken, and then leeches applied. Remarkably, he survived and the doctor celebrated his treatment, convinced that without his bloodletting the man would surely have died.

The practice of bloodletting was reinforced by the much-valued experience of older wise practitioners. It rested securely on their endless store of anecdotes. The practice was widespread, as illustrated by the records which show that England imported 6 million leeches from France in 1830. Historians speculate that President George Washington might have survived his bought of influenza, had he not been relieved of 6 pints of blood.

It took nearly a hundred years for doctors to abandon the practice even though evidence had been gathering since the 1850s. There was substantial resistance to any criticism based on numerical analysis, although there was statistical evidence that bloodletting was entirely ineffectual. Most physicians were quite scornful of the use of statistical methods which discredited bloodletting. Years of experience and tradition were stronger evidence than numbers. However, the challenges to bloodletting continued to arrive from other direction. From Louis Pasteur it was learned that it was bacteria which caused material to rot and ferment, not some bad vapor in the air. Joseph Lister found that surgical preparation of instruments and washing hands with carbolic prevented gangrene after surgery. Surgeons were impressed by Lister's success in preventing infection, but bloodletting was still practiced into the 20th century; a medical textbook published in 1930 still recommending it.

The history of bloodletting is a reminder that even hundreds of personal experiences and testimonies of intelligent learned men do not necessarily reveal the truth. The tide takes time to turn belief around, particularly when the alternative ideas are far less appealing. There were many scientists who were uncomfortable with the uncertainties inherent in the new ideas of quantum physics. They clearly preferred the familiar solid ground and reliable laws of the more plausible classical physics. "God does not play dice" complained Einstein. The old order lingers on, as there are some who still insists that occlusal equilibration reduces the symptoms of temporomandibular joint dysfunction.

H.4.3 Evidence-Based Knowledge

The alternative to anecdote is evidence. Evidence-based studies require a number of qualities. In short, they must be randomized, controlled, and double blind.

The randomized quality applies to the selection of the study population. It should be a population chosen without having been filtered or selected for any particular attribute.

The controlled quality applies to making comparisons between one treatment or drug with another. In order to be able to make fair comparisons, there has to be sufficiently large sample which receive no treatment at all.

The blind quality applies to both the subjects and the observers. When scoring or recording results, the observers should not be aware of which treatment each subject had. The subjects themselves should not be aware of which treatment they had, hence double blind.

Finally, the data arising from the study should be analyzed statistically. This process requires sufficient size of sample for each group and the appropriate use of statistical tests.

For example, imagine that a new analgesic has been produced by adding codeine to aspirin, and scientists want to test whether the combination tablet is really any better than aspirin alone. They could observe volunteer patients with toothache taking either one of the two tablets (aspirin or aspirin plus codeine). They could watch carefully, listen to patient reports, and get a feeling or even speculate on what is probably the better analgesic. If there was a small team of scientists, they might find opinion was divided, their competitive instincts might arise, and their voices become raised in debate, or even argument. Some might claim that they have evidence of having actually witnessed the dramatic improvement after a patient had taken a particular tablet. This is an example of anecdotal evidence, and it is very weak.

The evidence-based method requires that first of all the investigators are evenly prepared for either result. They must not bring any prejudice to the trial. They will have to ask for volunteers and explain the procedures. They must be careful to avoid collecting a population that is biased in any way such as gender or age. They have to devise some measurements of the reduction in pain achieved by each analgesic. Pain is difficult to measure but a 10-point scale (0 is no pain and 10 is unbearable) might be used, or even a visual analogue scale.

The investigators will want to set up a clinical trial on a group of patients who have similar levels of pain. There has to be some control with which to compare the new drug, so some of the patients need to be given an analgesic whose effectiveness is known, and some need to be given a tablet with no active ingredient at all. This is called a placebo, and it is a very important component of all experiments to test drugs. The reason is that as much as 40% of the patients who receive a placebo will report a reduction in pain. This is not because they are having "imagined" pain, as all pain is real, but because pain is a complex experience, and even the promise of its control brings relief. It is also essential that patients are not told whether they are to receive a placebo or a tablet containing the active ingredient.

The scientists will want to keep the manufacturers of this new analgesic at arm's length during the assessment, certainly, they should not interview the patients. If the manufacturers have funded the study, this must be acknowledged.

The allocation of active tablet and placebo must be made in a randomized way and not by selection. Patients will report their experience of pain relief to someone who does not know which tablet they received. Both the patient and reporting clinician are "blind" to the "code" of who has an active tablet.

All the information must be decoded, listed, and compressed using statistical methods to discover whether any slight differences might be due to chance or can be confidently attributed to differences in the analgesic. The principle is the *null hypothesis.* This means that any differences observed are *understood to be due to chance alone.* Unless it can be shown, that differences are so greater than could be explained as chance. This attempt to avoid bias may seem very long winded and unnecessarily pedantic. However, it is clearly crucial to discovering the real influence of treatments. A recent survey of published clinical trials which tested the analgesic power of acupuncture in comparison with controls revealed the value of double-blind trials. Those acupuncture trials which were not randomized and blind overestimated the beneficial effect of acupuncture.

This example serves to validate the process of careful method in teasing out the influence of a single factor on a complex process. Scientific method, following Bacon's rules of induction is a well-proven approach to getting reliable answers to questions of this sort where we want to make accurate comparisons. In this particular example, nothing less rigorous would be appropriate if we wanted to get close to the truth about the comparative effect of those two tablets. This method of induction searches for truth, not speculation.

It is these research methods of randomized and controlled trials which are lacking when evaluating the research evidence to support the use of occlusal equilibration as an elective intervention for prevention of TMD. Even the use of equilibration as a treatment is controversial.

It is incumbent on the student and practitioner to apply the most stringent assessments of what may be on offer as clinical evidence. However compelling the anecdotes and however loud the voices of consent, we must always remember how long it took for our medical forefathers to question and reject anecdotal evidence for bloodletting.

H.4.4 The Deficiencies of the Process of Induction

The methods used in the study design set out above do not take into context a wider understanding of pain control. In reducing pain to some "thing" we can measure, we reinforce a perception that pain is a predictable sensory response to tissue damage. This reduction brings with it the expectation that there is a linear chain of causes which determine events. However, pain is not a linear process. Sometimes, tissue damage causes no pain, and sometimes, pain is experienced without any sign of tissue damage. Many factors converge to produce pain, such as past experience, cultural attitudes, levels of understanding, anxiety or fear, meaning, emotions, and so on. Those rather fuzzy, difficult-to-measure factors are less often the subject of research. I am not suggesting that they bias the results of our random study, they are in fact one of the main reasons such studies have to be randomized. However, those less measurable influences on pain, such as emotions, may be the most important to identify and control. Clearly, if I have a dental abscess, I want appropriate treatment which may be an antibiotic and drainage of the abscess. There is no call for a psychologist. Chronic pain, however, is a different matter. Drugs and surgery are not that effective. We would want to spend more effort in understanding the influence of depression, stress, anger, despair, all of which have profound influences in stirring up the whole pain process. We need to see pain as the subjective experience of a network of interacting agents, rather than a linear chain of causal links. ▶ Fig. H.1 attempts to illustrate the difference between a linear chain and a network.

It is challenging to design studies which have to contend with many interactive agents, each of which is difficult to measure. A research project which sets out to test one measurable variable is easier to plan and more likely to yield results. I have used an imagined study on pain to illustrate the need for inductive scientific method, just as Bacon recommended in order to obtain reliable results where comparison is required. However, while clinical trials are the real test of effectiveness of treatments, they are not research methods which lead to the fresh understanding or making real discoveries. An inductive process would not have led to Darwin's theory of evolution.

Suggested Readings

Cracks, Composites, and Teeth

Walker J. Cracks propagation and fracture. Sci Am 1986; Oct:178

Chou TW, McCullough RL, Pipes RB. Composites. Sci Am 1986; Oct:167

French M. Invention and evolution—design in nature and engineering. Cambridge: Cambridge University Press; 1988

On Growth and Form

D'Arcy WT. On growth and form. Cambridge University Press, Cambridge, UK; 1942

French MJ. Invention and evolution—design in nature and engineering. Cambridge: Cambridge University Press, Cambridge, UK; 1988

Gould SJ. Hutton's purpose. Hens Teeth and Horses Toes. Penguin Books; 1987

Goodwin B. How the Leopard Changed Its Spots. Spryger; 1996

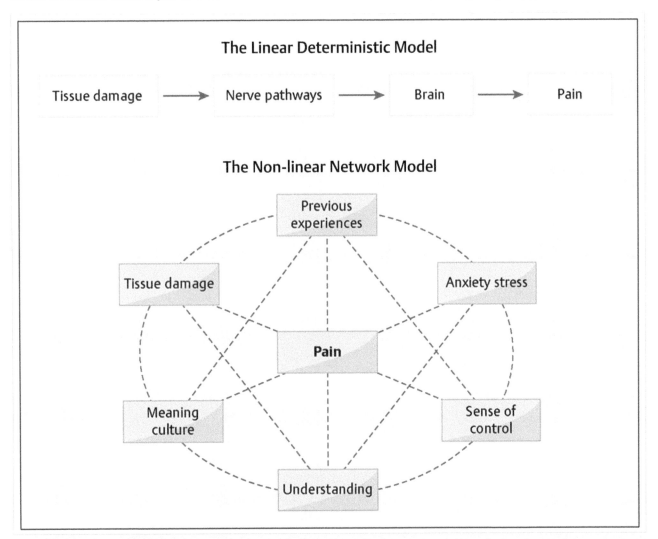

Fig. H.1 Difference between a linear chain and a network.

The Heritage of Fibrous Polymers

Baer E. Advanced polymers. Sci Am 1986; Oct:156–161

French MJ. Invention and evolution—design in nature and engineering. Cambridge: Cambridge University Press; 1988

Anecdotal Evidence; a Poor Substitute for Science

Sheldrake R. The sense of being stared at and other aspects of the extended mind. Arrow Books; 2003

Türp JC, Schindler H. The dental occlusion as a suspected cause for TMDs: epidemiological and etiological considerations. J Oral Rehabil. 2012 Jul;39(7):502–512

Glossary of Terms in Biology

A

Abductors—Muscle taking a limb or the jaw away from the body.

Acetylcholine—A neurotransmitter substance found at all cholinergic synapses including those of motoneurons at the neuromuscular junction.

Acini—The secreting units of a gland. Each acinus is a sack-like structure, lined by secreting cells. The sack opens out into a tubule.

Acute necrotizing ulcerative gingivitis—Abbreviated to ANUG, a painful and destructive infection of the gingiva caused by a shift in the normal balance of bacteria in the gingival sulcus, in which fusobacteria and spirochetes become dominant.

Adapt—To modify in response to change. When used in regard to evolution, it means that some structure or behavior of an organism may over time appear to change in response to a new threat or opportunity in the environment. The bacterium which causes tuberculosis has developed certain strains which have adapted to the antibiotics used to treat the disease which is now becoming more difficult to treat.

Adductors—Muscle bringing a limb or the jaw toward the body.

Adhesion—To form a chemical bond of attachment between two surfaces (see Ligand and Lectin).

Adrenalin—See epinephrine.

Aerobic respiration—A type of respiration which requires oxygen and in which glucose is broken down to release energy in a series of steps. The end products are carbon dioxide and water. Step 1: Glucose is broken down to pyruvic acid in the cell cytoplasm with the release of four hydrogen atoms. Step 2: Pyruvic acid is oxidized to acetyl coenzyme A (acetyl-CoA), with the release of four further hydrogen atoms. Step 3: In the KREB cycle, 16 atoms of hydrogen are released. At all stages, the hydrogen atoms are used to form the high-energy molecule adenosine triphosphate (ATP) via the electron transport system. See also Anaerobic respiration.

Affected dentin—Dentin which has been demineralized by acids in advance of invading caries bacteria. A distinction is made between affected dentin and infected dentin, because affected dentin is able to remineralize and should not be removed during cavity preparation.

Aggregate—Clumps or collections of small particles or bacteria.

Alkaline phosphatase—An enzyme which removes phosphate groups from organic compounds at an alkaline pH. It is found in high concentrations in matrix vesicles which are about to form new bone mineral. Alkaline phosphatase activity is a good indicator of bone formation.

Alveolar bone—Bone which develops around the roots of the teeth to hold them firmly in place. See Gomphosis. If the teeth are extracted, the alveolar bone resorbs away. Alveolar bone consists of both trabecula and cortical types of bone.

Ameloblasts—Cells which differentiate from ectoderm and secrete enamel during tooth development.

Amino acids—Building blocks of proteins containing a carboxyl group (COOH) and an amino group (NH^2) both attached to the same carbon atom. The difference between the 20 common amino acids lies in the nature of a side chain, the "R" group. Each amino acid has a code of three adjacent nucleotides on the DNA molecule. Amino acids are joined together by peptide bonds to form polypeptides and proteins.

Amorphous calcium phosphate—A noncrystalline form of apatite which may form as much as 30% of bone mineral.

Amygdala—Part of the limbic system, which seems to provide the emotional assessment of a new sensation with the memory of a similar sensation.

Anaerobic respiration—The first step in the production of ATP is to break down glucose. This process of glycolysis is a 10-step series of reactions leading finally to the smaller molecule pyruvate. The energy derived from this process is a hydrogen ion and an electron, which are both placed onto the carrier molecule as nicotinamide adenine dinucleotide ($NADH^+$). As the pyruvate and $NADH^+$ are produced, they could move into the mitochondria for the next stage of aerobic respiration, provided oxygen is available. If there is no oxygen, $NADH^+$ is used in a process of substrate phosphorylation to form ATP. However, the pyruvate builds up. It is then converted to lactic acid and removed to the liver. If lactic acid is not removed fast enough, it causes muscle weakness and pain. Anaerobic glycolysis does not produce a high yield of energy. There are still high-energy bonds remaining in the pyruvate, and there is no benefit from the large yield of ATP made possible by the electron transport system in the mitochondria.

Angiogenesis—The development of blood vessels, a key event in embryology and healing.

Ankylosis—Bony fusion of the two surfaces of a joint to each other, which prevents movement. Ankylosis of the tooth root to its bony socket may causes root resorption.

Antibacterial—Inhibiting the growth of bacteria.

Antibodies—They are proteins called immunoglobulins which circulate in the blood and body fluids. They bind specifically to antigens that have induced them. Antibodies are able to inactivate bacterial toxins and viruses and help phagocytes to engulf whole bacteria. They have a vital role to play in the body's immune response to foreign proteins.

Antigens—Proteins, usually foreign, which cause the bodies defense system to produce an antibody. Antigens may be food proteins, bacteria, viruses or protozoa, or cells from another individual (transplant).

Antrum—A hollow cave or sinus inside the maxillary bone which is lined by respiratory epithelium.

Apatites—A family of calcium phosphate salts which are found in hard tissues like bone, teeth, and shells.

Apoptosis—Death of a cell which is programed by a set of specific genes. Apoptosis of chondrocytes allows osteoblasts to attach to their calcified matrix and the epithelial cells forming webs between the fingers to die.

Articular—One of the bones which together with the quadrate bones and the dentary made/make up a reptile's jaw. In mammals the quadrate bone is incorporated into the middle ear as the malleus.

Artificial mouth—A laboratory device for keeping bacteria growing in a controlled environment. It allows for observing bacteria and their growth under different experimental conditions.

Ascorbic acid—Ascorbic acid or vitamin C is a dietary requirement for the proper formation of collagen. Deficiency causes scurvy.

ATP or adenosine triphosphate—ATP is a convenient packet of energy used by both animals and plant cells. The energy in ATP is stored in its three negatively charged phosphate groups which are held close together, in spite of their repulsion for each other. This energy, multiplied many hundreds of thousands of times, for each cell is able to move our muscles, transport molecules across membranes, and power all the cells other energy requirements. Once the energy has been used, the ATP molecule now only has two phosphate groups. It needs energy now from either aerobic or anaerobic respiration to charge it up again, a process known as phosphorylation. Large stores of ATP are not kept as it is highly reactive. The long-term storage of energy in animals is in carbon-rich molecules, such as glycogen or fatty acids. In plants, energy is stored as starch.

Attachment—See epithelial-attachment.

Autocrine—Cell messengers which are produced by the cell itself and regulate the expression of genes.

Autonomic nervous system—It controls routine body functions such as gut activity, respiration, blood pressure, and heart rate. There are two main divisions: the sympathetic nervous system and the parasympathetic system.

Axon—The extension of a nerve cell as a thin tube which may be as long a meter or a few short microns in length. The axon like the cell body is able to depolarize and carry impulses along its length. The impulses from one axon to another nerve cell are transmitted at a synapse. Axons may be myelinated or unmyelinated, and they may vary in diameter. Thicker, myelinated axons transmit impulses faster than thin unmyelinated axons.

B

Bacteriocins—Toxins produced by bacteria to inhibit the growth of similar or closely related bacterial strains.

Basal lamina—A term used to describe the different layers which make up the basement membrane. These different layers of the basement membrane, the lamina lucida and lamina densa, are only visible with electron microscopy. Into the lamina, dense collagen fibers of the lamina propria are anchored. And on the epithelial side are anchored bundles of tonofilaments from the hemidesmosomes which anchor the basal epithelial cells to the basement membrane.

Basement membrane—A thin sheet of proteins held together by type IV collagen. On this sheet, epithelial cells attach with hemidesmosomes. All epithelia, whether simple cuboidal cells such as found in the salivary glands or endothelial cells lining capillaries or thick stratified squamous epithelia of the skin, are all anchored to a basement membrane.

Benign—Not harmful. In the sense of tumors, not malignant. When referring to parasites, quite harmless.

Biofilm—A layer of microorganisms on a surface which is kept constantly wet. Dental plaque is an oral biofilm.

Biosurfactants—Products of bacteria which increase the hydrophilic nature of a surface so as to allow for better adhesion.

Blastocyst—An embryo which has been growing only a few days and is formed of a clump of about 200 cells. These cells are *stem cells*; they will form the three primary germ layers of the future fetus.

Blood clotting—One of the three key processes in hemostasis, the prevention of blood loss. After 3 minutes of rupture of a small blood vessel, the entire cut is filled with a blood clot. After an hour, the clot has retracted inside the vessel making the plug even more effective. Within a few more hours, fibroblasts have moved into the clot, followed by capillary-forming endothelial cells. Within 10 days, the clot is replaced by fibrous scar tissue. Clotting takes place in three steps. (1) In response to damage to the blood vessel prothrombin activator is formed. (2) This activator converts prothrombin into thrombin. (3) The thrombin acts as an enzyme-converting fibrinogen into fibrin threads which adhere to the damaged walls of the blood vessel, trap platelets, blood cells, and plasma to form a clot.

Blood groups—Blood cells from different people do not always have the same cell surface antigens. A transfusion of blood whose antigens do not match the recipient evokes an immune response and the donor cells are broken down. Two of the common blood groups are the A, B, O group and the Rh group. The blood group antigens are glycoproteins or glycolipids.

Bolus—A piece of food which is being chewed to break it down into small pieces.

Bone membrane—A theoretical membrane separating the fluid surrounding bone crystals from the fluid of the surrounding connective tissue. The membrane would be formed by the endosteum.

Bone morphogenic proteins (BMPs)—Part of the cytokine family of transforming growth factors. BMPs have a powerful ability to cause differentiation of stem cells into osteoblasts and to initiate bone formation.

Bradykinin—One of several substances, all known as kinins, which cause vasodilation and increased capillary permeability, both events associated with inflammation.

Buffers—Chemicals which are able to keep the pH of a solution within a normal range, neither acid nor alkali. Salivary buffers are important in reducing the progress of caries by neutralizing plaque acids.

Buttress—An arch-shaped support used by builders of bridges and churches in the days before steel.

C

Calcium-binding proteins—Proteins which have the ability to store calcium ions and to bind onto calcium in the hydroxyapatite of the enamel surface.

Calculus—A hard deposit of calcified plaque which is found around the neck of the tooth. When it is above the free gingival margin (supragingival), it is white and chalky. When it is below (subgingival), it is dark and hard.

Candidiasis—An infection caused by *Candida albicans*, a normal commensal of the mouth, also called "thrush."

Capsule—A fibrous casing surrounding an organ or gland; also, a coating for some bacteria which protects them, from the body's immune system. It is only the variety of pneumococcus species which has a capsule which is able to pass the immune barrier and cause pneumonia.

Caries—The demineralization and breakdown of tooth structure by plaque acids.

Cariogenic—Likely to cause caries. Sugar is cariogenic because it supports the growth of plaque.

Carious plaque—Types of plaque which are associated with caries.

Carnivorous—An animal whose diet consists of animal tissue.

CEJ—See cementoenamel junction.

Cell junctions—Sites on the cell membrane where cells attach to neighboring cells. There are three main types. (1) *Adhering junctions*, which anchor cells to each other to resist separation. They may form a belt of adhesions between cells (as between muscle cells) or spot attachments like desmosomes which hold epithelial cells together. (2) *Tight junctions* have no space between the membranes and allow no leakage between cells. They are found between cells of a secreting glands and between endothelial cells of blood vessels to prevent fluid leaking out. (3) *Gap junctions* are channels which allow transfer of small molecules like ions, sugars, and amino acids between cells.

Cementoenamel junction—The junction between the enamel covering the crown of the tooth and the cementum covering its root. Often referred to as the CEJ.

Cementoblasts—Cells of mesenchyme origin induced by proteins from cells of ectodermal origin to form a layer of cementum around the roots of teeth.

Cementum—A thin layer of bone-like material covering the roots of teeth and sometimes the enamel surface, containing both extrinsic and intrinsic fibers.

Central nervous system—The brain and spinal cord. The nerves which leave the spinal cord and brain comprise the peripheral nervous system.

Chemotaxis—The movement of cells in response to chemical messengers. The movement of neutrophils and macrophages into damaged tissues is brought about by signals released by damaged tissues and bacterial products. The term applies to the movement of any organism attracted by a specific chemical, which may be a suitable nutrient.

Cholinergic—Cell receptors specific for the neurotransmitter acetylcholine. Cholinergic receptors are found at neuromuscular junctions of muscle fibers and at all the synaptic junctions of the parasympathetic nervous system. They are also found at the preganglionic synapse of the sympathetic nervous system.

Chondroitin sulfate—The major glycosaminoglycan of cartilage, the other being keratan sulphate.

Chromosomes—Structures in the nucleus of a cell which appear visible during cell division. Each chromosome (humans have 24) is a tightly coiled string of DNA wound round a protein.

Clearance—The removal by swallowing of substance in the mouth. Clearance is dependent on the completeness of swallowing and the rate of flow of saliva.

Clones—A family of cells, or organisms, which are all identical to a single parent. They are produced by asexual reproduction. When a B lymphocyte has recognized a foreign antigen, it provides millions of identical daughter cells in order to produce the specific antibodies in large quantities.

Clotting—See blood clotting.

Code—The code of nucleotides is written in "words" of three letters using an "alphabet" of four "letters." These four components of the code are adenine, thymine, cytosine, and guanine.

Collagen—The most common protein found in the body. It has a fibrous structure and makes up the main organic component of bone and dentin, and the fibers of tendons and ligaments.

Collagenase—An enzyme produced by fibroblasts which breaks down collagen fibers. The fibroblast recycles the component amino acids, and secretes new collagen fibers. This process of remodeling occurs throughout life. Osteoclasts also secrete collagenases in order to remove bone matrix. Several bacteria are able to secrete collagenases and are thus able to break down and penetrate through collagen fibers in the periodontal ligament.

Colonies—Communities of organisms which have taken up residence in a habitat.

Commensalism—Members of one INK "https://en.wikipedia.org/wiki/Species" \o "Species" species gain benefits while those of the other species neither benefit nor are harmed.

Competency—The ability of a cell to respond to messengers which could cause it to differentiate into a more specialized cell. Some cells like pericytes remain competent throughout life, whereas others, such as the oral epithelium, are only able to form a tooth bud during the 12th to 16th week of fetal development.

Composite—A material made from two or more different types of material which contribute different properties. For example, bone is a combination of a resilient fibers of collagen in a brittle matrix (hydroxyapatite).

Compressive strength—Ability to withstand a crushing force.

Condylar process—The vertical extension of the mandible which ends in the condyle head, the moveable part of the temporomandibular joint.

Connective tissue—One of the four main types of collections of cells (tissues) which consists of cells in a matrix of ground substance and fibers. Some connective tissues support structures like blood vessels and glands. Others are more structural, like bone, tendons, and cartilage.

Contralateral—The opposite side as distinct from ipsilateral. Often used to refer to the teeth, joint, or muscles on the opposite side from the chewing side.

Coronal section—A plane view through the body which is parallel to the ground and divides the body into dorsal and ventral parts.

Coronoid process—The vertical extension of the mandible anterior to the condyle to which the temporal muscle attaches.

Cortical bone—The outer layer of bone which is dense and made up of lamellae.

Covalent bond—A strong bond between atoms formed by sharing outer electrons. When an atom has eight outer electrons, it is stable. Those which naturally have eight, like neon and argon gasses, are quite unreactive. The carbon atom has four outer electrons and therefore needs four extra electrons to be stable. Four hydrogen atoms make a good partnership for carbon (CH_4, C_2H_6 ... etc.), hence hydrocarbons (saturated with hydrogen atoms) are quite stable, insoluble, and unreactive. One oxygen atom (outer shell has six electrons) and two hydrogen atoms (H_2O) also make a stable arrangement, although not as stable as the hydrocarbon family as the water molecule is a little unbalanced, providing hydrogen bonds and other unusual properties of biological importance, such as its ability to hold other molecules in a solution.

Cusps—Peaks or raised areas of a tooth which usually fit into a fossa on the opposing tooth.

Cytokines—Chemical messengers that allow neighboring cells to communicate with each other. They are paracrine messages as distinct from endocrine or hormonal messengers. There are several main families of cytokines including growth factors, neurotransmitters, lymphokines, and many others. The method of communication involves detection of the chemical message, a ligand, by receptor proteins (e.g., an integrin on the cell membrane of the receiving cell). The result of the message is a shift in the level of gene expression or the expression of new genes and altered cell behavior. Cytokines are complex as they sometimes inhibit and/or facilitate the actions of each other.

Cytoplasm—The contents of the cell, not including the nucleus.

Cytoskeleton—A system of fine filaments which cross the cell in all directions, helping to keep or change its shape. There are three main types of filaments; in order of decreasing size they are microtubules, microfilaments, and intermediate filaments.

Cytotoxins—Products released by bacteria which are toxic to other living cells.

D

Darwinian medicine—An approach to the treatment of infective diseases which takes account of the coevolution between the host and its parasite.

Deciduous—From the Latin "falling" it applies both to trees which lose their leaves in winter and teeth which are lost to make way for the permanent set.

Demineralization—Reduction in amount of mineral in tissue. This reduction occurs when the crystals of apatite are dissolved, usually in an acid environment.

Dental abscess—An abscess around the apex of a tooth due to spread of infection from the pulp.

Dental papilla—The condensation of dental mesenchyme which provides the stem cells from which odontoblasts, cementoblasts, and osteoblasts will form the pulp–dentin, cementum, and alveolar bone of the tooth socket.

Dentary—One of several bones which together made up the lower jaw in early reptiles. During evolution the other bones, the articular and quadrate bones, became part of the inner ear, and the dentary became the single mandible of mammals.

Dentin—A hard material like bone which forms the root and inner core of the crown of teeth. Unlike bone, dentin has fine tubules which contain the elongated process of odontoblasts, the dentin-forming cells.

Dentin–pulp—A term used to describe the unity between dentin and pulp, and to view it as one integrated tissue.

Depolarization—All cells have a slight difference in electrical potential between the inside and outside of the cell membrane. This difference is called a membrane potential and is due to a greater number of sodium ions (positively charged) outside the cell than inside. This imbalance is maintained by a membrane pump which pushes sodium ions out of the cell. Another pump also pushes potassium ions into the cell, so there should be no difference in the balance of positive ions. However, the potassium ions leak back out again, so there is always a potential difference across the membrane. Nerve cells have the ability to depolarize or reverse the membrane potential, so that the inside is positive and the outside negative. This reversal is short lived and is soon corrected, but it is long enough to influence the adjacent parts of the membrane and to be carried, like a wave, all the way along a nerve axon to the next nerve where it reaches a synapse The reversal is caused by a sudden opening of cell membrane gates which allow a flood of sodium ions into the cell. This flood causes the inside to become positive, but the gates are soon shut and potassium gates opened, which allow potassium ions to flood out and restore the membrane potential. This can all happen several times in 1 second, but after a while there is no flood, and the sodium pump has to get to work to build up enough pressure for the depolarization to work again.

Dermatan sulfate–A glycosaminoglycan found in skin, tendon, blood vessel, and heart valves.

Desmosomes–One of the types of cell junctions by which cells join or communicate with each other. Desmosomes consist of a round plaque of protein, desmoplakin on the cell membrane. Into the plaque are attached fine filaments which are part of the cell's cytoskeleton. So, the plaque is attached to the skeleton of the cell. Where the filaments enter the plaque, they are so dense as to be visible with a light microscope. They are then called tonofilaments. The plaque of one cell adheres to the plaque of another. This system of joining cells is designed to resist mechanical separation, so we see desmosomes joining epithelial cells which hold tightly to each other. If epithelium is processed for histology, some shrinkage occurs, and the epithelial cells separate from each other, except where the desmosomes hold them together. The pulled-out tags of cell membrane give these cells a star-like shape, and so they are called the stellate cells.

Desquamation—The detachment of cells from the surface of an epithelium.

Dextrans—Polysaccharides made by bacteria. They have a slimy consistency and contribute to the sticky nature of plaque.

Differentiate—Change in the pattern of genes expressed by a cell resulting in altered function, from a more primitive parent cell to a more specialized group of daughter cells.

Diphyodont—Only two sets of teeth, one deciduous and one permanent (from "di" = two," "phyo" = generation, and "dont" = teeth). See also Polyphyodont.

Displacement—Displacement of a tooth refers to its movement within the confines of the tooth socket. A tooth can be displaced more easily when forced in a lateral direction than when forced into the socket. Continual or frequent displacement of a tooth may lead to it repositioning itself in the socket.

DNA—Deoxyribose nucleic acid, a complex nucleic acid molecule which is used by cells to store genetic material as genes which control the structure of proteins and hence influencing all enzyme reactions. DNA is coiled in a single closed loop in prokaryotes, but coiled round other proteins to form a chromosome and stored in the nucleus of eukaryotes.

Dry socket—The infection of the socket of a recently extracted tooth due to the absence of the formation of a blood clot which would otherwise fill the socket.

Duct—A tube which carries a secretion onto the surface of skin or mucosa.

Dysbiosis—An imbalance in the microbiome, particularly of the gut, which is associated with disease such as inflammatory bowel disease and other gastrointestinal disorders.

E

Ecological balance—A stable balance in the numbers of each species in an ecosystem. In the ecosystem of the mouth, this balance is brought about by competition and cooperation between the different organism and the hosts defense, which tend to control population size.

Ecosystem—A stable environment in which live a large number of different forms of life, each affecting the other. Example are a forest, desert, tidal area, soil, oral cavity, gut.

Ectoderm—The outer of the three cell layers which form as the clump of early embryonic cells begins to differentiate. The ectoderm will form the epidermis of the skin and the nervous system. The other two layers are the mesoderm and the endoderm.

Ectomesenchyme—A name given to dental mesenchyme which reflects its partly ectodermal origin.

Eicosanoids—These are a class of hormones which are all made from phospholipids. They include prostaglandins, thromboxanes, and leukotrienes.

Elastic fibers—They are long, thin, ribbons-like fibers, sometimes even sheet-like. They are composed of a central core of elastin, a rubbery protein, surrounded by glycoprotein microfilaments. Elastin is found all over the body but particularly in the walls of blood vessels and in our vocal cords.

Electron—The negatively charged elements of an atom which circle the nucleus. If an electron is lost, the atom becomes a relatively positively charged ion. It has been ionized.

Electron transport system—Hydrogen ions produced during the three preparatory steps of aerobic respiration are carried by nicotinamide adenine dinucleotide (NAD). The hydrogen ion plus one electron form NADH, which is taken to the electron transport system. This transport system is run by a series of five molecules. The first removes the two electrons from NADH (one comes from the hydrogen atom, leaving behind a hydrogen ion). These two electrons bounce from the first molecule in the transport system to the second, third, fourth, and then last one, cytochrome oxidase, which finally places the electrons onto oxygen gas O_2. The electron-rich oxygen atoms are attractive to the hydrogen ions, and they combine to form water. (Oxygen in the process of aerobic respiration acts therefore as an electron acceptor). In the process of bouncing "downhill," the electrons have released sufficient energy to power up a small battery. This battery has been made by pumping hydrogen ions out of the inner membrane of the mitochondria. The collection of hydrogen ions outside piles up and their electrical pressure mounts. They want to get back across the membrane and are allowed one at a time to pass back through the enzyme ATP synthase. This enzyme sits like a water wheel in the cell membrane, turned by the passage of hydrogen ions. Its turning wheel builds an ATP molecule in every turn. The wheel may be going at about 200 revolutions per second, powering the synthesis of an ATP molecule with each turn. ATP formed in this way takes a while but can be sustained to fuel the body during aerobic exercise. When the demand for power exceeds this rate, the cells have to rely on anaerobic respiration.

Electrostatic—A force generated by differences in electric charge of two particles.

Enamel prisms—Rod-like bundles of hydroxyapatite crystals which are orientated at right angles to the tooth surface. Each prism can be traced from the outside of the enamel all the way to the dentin junction.

Enamel—The outer hard layer which covers the dentin around the crown of a tooth. Enamel consists of closely packed crystals of hydroxyapatite with very little organic material. A recognizable unit of structure in enamel is the enamel prism.

Enameloid—A type of enamel found in fish and reptiles in which the enamel prisms are haphazardly arranged; in contrast, enamel prisms are parallel to each other and orientated at right angle to the tooth surface.

Endocrine glands—The secretion passes into the bloodstream, like insulin, epinephrine.

Endoderm—The inner of the three cell layers which form as the clump of early embryonic cells begins to differentiate. The endoderm will form the gut system and its associated organs. The other two layers are the mesoderm and the ectoderm.

Endoplasmic reticulum—A system of inner cell membranes which is continuous with the nuclear membrane. It transports products of cell synthesis to the Golgi apparatus. Described as rough endoplasmic reticulum when there are many ribosomes attached.

Endorphins—A neuropeptide which has specific binding sites on nerve cells called opiate receptors. When the receptor is activated by endorphins or morphine, it reduces the excitability of the postsynaptic cell. Peptide receptors are also found on lymphocytes which suggest an association between neuropeptides and the regulation of the immune response.

Endosteum—A layer of bone-forming cells, osteoblasts, which covers the entire surface of the internal aspect of cortical and spongy bone, separating it from the surrounding connective tissue. see also Bone Membrane.

Endothelial cells—The epithelial cells of the endothelium which lines blood vessels. The cells are flattened into a pavement stone shape and are usually two or three layers thick.

Endotoxins—The contents and cell walls of dead bacteria which may be toxic to the host.

Enkephalins—Similar in structure and action to endorphins.

Environment—Describes the surroundings in which organisms live. Some physical features of an environment are fairly stable, like trees, rivers, mountains, houses, soil, teeth. Some physical features are changeable, like wind, water, light, pH, food supply. Other features are less predictable, such as the balance in the community of collaborators, competitors, and parasites. All forms of life including bacteria in the mouth have an environment, which has an important influence on their survival. Successful organisms manage to exploit their environment to the best advantage or to adapt to it, perhaps only after several generations, if it becomes a serious challenge to the species.

Enzyme—A protein that controls and helps a chemical reaction to take place but is not used up in the process. Usually, each enzyme is specific for a particular step in a reaction. Enzymes are sensitive to their environment, especially to excessive temperature or pH.

Epidermal growth factor—A cytokine that stimulates epithelial cell proliferation.

Epigenetic—Means "above" genes. Epigenetic modulators influence the way a gene is read by the cell by turning the gene "on" or "off". Genes are read and interpreted by the cell rather than being determinants of cell function. They may play a major role in control of disease and many drugs work as genetic modulators.

Epinephrine—A neurotransmitter substance found at all adrenergic synapses (norepinephrine or epinephrine). It is the most common neurotransmitter in the nervous system, in particular, at ganglion cells of the sympathetic nervous system.

Epitaxy—The initiation of crystal formation in a saturated solution by providing a template against which crystal can form. There are specific sites on collagen molecules which appear to function as templates against which hydroxyapatite crystals form.

Epithelial attachment—The cuff of junctional epithelium which joins the gingival sulcus epithelium to the enamel of the tooth. Apical migration of the epithelium down onto the cementum may occur due to ageing or periodontal disease. Loss of attachment produces a periodontal pocket and a new habitat for anaerobic oral bacteria.

Epithelium—A layer of cells which forms aligning for a tube or the covering for an organ or the whole body.

Eukaryote—A cell in which the genetic material is confined to the nucleus, in distinction to a prokaryote in which the genetic material is dispersed throughout the cell. Other distinctions of eukaryotic cells are the presence of organelles such as the Golgi apparatus, endoplasmic reticulum, lysosomes, and mitochondria.

Exocrine glands—The secretion passes into a duct like sweat, saliva, and mucous.

Extinct—A plant or animal species may entirely cease to exist. Recent examples are the dodo, a large flightless bird which used to live as recently as 200 years ago on the island of Mauritius. There are today many species of birds, flowers, fish, insects, large mammals, including certain types of whale, which are threatened with extinction, most as a result of human activity. Happily, the smallpox virus is about to become extinct.

Extracellular matrix—The supporting surrounding material of a cell including ground substance and fibers.

Extrinsic fibers—Refers to those fibers of cementum which are continuous with periodontal ligament fibers. Extrinsic fibers have been trapped in cementum during its formation in order to anchor them. see also intrinsic fibers and Sharpey's fibers.

Exudate—The fluid plasma which leaks out of blood vessels due to an increase in capillary permeability. The increased permeability is caused by histamin, and bradykinin, which are released in response to tissue damage. The formation of an exudate is the first step in the process of inflammation.

F

Fatty acids—Long straight chains of carbon and hydrogen ending with an acid group at one end. Saturated fatty acids have no capacity to absorb more hydrogen atoms. Animal fats are mostly of this type and are considered less healthy as they end to accumulate in the linings of arteries.

Feedback—A system of control, where work being done is modified by the product. For example, the blood pressure is maintained by the strength of the heartbeat and the muscle tone of the arterioles. In the walls of the large arteries are receptors sensitive to the degree of stretch in the muscle wall. As the blood pressure increases, the walls are stretched, and the receptor sends signals via the brain to the sympathetic nervous system back to the heart and blood vessels, causing decreased pumping effort and more relaxed muscle tone in the arteries. In chemical reactions, the accumulated product slows down the rate of production. For example, if the oxygen level of the body falls, the rate of respiration increases to restore the levels to normal. These control systems are thus circular; what is produced returns to control the further production. They are examples of negative feedback and are common in maintaining stability or homeostasis. Positive feedback is less common as it tends to be unstable. An example is the release by platelets of thrombotaxin. When the levels of thrombotaxin are high, they do not inhibit further production as occurs in a negative feedback system but actually stimulate more platelets to produce more thrombotaxin and so on until there is an explosive increase in the number of sticky platelets. This is useful in an emergency to stop bleeding, but very dangerous when a clot forms inside a blood vessel.

Fiber—A long thin string-like structure constructed of smaller fibrils and even smaller microfibrils. Examples are collagen, elastic, and keratin fibers. Collagen fibers are arranged parallel to each other in a tendon to give it great resistance to tension (pulling).

Fibrinogen—A large soluble protein found in blood which is converted into fibrin during blood clotting.

Fibroblasts—Cells of connective tissue which form both the intercellular matrix and fibers.

Fibronectin—A glycoprotein which is found in the extracellular matrix and is important for the attachments and therefore the movement of cells.

Filamentous—Long, thin, hair-like.

Fimbria—An appendage found in some bacteria which is thinner and shorter than a flagellum. It may be a site of attachment to a lectin which binds onto other organisms or salivary pellicle.

Fluorapatite—An apatite crystal in which fluoride has replaced hydroxyl ions.

Fluorosis—Mottling of the teeth caused by an excess of fluoride in the drinking water. A fluorosis index recognizes four stages of severity.

Foramina—The plural of foramen, which is a hole, for example, foramen ovale.

Fossils—Dead plant or animal remains which have become infused with minerals over many millions of years and are now hard and rock-like. The original shape of the animal or plant may be very well preserved.

Fractal dimension—A dimension which is some fraction in between a line (1) and a plane (2), or a plane and a solid (3). These fractal dimensions are useful in describing the quality of natural lines and surfaces, such as coastlines, trees, vascular branching, and the patterns of trabecula bone.

Freeway space—The space between the teeth when the jaw is in a rest position.

Frontal plane—An imaginary plane through the body which divides it into left and right sides.

G

Gangrene—The death of tissue on a large scale. May be caused by certain bacteria which spread rapidly through tissues or by an inadequate blood supply.

Ganglion—A collection of nerve cells usually found outside the central nervous system, from which axons arrive from the periphery and proceed to the spinal cord or brain.

Gene cloning—A technique which uses recombinant DNA, inserted into a host cell as a plasmid, which reproduces copies of itself, and hence the inserted gene, many times.

Gene regulation—A wide range of controls on the expression of a gene's products, whether proteins or regulatory molecules of other genes. See also Upregulation.

Generic—Belonging to the same main group. For example, generic medicines are identified by the main group they fall into rather than by their trade names.

Genes—The unit of inheritance that transmits information from one cell to its daughters and hence to the next generation. A gene consists of a specific series of DNA nucleotides. Each group of three nucleotides is the code for an amino acid. Humans have about 200,000 genes which collectively are known as the genome.

Genetic engineering—See Recombinant DNA.

Genome—The complete complement of genetic material in a species.

Gingival crevice fluid—A secretion found in the gingival sulcus, formed by the cells attaching the gingival epithelium to the tooth.

Gingival sulcus—A potential space between the gingival margin and the tooth lined by nonkeratinized epithelium. The depth of the sulcus is normally between 1 and 2 mm in health.

Gingivitis—An inflammation of the gingival mucosa, due to the increase in the virulence or mass of bacteria in the gingival sulcus, or to reduced resistance of the host.

Glands—A collection of cells secreting a specific product such as insulin or sweat.

Glucocorticoids—One of the two major hormones secreted by the adrenal medulla. The most common glucocorticoid is cortisol (hydrocortisone), but they all share the common effect of increasing blood glucose concentration. They may achieve this at the cost of body protein stores by converting amino acids into glucose. Cortisol also converts fatty acids into glucose. Any type of stress, including trauma, infection, fear, anxiety, or malnutrition causes an increase in cortisol secretion. Cortisol stabilizes the membrane of lysosomes, which are then unlikely to rupture, a process which stimulates inflammation. Cortisol therefore inhibits inflammation. Cells like neutrophils are less able to protect the body from foreign proteins. Stress therefore reduces the body's ability to cope with infection. Malnutrition not only stunts mental and physical development but also allows viral, bacterial, and parasitic infections to flourish.

Glucosamine—A glucose or galactose molecule with an amine group attached. See also Glucuronic acid.

Glucose—A molecule of great importance to life as it provides a ready source of energy for both plant and animal cells. Glucose can only be formed in plants with the aid of sunlight. This process of photosynthesis sustains all animal life on earth. The glucose molecule is formed by a ring of six carbon atoms. It is progressively broken down in a process called glycolysis during both aerobic and anaerobic respiration into ATP.

Glucuronic acid—A glucose molecule with an acid carboxyl group. One of the two molecules which makes up the repeating disaccharide unit of glycosaminoglycans, other molecule is a glucosamine.

Glycine—One of the 20 amino acids commonly found in proteins.

Glycogen—A polysaccharide made up of repeated glucose units. Animals make glycogen and store it in liver and muscles.

Glycolysis—The breakdown of glucose in a series of metabolic steps. Energy in the form of ATP is released even if there is no oxygen available as in anaerobic respiration. In the presence of oxygen as in aerobic respiration the breakdown is more complete and yields more energy.

Glycoproteins—These are proteins which have many sugar molecules attached to them. They are an important component of saliva where they provide lubrication for the teeth. They also have a wide range of other functions in connective tissues. Examples are fibronectin, osteonectin, osteopontin, and interferon. Glycoproteins are also found in cell membranes where they define part of the cell's identity. The four major blood groups are defined by glycoproteins on the cell membranes of red blood cells.

Glycosaminoglycans (GAGs)—Large to huge molecules of the connective tissue matrix made up of repeating disaccharide units linked to a protein core. The disaccharide units are made of glucosamine and glucuronic acid. The position of a sulphate molecule on the glucosamine determines the type of GAG.

Golgi apparatus—A cell organelle which is part of the inner cell membrane. It collects and stores the products from the endoplasmic reticulum. It is prominent in actively secreting cells.

Gomphosis—A form of tooth attachment in which the root is held in a bony socket by a fibrous ligament.

Gonial angle—The angle made by the posterior part of the ramus and the lower border of the mandible.

Ground substance—A jelly-like substance which surrounds cells and provides with fiber, a supportive matrix around each cell. It consists of water and huge molecules which help transport nutrients to cells and carry away cell products.

Guided tissue regeneration—A surgical technique designed to exclude epithelium and connective tissue from a site where new cementum formation or new alveolar bone formation is desired. The healing site is protected by a membrane or mesh which may resorb after healing or require surgical removal.

H

Habitat—A location which has a suitable environment for an organism to live in. Caves are natural habitats for bats, trees for birds, oral surfaces and crevices for some bacteria.

Hemostasis—The prevention of blood loss through a damaged vessel wall. There are three main mechanisms: vasoconstriction, formation of a platelet plug, and blood clotting.

Heparin sulfate—A glycosaminoglycan which is unusual in that it is stored inside the cell (mast cells) surrounding the liver. Heparin prevents blood clotting.

Herbivorous—An animal whose diet consists of grass, leaves, roots, or other plant matter.

Heterodont—A dentition in which some of the teeth have different shapes and special functions (from "hetero" = different). See also Homodont.

Hierarchy—An order of power between individuals. A ranking of most dominant to least dominant.

Hippocampus—Part of the limbic system, it seems to provide a spatial map useful in the event of a sudden need to escape from an unpleasant sensory experience.

Hypothalamus—This small body of nerve cells controls the activity of the pituitary gland, the source of several hormones which controls the activity of other hormones, including adrenocorticotropic hormone (ACTH), which in turn controls the level of glucocorticoid secretion. The hypothalamus also has powerful connections with the other members of the limbic system, from which nerve pathways descend to control nerves in the spinal cord. The influence of the limbic system on the hypothalamus explains the raised levels of glucocorticoids in response to emotional stress. This bridge with the peripheral nervous system provides a link between the emotional state of a person, as influenced by the activity of the limbic system, and the excitability of neurons in the spinal cord to incoming pain impulses.

Histamine—It is a product of the amino acid, histidine and is released by damaged cells. Histamine causes an increase in capillary permeability and vasodilation, two vascular events which are the first stages of inflammation. Histamine is also a neurotransmitter substance released at nerve synapses mostly in the hypothalamus.

Homeostasis—Control of an organism's internal environment. Water content, temperature, acid–base balance, level of oxygen and carbon dioxide, adequate supply of energy are some of the many factors in the organism which require monitoring and control. A common form of control is feedback.

Homodont—A dentition in which all the teeth are the same shape (from "home" = same) see also Heterodont.

Hyaluronic acid—The largest glycosaminoglycan known, it plays an important role of restricting the flow of water in tissues, particularly in synovial fluid, where it acts as a lubricant.

Hydrogen bonds—A weak force holding two molecules containing hydrogen together, each of which has a covalent bond with another atom. For example, water is a molecule made up of two hydrogen atoms attached covalently to an oxygen atom. The hydrogen proton is, however, not completely balanced and is still attracted to the oxygen atom of a neighboring molecule. Molecules of water are thus held together by hydrogen bonds, which account for the unusually high boiling point of water considering its low molecular weight. Hydrogen bonds hold protein molecules in shape by linking up various sections. When proteins are heated, these bonds collapse and the protein is physically altered, even though its chemical composition remains unchanged. When an egg is heated, the white part rapidly gels, indicating a change in the shape of the protein. The process is not reversible. So, an egg cannot be uncooked.

Hydroxyapatite—One of the apatites which is the main salt of bone and teeth.

Hydroxyl ion—A negatively charged ion of hydrogen and oxygen written as OH^-.

Hyperplasia—An increase in the size of an organ due to an increase in the number of cells. The developing embryo increases in size due to cell division. The cells of some tissues retain the ability to divide throughout life, like the epithelium and connective tissues, but muscle and nerve cells lose their ability to divide soon after birth. When hyperplasia is uncontrolled, it produces a tumor, which may be benign if it is well contained, not destructive and does not spread. However, it may be malignant, destroys normal tissue, and spreads all over the body.

Hypertrophy—An increase in the size of an organ due to an increase in the size of each cell. Muscles increase in size due to hypertrophy.

Hypoplasia—Reduced formation of a tissue during development. Enamel hypoplasia may be recognized as pits and depressions in the enamel and may be caused by fluorosis.

Hypotonic—A comparison between two solutions indicating that one has a lower osmotic pressure or is less salty than the other.

I

In vitro—Experiments which are carried out in a laboratory as distinct from in vivo experiments.

In vivo—Experiments which are carried out in live animals as distinct from in vitro experiments.

Immunity—The body's response to a foreign antigen either ingested as food or as part of a foreign organism. There are two major ways the body defends itself; one is by antibody production, the so-called humeral response, as the antibodies circulate in the blood and the fluid between cells. The other is the cellular response, as it involves the cells of the immune system, the family of leucocytes. The particular leucocyte responsible for immune specificity is the lymphocyte. In total cell mass, there are as many lymphocytes as there are liver or brain cells. During development, there are millions of B (from the bone marrow) lymphocytes made, each with a different cell membrane ligand, specific for any one of millions of antigens. The lymphocytes are circulating all the time so that they can have the chance to meet up with a foreign antigen. As soon as an antigen has been recognized by one of these cells, and bound to the cell ligand, it stimulates the cell to reproduce millions of copies of itself. All the daughter cells are clones of the original cell. These B-lymphocyte daughters migrate to the site where the antibody is needed. Instead of making an antigen for the membrane these cells make large amounts of soluble antibody. They are now recognizable as plasma cells. T lymphocytes (having spent time in the thymus) comprise the cell-mediated response to an antigen. They are of two types: killer T cells and helper T cells. Most T lymphocytes are helpers, and they regulate the response of the B lymphocytes. The killer T cells are, however, capable of recognizing the foreign antigen on the surface of a cell, and then killing the entire cell. The immune response is part of a less specific defense and healing response of the body known as inflammation.

Indirect pulp cap—A dressing, usually calcium hydroxide, placed against the pulpal wall of a deep cavity in order to encourage affected dentin to remineralize. The cavity is closed with a temporary filling material and reopened after 6 weeks to assess the state of the pulp.

Induction—Cell differentiation which is brought about by the influence of cytokines released by cells of another type.

Infected dentin—Dentin which has been damaged beyond repair by caries and is infected by large numbers of caries bacteria.

Inflammation—It is a whole complex of events which occur in sequence in response to injury. Tissue damaged by bacteria, chemicals, heat, trauma, etc. release histamine and bradykinin and serotonin, which cause an increase in capillary permeability and vasodilation. Both these factors contribute to the formation of a fluid exudate in the damaged tissue, which includes fibrinogen and therefore soon clots into a firm gel. This process has the effect of walling off the bacteria or toxic substances causing the damage, or at least it slows down their spread into surrounding tissues. Local macrophages begin their phagocytic activity, but their numbers are small. Damaged tissues also release interleukin, messengers which are transported all the way to the bone marrow, where millions of leucocytes are stored. These stores now release leucocytes, mostly neutrophils into the blood. The neutrophils gather at the site of damage, because the endothelial cells of the local capillary walls have become sticky to leucocytes. This stickiness is specific for leucocytes and is the work of selectins expressed on the cell membrane of the endothelial cell. The leucocytes begin to catch and roll along the endothelium until they are brought to a standstill. The increased permeability of the endothelial cells allows leucocytes to wriggle out of the capillary and migrate into the damaged area. This migration is also dependent on a process known as chemotaxis, in which cytokine messages from the damaged cells attract the leucocytes to come to their aid. After several days, the battle zone is filled with dead bacteria, dead tissue cells, dead neutrophils, and macrophages. This dead mass of tissue is called pus. The end of the event may be the gradual resorption of pus by fresh macrophages, or the pus, now under some pressure, may force its way somewhere else. Pus from the apex of a tooth may escape laterally through the alveolar bone and mucosa, where it is recognizable as a "gum boil." Ten days after a foreign protein is detected for the first time, the body's immune system has mounted a more specific defense. Antibodies are produced by B lymphocytes, and T lymphocytes have been alerted to the invasion.

Insulin—An endocrine hormone produced in the spleen which controls the amount of sugar in the blood by (1) transporting it into cells and promoting glycolysis, (2) converting it into glycogen for storage in the liver and muscles, and (3) converting it into fats. Without sufficient insulin, glucose accumulates in the blood and urine, and the cells of the body are starved, a condition known as diabetes. The control of insulin production is another example of a feedback system.

Insulin-like growth factor (IGF)—A cytokine that influences growth hormone activity.

Integrins—These are the cell surface receptor molecules which match up with parts of the matrix protein ligands to allow adhesion of the cell to the matrix. The attachment of cells to matrix proteins also influences the cells behavior by the expression of genes. The integrins are a family of proteins found doing the same job on all animal cells. Their importance in maintaining the structural integrity of cells led to the name integrins.

Intercalated ducts—Ducts which carry saliva between the tubules and the striated ducts.

Interferon—A glycoprotein produced by cells which mobilizes the T lymphocytes to inhibit viruses and the growth of cancer cells.

Interleukins—A variety of compounds (about 20) that are produced by lymphocytes, macrophages, and monocytes. They regulate the cell-mediated response of the immune system. *Interleukin-1* is involved in the triggering of the immune response, starting acute inflammation and maintaining chronic inflammation. *Interleukin-2* is produced by helper T cells and induces proliferation of immune cells, both T and B. *Interleukin-3* promotes the differentiation and proliferation of stem cells of the leucocyte family. *Interleukin-6* produced by various cells including tumor cells and acts as a stimulant of plasma proteins and B and T cells. *Interleukin-12* is produced by a range of cells. It activates T cells and natural killer cells. It promotes the response to a range of pathogens including HIV of interleukin-2. It appears to be one of the most promising interleukins for the control of viral, bacterial, and protozoal infections.

Intermediate filaments—Unlike microfilaments and microtubules, they are very stable. Instead of being stacked proteins, as in actin, intermediate filaments are built of interlocking proteins. A dense sheet of intermediate filaments strengthens the nucleus. Skin cells are filled with keratin, which at the last moment, just before they die. They cross-link to provide a really insoluble barrier layer of the skin. The cross-linkage is between the sulfur atoms of cysteine, one of keratin's amino acids.

Interproximal wear—Loss of enamel on the adjacent surfaces of teeth which is due to continual friction between the two surfaces as teeth move against each other.

Intratubular dentin—Dentin formed inside the tubule by the odontoblast process in response to tooth wear, aging, or arrested caries.

Intrinsic fibers—Refers to those fibers of cementum which were laid down by cementoblasts. See also Extrinsic fibers.

Ionized—The loss or gain of an electron from an atom which makes it no longer neutral but an electrically charged *ion*. If the electron leaves the atom, it becomes a positively charged ion, such as when calcium or sodium becomes ionized (Ca^+, Na^+). If the electron is gained, the atom becomes relatively negatively charged such as when chlorine or a phosphate group of atoms lose an electron (Cl^-, PO_4^-). Ionized atoms or groups of atoms are more reactive than when they are neutral.

Ions—An atom or molecules which has a net electrical charge. This may be caused by the temporary loss (positive ion) or gain (negative ion) of an electron. A calcium ion is written Ca^+.

Ipsilateral—The same side as distinct from contralateral. Often used to refer to the teeth, joint, or muscles on the same side as chewing is occurring.

J

Junctional epithelium—The epithelium which seals the base of the gingival sulcus against the tooth.

K

Keratan sulfate—A glycosaminoglycan found in cartilage with chondroitin sulfate.

Keratin—A fibrous polymer which is not as strong as collagen but less soluble. It forms the strong and water-resistant properties of skin, nails, hair, horn, and beaks.

Keratinized—An epithelium in which the superficial cells have lost their nuclei and become filled with intermediate filaments of keratin.

Keratinocytes—Cells of the epidermis which secrete the protein keratin. They become progressively flattened as they mature and eventually are off.

Keystone species—A species that has a disproportionately large effect on the environment relative to its abundance.

Krebs's cycle—The end stage of aerobic respiration. Krebs's cycle is a circular series of reactions taking place in the matrix of mitochondria in which acetyl-CoA is broken down into carbon dioxide and hydrogen atoms. The hydrogen atoms are used to produce ATP via the electron transport system.

L

Lacuna—A cavity in which a cell lies surrounded by a hard connective tissue. Chondrocytes lie in a lacuna of cartilage. Osteoclasts lie in a lacuna of bone which they have resorbed.

Lamella bone—The microscopic structure of cortical bone gives it the appearance of concentric or parallel plates (from Latin, lamella, the diminutive of lamina, meaning a plate or leaf).

Lamina propria—The layer of loose connective tissue underneath the epithelium of mucosa, which provides physical and nutritional support.

Lamina dura—The name given to the radiographic appearance of a dense layer of bone around the tooth root. It represents the dense cortical bone lining the tooth socket.

Laminin—An adhesive molecule of connective tissue related to fibronectin and tenascin.

Langerhans' cells—These cells are active in the immune response of the skin and mucous membrane. They act as sentries, detecting the presence of foreign antigens on the surface of the epithelium. They do not contain keratin and are thus sometimes called clear cells.

Lectin—A protein molecule which binds onto a specific sequence of sugars. Bacteria may use lectin attachments to bind onto each other or oral surfaces.

Leucocytes—Unpigmented (white) cells of the blood. Those with granular cytoplasm are neutrophils, eosinophils, and basophils. The agranulocytes are lymphocytes and monocytes.

Leukotrienes—Concerned with signaling between cells of the immune system and a member of the eicosanoid family of hormones.

Ligand—A protein molecule which binds to another specific protein molecule. The forces of the bond are week and thus protein–ligand bonds depend on close fit of one molecule to the other so as to capture as many bonding sites as possible. Ligands are specific for a particular protein. They are found on cell surfaces of microorganisms where they assist in cell adhesion. They are also sites on cell membranes onto which protein messengers attach such as cytokines. See also Lectins.

Limbic system—A ring of structures around the thalamus which plays a major role in pain as well as other types of behavior. The limbic system includes the hypothalamus, hippocampus, amygdala, septum, and cingulum. The limbic system plays an important role in pain at the level of motivation to avoid it. It thus operates at a slightly higher level than the reticular formation with strong connections to the thalamus and cortex.

Lipid—Large molecules containing hydrogen and carbon which are insoluble in water. Simple lipids consist of long chains of fatty acids. Compound lipids contain phosphoric acid, sugars, nitrogenous bases, or proteins, and include the phospholipids, glycolipids, and lipoproteins. Steroids may also be classified as lipids.

Lubrication—Helps two surfaces to slide over each other.

Lysine—One of the 20 amino acids common in proteins. It is a common amino acid of collagen and like proline must be hydroxylated by ascorbic acid in order to allow the formation of bonds which will hold the triple helix together.

Lymphocytes—White cells involved in the immune response. B lymphocytes are so called because they mature in bone, while T lymphocytes mature in the thymus. Both cells look alike until they recognize a foreign antigen. The B cell starts to make antibodies while the T lymphocytes accumulate vesicles loaded with cytotoxic agents. On contact with a foreign cell, the lymphocytes change shape so that all its vesicles are pointed at the enemy. The release of cytotoxic agents needs to be carefully controlled. One of the methods by which the enemy cell is killed is by agents which make holes in its cell membrane. Enemy cells maybe bacteria or the body's own cells which have ingested viruses, or they may be cancer cells or the cells of transplanted organs.

Lymphokines—A variety of cytokines released by lymphocytes which coordinate the proliferation of T and B lymphocytes. They also regulate the brain's contribution to the immune response via the hypothalamus, adrenal cortex axis.

Lysosomes—Small membrane-bound vesicles in the cytoplasm of cells which contain toxic enzymes. When a cell dies, these membranes rupture and the enzymes are released. They break down the cell structure, and the debris is removed. The lysosome also contains cytokines, which summon inflammatory cells and stimulate inflammation. The contents of lysosomes can be released by macrophages and neutrophils both to kill bacteria and viruses and to stimulate inflammation.

M

Macrophages—Cells derived from monocytes which have the ability to phagocytose foreign particles and dead tissue and to move through tissue or to remain fixed in one place. There are many macrophages in the spleen where they remove dead red blood cells from the circulation.

Major salivary glands—There are three large glands on each side of the face: the parotid, submandibular, and submaxillary.

Malleus—One of the three bones of the inner ear. The others are the stapes and the incus.

Mastication—The process of preparing food for swallowing and digestion by chewing it.

Matrix—Comes from the Latin word "mater," meaning mother. It is a structure which encloses or holds something within it.

Cells are held or enclosed in a matrix of fibers, water, and large molecules called the ground substance.

Matrix vesicles—Small bubble-like structures containing calcium-binding phospholipids and alkaline phosphatase. Crystals of hydroxyapatite from inside the vesicle which ruptures and releasing crystals into the surrounding osteoid or predentin so as to start mineralizing it.

Mechanoreceptors—Sensory receptors which respond when mechanically deformed by pressure, tension, vibration, or touch.

Mesenchyme—Dental mesenchyme is tissue derived from the mesoderm of the embryo and which has been infiltrated and highly influenced by migrating cells from the neural crest.

Mesial drift—A gradual movement of all the posterior teeth in a mesial direction. It occurs only if there has been interproximal wear between the teeth. The drift is not a passive one, however, as it has been shown that during chewing the bite force has a mesial component.

Mesial—Toward the midline.

Mesoderm—The middle of the three cell layers which form as the clump of early embryonic cells begins to differentiate. The mesoderm will form the muscles, blood system, connective tissue, including bone and dentin, the kidneys, and the dermis of the skin. The other two layers are the ectoderm and the endoderm.

Messenger RNA—A ribose nucleic acid which carries the DNA code in matching nucleotides from the nucleus to the ribosome of the cell.

Metabolize—To obtain energy by breaking down a molecule into smaller components as in respiration or to store energy by building a more complex molecule out of smaller components. It always takes place in a number of stages, controlled by enzymes. Each step in the process follows a predictable "metabolic" pathway for that reaction.

Microbiology—The study of the microscopic forms of life.

Microfilaments—These are the smallest filaments of the cytoskeleton. The filaments are made of hundreds of actin molecules stacked in a line. They can be quickly broken down or extended. Actin filaments give the cell its shape and help to change it. When cells move, in embryology and repair, or just during the continual patrol of lymphocytes, they must hold on to something in order to crawl. The filaments serve to anchor one part of the cell via fibronectin to the cell matrix, so the rest of the cell can pull itself toward the anchor. Lymphocytes move and scavenge by sticking out arms and feet to help them crawl and engulf foreign particles. Muscle cells change their shape by using stacks of actin filaments as a ladder on which myosin climbs.

Micron—1,000th part of a millimeter.

Microorganisms—Single-celled animals which may range from the very small viruses through bacteria and fungi to almost visible protozoa.

Microtubules—These are the largest filament in the cytoskeleton. They are the hollow tubes along which cell products are conducted long distances. The system is not unlike a railway network around the cell, sometimes involving long distances. For example, neurons transport out neurotransmitter substances along the axons to distant synapses inside microtubules.

Minor salivary glands—These are microscopic glands under the surface of the oral mucosa. They are found throughout the lining mucosa of the mouth including the tongue.

Mitochondria—A cell organelle found in eukaryotic cells which produces ATP as a product of Krebs's cycle and the electron transport system. Cells requiring large amounts of energy, such as secreting odontoblasts, have large numbers of mitochondria. Mitochondria are self-replicating and contain their own DNA for this purpose.

Mitosis—The division of a cell into two daughter cells, each of which is identical.

Mitotic activity—The rate of mitosis, and hence cell division. The mitotic activity of basal cells in an epithelium must match the rate of desquamation.

Molecules—A combination of atoms joined together in fixed proportions.

Monocytes—They remain in the blood only a short time before they migrate into the tissues particularly where dead tissue must be removed, where they are called macrophages.

Morphogenesis—The process in which tissue shapes and organ structures are developed during embryology.

Morphogenic field—An environment in which the shape or pattern of a developing organ is determined.

Motoneuron—Nerve cells with their cell bodies in the brain stem or spinal cord, which transmit impulses along their axons to effector organs, including endocrine, exocrine glands and muscles fibers. The axons of most motoneurons have many branches, each of which ends at a neuromuscular junction. The group of muscle cells innervated by one motoneuron is called a motor unit.

Mucoperiosteum—A type of oral mucosa which has a fibrous lamina propria, no submucosa, and is attached to the underlying periosteum of bone. The attached gingiva is a mucoperiosteum.

Mucous—A secretion which is viscous and slimy due to the presence of glycoproteins.

Mutation—A change in the order of nucleotide bases on a gene, which alters the configuration of the protein produced, and thus may alter the behavior of the cell. A mutation may cause a cell to die or become cancerous. Mutations in bacteria and viruses help them to evade detection by their hosts.

Myelin—The fatty covering of myelinated nerves which appears white to the naked eye. The parts of the brain and spinal cord in which myelinated nerves run have therefore been called the "white" matter as distinct from the "gray" matter composed of nerve cells. Myelin also contains about 20% of proteins whose prime role is to mediate adhesion between adjacent Schwann cells. These cell membrane glycoproteins are also members of the immunoglobulin family of cell surface proteins. Defects in these surface proteins may cause them to act as antigens to the immune system. The disease multiple sclerosis is caused by antibodies to the myelin proteins, which results in inflammation and loss of myelin.

Myelinated—Nerve axons which are completely wrapped in a sheath of myelin by Schwann cells. One cell wraps about a millimeter of nerve axon. Myelinated nerve axons carry impulses faster than unmyelinated nerves as the impulse jumps across the myelin sheath of each adjacent Schwann cell to that of the next.

N

Nerve growth factor—A cytokine that promotes the growth and repair of sensory nerves and maintenance of sympathetic nerves.

Neural crest cells—Cells derived from the ectoderm layer in the embryo. This layer folds to form a neural tube which will later become the spinal cord of the animal. Cells from the crest of this fold leave the ectoderm and migrate into the mesoderm layer. These neural crest cells are thus of ectomesenchymal origin. They migrate to form the dental mesenchyme, supportive cells of the nervous system, the adrenal cortex, and melanocytes of the skin.

Neuromuscular junction—The synapse between the axon terminal of a motoneuron and a skeletal muscle fiber. The release at this synapse of the neurotransmitter substance, acetylcholine causes the muscle to contract.

Neuropeptides—Compounds which have extremely potent affect to excite or depress nerve cells in very low concentration. In this regard, they are distinctly different from neurotransmitters. They include substances such as prostaglandins, substance P, endorphins, and enkephalins. Neuropeptides also have receptors on lymphocytes and thus influence the immune response.

Neurotransmitters—Chemicals which are secreted into a synapse in order to transmit an electrical nerve impulse from a nerve axon of one cell to the cell body of another nerve cell. They bind to receptors on nerve cells and are produced rapidly in high concentrations at nerve synapses. In these respects, they differ from neuropeptides. There are many different neurotransmitter substances. They include acetylcholine, epinephrine, histamine, serotonin, GABA, and glutamate.

Neutrophils—Members of the family of white blood cells which are involved in nonspecific phagocytosis of bacteria and foreign material. Neutrophils are also called polymorphonuclear leucocytes (PMN) because of their multilobed nucleus. Neutrophils also release toxic enzymes stored safely in their cytoplasm as lysosomes and released in the presence of foreign proteins. These toxic enzymes may do more harm to the host tissues than the bacteria they were released to kill.

Niche—An opportunity which can be exploited in order to make a living or survive in an ecosystem.

Noma—A highly destructive and usually fatal infection of the teeth and jaws which is a progression of ANUG, only found in malnourished children. It is also called cancrum oris.

Nucleic acids—They occur as chains of nucleotides, either as DNA (two chains) or RNA (one chain) and make up the genetic material of a cell.

Nucleotides—They are made up of three components: a pentose sugar (ribose or deoxyribose), a phosphate group, and an organic base, which may either be a purine (adenine or guanine) or a pyrimidine (cytosine thymine or uracil). This basic structure is found in many important cell molecules such as in ADP, ATP, and coenzymes. Nucleotides also form the subunits from which nucleic acids (DNA and RNA) are built.

Nucleus—A cell organelle which contains the chromosomes whose genes control the structure of proteins within the cell. The nucleus is also a term used to refer to the mass of nerve cell bodies connected by tracts of nerve fibers, which occur in the brain.

O

Occlusal wear—Loss of enamel on the biting surface of the teeth due to the abrasive action of chewing natural unprocessed food.

Odontoblast process—The extension of the cytoplasm of an odontoblast which remains surrounded by dentin during tooth formation. The process is still an active part of the cell and contributes to the production of intratubular dentin in response to aging, tooth wear, or arrested caries.

Odontoblasts—Cells lining the dental pulp derived from the dental papilla, which form the dentin of the tooth crown and root. New odontoblasts may become differentiated from less specialized pericytes in the pulp.

Occlusal interference—Contact between opposing teeth during chewing, which prevents the other teeth touching. In extreme lateral and protrusive positions of the jaw, this would happen in most dentitions and be of no concern. When occlusal interference occurs close to the area of maximum tooth contact, it may be troublesome.

Oncogenes—Genes which have the capacity if expressed to cause tumor formation.

Organelle—A structure within a cell which has a specific structure or function, such as the nucleus, endoplasmic reticulum, Golgi apparatus, lysosomes, and mitochondria. Cell organelles are a feature of eukaryotic cells.

Osmotic pressure—Water tends to move toward dense concentrations of ions. Sugar solutions on the surface of exposed dentin cause water to be drawn out of the dentinal tubules causing which distorts the odontoblast causing pain.

Osseous integration—A term used to describe the desired adhesion between an implant and the bone which holds it in place.

Osteoblasts—Cells which differentiate from pericytes and secrete both the matrix and mineral of bone.

Osteocalcin—A calcium-binding protein, synthesized by the osteoblast and secreted into the matrix at the time of bone mineralization. Mice bread without the osteocalcin gene develop heavy bones suggesting that osteocalcin is a negative regulator of bone formation.

Osteoclast—A multinucleate cell capable of removing both the organic and mineral component of bone. Osteoclast activity is controlled by nearby osteoblasts.

Osteoid—The extracellular matrix in which bone forms. It is high in collagen and other bone proteins but lacks any crystal formation.

Osteonectin—A bone glycoprotein which has the property of binding to both collagen fibers and the hydroxyapatite crystals and thus may be important in initiating bone mineralization by acting as a template for nucleation. Osteonectin is also produced by endothelial cells and platelets and is able to bind fibrinogen.

Osteopontin—An adhesive glycoprotein related to sialoproteins, which is secreted by osteoclasts to assist in their adhesion to the bone surface. After bone resorption, it may then act as a signal to stimulate osteoblast activity.

Osteoporosis—A reduction in bone mass which occurs commonly in postmenopausal females, but also in older men. It is due to a reduction in the activity of the ovaries and a decreased secretion of estrogen. Bone formation and bone healing are not affected, but more bone is resorbed by osteoclasts than is replaced. Lack of exercise is also a factor in bone loss.

Oxytalan fibers—These are related to elastic fibers, though they have a smaller core of elastin. They are found in the periodontal ligament and in the epidermis of thin skin but not in the oral mucosa.

P

Paracrine—Cell messengers also called cytokines which are locally acting, produced by neighboring cells or the extracellular matrix, as distinct from endocrine or hormonal messengers.

Parakeratinized—An epithelium in which the superficial cells have not lost their nuclei but have become filled with keratin. See also Keratinized.

Parasympathetic—Part of the autonomic nervous system concerned with maintaining routine functions. Always acts as a balance to activity of the sympathetic nervous system.

Pathobiont—A normally harmless symbiont that can become pathogenic under certain environmental conditions.

Pathogenic—Able to cause disease.

Pellicle, salivary—A thin layer of salivary proteins, which forms on the surface of enamel.

Peptide bonds—A covalent bond made between the carbon atom of the carboxyl group of one amino acid and the nitrogen atom from the amine group of another. In the process, a molecule of water is removed. Peptide bonds allow chains of amino acids to form polypeptides and proteins. When peptide bonds are broken apart, they need water to reform the amino acids. This process is known as hydrolysis and occurs during cooking and in digestion.

Periaqueductal gray—It is an integrative center for inputs from the autonomic nervous system, the limbic system, and from sensory and motor pathways. It has an inhibitory effect on pain transmission due to descending connections through the raphe nucleus along the corticospinal tract to the cells of the dorsal horn.

Pericytes—Small cells lying next to the endothelial cells of capillaries which have the capacity to differentiate into osteoblasts.

Periodontal pocket—Loss of epithelial attachment to the tooth producing an increase in gingival sulcus depth beyond the normal 1 to 2 mm.

Periosteum—A connective tissue layer containing osteoblasts on the external aspect of all bones. See also Endosteum.

Peritubular dentin—See Intratubular dentin.

pH—A measure of how acid or alkali a solution is. As the pH gets lower, the solution is more acid. At a pH of 7, the solution is neither acid nor alkali. pH is the inverse of the logarithm of the concentration of hydrogen ions.

Phagocytosis—The ingestion of small particles, bacteria, or viruses into the cell by engulfing it in a vacuole.

Phosphate—A salt in which the negatively charged part is a phosphorus molecule joined to four oxygen molecules as PO_4.

Phosphoproteins—Proteins which contain available phosphate groups.

Phospholipids—These are the most common lipids in our cell membranes. The head group contains a phosphate and is readily soluble in water. Phospholipids are also found in the cell matrix, and they provide the first step in the synthesis of prostaglandins.

Planktonic—A form of lifestyle in which an organism floats freely in a fluid without significant attachment or association with other living forms.

Plaque—It is a film of bacteria in a matrix of salivary and bacterial polymers. It can be called a biofilm, as it has a complex population of organisms, which when mature reach an ecological balance with one another.

Plasma—The fluid part of blood, containing proteins and salts, from which the blood cells have been removed. See also Serum.

Plasmid—A circular piece of DNA found in the cell cytoplasm of bacteria which is able to reproduce itself independently of its host. Plasmids may transmit a resistance to antibiotics from one bacterium to another. They are of great importance in techniques using for recombinant DNA.

Platelet-derived growth factor—A cytokine found especially in platelets. It stimulates cell proliferation and encourages wound healing.

Platelets—These are small colorless disks of cytoplasm found in blood. When platelets come into contact with a damaged vessel surface, they change in several important ways. They begin to swell, their shape becomes irregular with protruding processes, they become sticky, and they release an enzyme which causes the formation of thromboxane, one of the precursors of thrombin. Thromboxane also activates nearby platelets, thus starting a positive feedback which rapidly increases the mass of sticky platelets, which form a platelet plug. This process accounts for daily damage to capillary walls. Damage on a larger scale requires other mechanism for hemostasis. Platelets also release serotonin, which acts as a powerful vasoconstrictor.

Polymers—Large molecules made up of many joined units of a simpler molecule. Examples are polysaccharides and polypeptides.

Polypeptides—Chains of amino acids joined by peptide bonds. They are not the size of proteins but may be biologically very active. Some hormones are peptides, such as insulin, which has 51 amino acid residues. Peptides may also be powerful neurotransmitter substances.

Polyphyodont—Continuous replacement of teeth with many generations (from "poly" = many, "phyo" = generation, and "dont" = teeth). See also Diphyodont.

Polysaccharides—Long molecules made of chains of sugars linked together. Examples are starch, glycogen, and dextrans.

Predentin—The extracellular matrix produced by odontoblasts, which becomes mineralized to form dentin. Similar in structure to osteoid.

Prokaryote—A cell in which the genetic material is dispersed throughout the cell in distinction to a eukaryote which has a nucleus and other organelles. Bacteria and blue–green algae are prokaryotes.

Prognathic—A prominent lower jaw which may bring the lower teeth ahead of the upper teeth.

Proline—One of the 20 amino acids common in proteins. It is a common amino acid of collagen and like lysine must be hydroxylated by ascorbic acid in order to allow the formation of hydrogen bonds which will hold the triple helix together.

Proline-rich proteins—A group of proteins in saliva which have the ability to bind to calcium. They provide the protective layer of pellicle on the tooth surfaces by binding to the calcium in enamel. They also bind onto microorganism providing a link between organism and the tooth surface. Proline-rich proteins help to detoxify tannins, which are potentially poisonous plant substances found in tea and unripe fruit.

Prostaglandins—These are members of a class of hormones known as the eicosanoids. They are released by cells which have been damaged and have a powerful ability to sensitize nerve endings causing tenderness to the damaged area and to cause vasoconstriction by contracting the smooth muscle of arterioles. They belong to a group of compounds which have a similar effect on nervous tissue known as neuropeptides.

Proteins—Usually very large molecules, from 10,000 to 200,000 amino acids, which form the structural component of a cell's matrix and cytoskeleton. All enzymes are proteins.

Proton—The positively charged elements of the nucleus of an atom. A hydrogen atom without its electron amounts to a single proton charge.

Pulp—The dental pulp is a connective tissue trapped inside the fully formed tooth with just one entry and exit for nerves and vessels at the apex of the root. The characteristic cell of the pulp is the odontoblast, which lines the walls of the pulp chamber and is able to form dentin throughout life.

Pulpitis—Inflammation of the dental pulp caused by irritation from chemical, physical, or bacterial injury usually transmitted to the pulp via the dentin. It is important for the clinical management of the tooth to decide whether the pulpitis is reversible, that is, will it resolve if the irritation is removed, or whether it has been damaged beyond its capacity to repair.

Pyrophosphate—Inhibitors of mineralization, they may offer phosphate ions in the presence of alkaline phosphatase. Crystals of calcium pyrophosphates are found in abnormal calcification of soft tissue, such as the disk of the temporomandibular joint.

Q

Quadrate—One of the bones which together with the articular bones and the dentary made/make up a reptile's jaw. In mammals, the quadrate bone is incorporated into the middle ear as the incus.

Quorum sensing—Organisms living in a community are able to signal to one another using signaling molecules. Bacteria use quorum signaling molecules to influence the expression of genes in other bacteria. They may influence other bacteria to form a biofilm, multiply more rapidly, or become pathogenic. Quorum sensing is also described as cross talk.

R

Ramus—The vertical part of the mandible which supports the coronoid and the condylar processes.

Recombinant DNA—It is DNA from a plasmid into which has been inserted a foreign gene. The plasmid is then introduced into a host cell, often the bacterium *Escherichia coli*. The host cell may then express the foreign gene and secrete the desired protein. This process, commonly known as genetic engineering, has been used to great effect in synthesizing proteins such as insulin and interferon.

Reduced enamel epithelium (REE)—The epithelium produced by the combination of the external and internal enamel epithelium. The REE remains covering the enamel crown until the tooth erupts when it fuses with the oral epithelium. The REE remaining on the enamel surface becomes the junctional epithelium.

Refined carbohydrates—Natural carbohydrates from which other bulk such as fibers have been removed. Granulated sugar is a refined form of sugarcane.

Remineralization—The replacement of mineral salts lost by demineralization of a solid salt.

Remodeling of bone—It refers to the constant removal by osteoclasts and rebuilding by osteoblasts. The mass of bone can be controlled constantly by altering the balance between removal and rebuilding. The shape of a bone can also be altered by removing in one place and building somewhere else without necessarily changing the total mass of a bone mass.

Repositioning of a tooth—It refers to its movement within the entire dentition which involves the remodeling of the tooth socket. Repositioning of teeth occurs naturally due to continued eruption and mesial (or distal) drift.

Rest position—A position the jaw adopts when at rest with the lips lightly together.

Reticular fibers—They are fine type III collagen fibers forming a net-like supporting framework or reticulum. They are found around small blood vessels, nerve cells, muscle fibers, and in particular, beneath epithelial membranes as part of the basal reticular formation.

Reticular formation—In the central core of the medulla, it consists of several structures, including the periaqueductal gray. The reticular formation integrates information from many sources and influences sensory motor and autonomic activity. It is involved in aversive drive (behavior which is an instinctive turning away from the unpleasant).

Retinoic acid—A product of retinol (vitamin A), which binds onto cell membranes and controls cell division and differentiation through gene expression.

Ribosomes—Structures in the cytoplasm of cells which attach onto messenger RNA (mRNA). At the ribosome, the code of nucleotides on the mRNA is translated into a series of amino acids.

RNA—Ribose nucleic acid. See Nucleic acids.

Root resorption—Resorption of cementum and underlying root dentin by osteoclasts. Temporary zones of root resorption may occur during orthodontic tooth repositioning. More extensive and irreversible root resorption may occur if the root becomes ankylosed.

Rugae—Raised ridges of epithelium, each with its core of lamina propria, found on the anterior wall of the hard palate.

S

Sagittal plane—An imaginary plane through the body at right angles to the frontal plane, which divides the body into anterior and posterior parts.

Salivary pellicle—See Pellicle, salivary.

Saturated solutions—Salts such as the apatites do not readily become ionized and dissolve in water. When no more ions can dissolve, the solution is said to be saturated. The concentration of ions in a saturated solution, its solubility product, is constant for each salt, at a neutral pH. If the solution becomes more acidic, more ions can dissolve from the solid. Saliva is a supersaturated solution of calcium phosphate.

Schwann cells—Members of a family of nerve-supporting (neuroglial) cells. The Schwann cell has an extensive cytoplasm which allows it to wrap a myelin sheath around nerve axons.

Sclerotic—Hardened, as in sclerotic dentin, which is hardened by intratubular dentin in response to tooth wear, aging, and arrested caries.

Secondary caries—Caries which has occurred after a primary lesion has been restored. It is most commonly due to failure of the restoration at its margins, which have broken down and allowed a leak to develop between the restoration and the wall of the cavity. Caries bacteria which have been left behind during cavity preparation are unable to produce secondary caries if the margins of the restoration have achieved a proper seal against the tooth.

Septa—The thin plate of bone between the roots of teeth (Latin septum = a wall). Also, the fibrous walls which separate sections of a gland. Septa separate sections of an orange or grapefruit.

Serotonin—5-Hydroxytryptamine is present throughout the body, especially in blood platelets and in the intestines. Its release from blood platelets contributes to the pain, vasoconstriction, and inflammation after injury. In nervous tissue, it functions as a neurotransmitter, mainly in the midbrain in clusters of cells called the raphe, and in the medulla. The fibers of these cells connect with the forebrain, cerebellum, and spinal cord. It therefore exerts a strong influence over arousal, sensory perception, emotion, and thought. Drugs which slow down the removal of serotonin can reduce depression and pain.

Serous—A watery secretion which resembles serum.

Serum—The fluid component of blood from which the clotting protein fibrinogen has been removed.

Sesamoid bone—A small bone which appears at the age of 13, adjacent to the carpometacarpal joint of the thumb and is of use in determining the skeletal age of a child.

Sharpey's fibers—These are collagen fibers which have been trapped in bone or cementum in order to anchor them. See also Extrinsic fibers.

Sialoproteins—A family of adhesion molecules which include osteopontin. Bone sialoprotein is formed by cells lining the root surface and influences cementoblast differentiation which encourages mineralization. Dentin sialoprotein appears to inhibit mineralization. Osteoclasts adhere both to bone sialoprotein and osteopontin.

Sinus—A curved-out hollow space inside the skull which is lined by respiratory epithelium and drains into the back of the throat. For example, maxillary sinus, ethmoid sinus, and sphenoid sinus.

Solubility product—A value found by multiplying the concentration of positive ions by the concentration of negative ions in a solution of a salt, hence $[Ca]^+ \times [PO_4]^- = K_{sp}$ (solubility product). The value for K_{sp} is constant when the solution of ions is saturated and in balance with its solid crystalline form. Acid helps increase the solubility of a weakly soluble salt.

Sphenomandibular ligament—A ligament which joins the lingula of the mandible to the spine of the sphenoid bone.

Spongy bone—The bone beneath the cortical bone which has been thinned out by bone remodeling to form a spongy inner core. Also called cancellous (lace-like) bone.

Stem cells—Cells of the blastocyst, an early stage of the embryo. They have the potential to differentiate into all the three primary cell types, ectoderm, endoderm, and mesoderm. These cells may in future be used to provide replacements of mature cells, such as neurons which have been lost or damaged by disease or injury.

Stippled—A pattern which is made of small dots. Gingiva has a stippled appearance due to small depressions caused by the attachment of clumps of fibers in the lamina propria to the basement membrane of the epithelium.

Striated ducts—Ducts which carry saliva from the intercalated ducts to a series of main collecting ducts. Striated duct cells are actively involved in secretion and absorption. Their striated appearance is due to the many long folds of the cell membrane.

Submucosa—A layer beneath the lamina propria of mucosa, which is loose and elastic. It may contain large blood vessels, nerves, glands, and lymphatic tissue.

Substance P—A neuropeptide with a particularly powerful ability to excite a postsynaptic cell. When substance P is released into a synapse of a sensory neuron, it causes severe pain.

Sulcus—See gingival sulcus.

Supersaturated solutions—When a solution is saturated and still more ions are added, they cannot be held in solution but precipitate as a solid deposit. The proline-rich proteins of saliva are capable of binding calcium. They hold a store of calcium ions which allows saliva to carry more ions in solution than is theoretically possible. Saliva is thus a supersaturated solution of calcium phosphate.

Symbiosis—A mutually beneficial interrelationship between two organisms, for example, between bees and flowers (pollen carrying in return for nectar). Also refers to any mutual coexistence which may not necessarily involve benefit to either organism. See also Pathobiont.

Sympathetic nerves—The sympathetic nervous system is one of the two main divisions of the autonomic nervous system. Sympathetic nerves make synapses at ganglia close to the spinal cord and have long postganglionic axons, which, in general, place the body on a state of alert. Always act as a balance to activity of the parasympathetic nervous system.

Synapse—The point at which one nerve cell connects with another. The nerve impulse is transmitted by the release of chemical neurotransmitter substances from the presynaptic cell membrane. The neurotransmitter substance diffuses across the synaptic cleft to the postsynaptic membrane which it depolarizes. When the postsynaptic cell is sufficiently excited by a number of incoming impulses and enough neurotransmitter substance, it discharges an electrical impulse along its axon membrane to the next neuron.

Synovial fluid—The lubricating fluid containing glycosaminoglycans which is held in the capsule of a synovial joint.

T

Template—An outline form which can be used to make many identical copies without being used itself. Metal templates can be used placed over a piece of clothing material, which is then cut according to the shape of the template. Many pieces can be made from the same template, and they will all be the right shape for that part of the garment. Molecular templates can guide the formation of crystals by providing a shape which is characteristic of, for example, an apatite crystal. The role of templates in crystal formation is called epitaxy.

Temporomandibular joint—The joint between the condyle of the mandible and the glenoid fossa of the temporal bone. The joint is divided into an upper and lower compartment by a fibrous disk and surrounded by a capsule.

Tenascin—An adhesive molecule of connective tissue related to fibronectin and laminin.

Thalamus—The major coordinating center or sensory information in the brain.

Threshold—The minimum level of a signal (sound, pressure, pain) which is detectable.

Thrombin—The final chain in the series of blood clotting forms fibrin from fibrinogen. Thrombin is formed from prothrombin by a prothrombin activator itself at the end of a series of reactions. This cascade of events may begin two ways. One is the release of tissue factors from damaged vessels. The other is the activation of factors in blood platelets which are altered by coming into contact with collagen or an artificial surface.

Thromboxanes—Concerned with platelet clotting and a member of the eicosanoid family of hormones.

Topical—In a local area, For example, application of medication to the affected part only.

Trabecula bone—A description of the radiographic appearance of spongy bone. Radiographs provide an unusual opportunity to see condensations within spongy bone. These condensations form lines or beams, which are orientated so as to give the best support to loads tending to crush or fracture the bone. The Latin word for a wooden beam was *trabes*, a small beam was a *trabecula*.

Transcription—A process which leads to the copying of a gene's code from a section of DNA onto a strand of messenger RNA, and which eventually leads to the synthesis of the peptide or protein which that gene codes for.

Transforming growth factor (TGF)—A superfamily of cytokines secreted by a variety of cells (monocytes, T cells, platelets, fibroblasts). The family includes bone morphogenic proteins, which stimulate angiogenesis, fibroblast proliferation, and inhibit T-cell proliferation.

Tropocollagen—The precursor to the collagen molecule secreted by the cell. The removal of terminal peptides on the tropocollagen allows each molecule to join end to end with another to make a collagen fibril.

Tubule—A small tube leading into a duct, or as in dentinal tubules.

Turnover—The replacement of cells by mitosis which keeps pace with cell loss, as in epithelia and blood cells. Also refers to the continual replacement of connective tissues like bone and fibrous tissue.

U

Upregulation—The increase in expression of a gene brought on by a signal arising outside or within the cell.

V

Vaccine—A planned exposure to an antigen in order that memory B lymphocytes can retain a memory for it. In practice, the organism carrying the antigen is either killed or modified so that it does not cause the disease. When encountered again, the antigen is recognized, and there will be a rapid production of antibodies. For example, smallpox, polio, measles. Influenza vaccines are less effective as new strains of the virus are always occurring which do not have recognizable antigens.

Vacuole—A sac-like structure within a cell lined by cell membrane containing material ingested by phagocytosis.

Vasoconstriction—A reduction in the diameter of small arteries (arterioles) which is caused by constriction of the smooth muscle fibers in the wall of the arteriole. Vasoconstriction is an important method of increasing the blood pressure. In local areas of damage, it prevents blood loss by hemostasis. Local vasoconstriction can be caused by nerve impulses to the smooth muscle from the sympathetic nervous system, by locally released prostaglandins, serotonin, and epinephrine.

Vasodilation—An increased reduction in the diameter of small arteries (arterioles), which is caused by relaxation of the smooth muscle fibers in the wall of the arteriole. While vasoconstriction prevents blood loss in damaged tissues, vasodilation follows in order to allow the blood flow to slow down and clotting factors and leukotrienes to seep into the damaged tissue. Local vasodilation can be caused by nerve impulses to the smooth muscle from the parasympathetic nervous system and by locally released bradykinins.

Viscoelastic—A property of a material which combines elasticity and viscosity. The suspension of a car and the periodontal ligament of the tooth are examples of viscoelastic support. Elasticity refers to the return of a material to its original shape after being stretched or compressed. Viscosity is the resistance of a fluid to flowing fast.

Viscous—A liquid which has a high viscosity or resistance to flow.

Index

Note: Page numbers set **bold** or *italic* indicate headings or figures, respectively.